ACNE
AND ITS
THERAPY

ACNE
AND ITS
THERAPY

Edited by

Guy F. Webster
Jefferson Medical College of Thomas Jefferson University
Philadelphia, Pennsylvania, USA

Anthony V. Rawlings
AVR Consulting LTD
Northwich, Cheshire, UK

informa
healthcare

New York   London

Informa Healthcare USA, Inc.
52 Vanderbilt Avenue
New York, NY 10017

© 2007 by Informa Healthcare USA, Inc.
Informa Healthcare is an Informa business

No claim to original U.S. Government works
Printed in the United States of America on acid-free paper
10 9 8 7 6 5 4 3 2 1

International Standard Book Number-10: 0-8247-2971-4 (Hardcover)
International Standard Book Number-13: 978-0-8247-2971-4 (Hardcover)

Library of Congress Cataloging-in-Publication Data

Acne and its therapy / [edited by] Guy F. Webster, Anthony V. Rawlings.
  p. ; cm. -- (Basic and clinical dermatology ; 40)
  Includes bibliographical references and index.
  ISBN-13: 978-0-8247-2971-4 (hardcover : alk. paper)
  ISBN-10: 0-8247-2971-4 (hardcover : alk. paper)
  1. Acne. 2. Acne--Treatment. I. Webster, Guy F. II. Rawlings, Anthony V., 1958- III. Series.
  [DNLM: 1. Acne Vulgaris. 2. Acne Vulgaris--therapy. W1 CL69L v.40 2007/WR 430 A187 2007]

RL131.A2568 2007
616.5′3--dc22   2007005325

Visit the Informa Web site at
www.informa.com

and the Informa Healthcare Web site at
www.informahealthcare.com

Introduction

During the past 25 years, there has been a vast explosion in new information relating to the art and science of dermatology as well as fundamental cutaneous biology. Furthermore, this information is no longer of interest only to the small but growing specialty of dermatology. Clinicians and scientists from a wide variety of disciplines have come to recognize both the importance of skin in fundamental biological processes and the broad implications of understanding the pathogenesis of skin disease. As a result, there is now a multidisciplinary and worldwide interest in the progress of dermatology.

With these factors in mind, we have undertaken this series of books specifically oriented to dermatology. The scope of the series is purposely broad, with books ranging from pure basic science to practical, applied clinical dermatology. Thus, while there is something for everyone, all volumes in the series will ultimately prove to be valuable additions to the dermatologist's library.

The latest addition to the series, volume 40, edited by Drs. Guy F. Webster and Anthony V. Rawlings, is both timely and pertinent. The editors are internationally respected for their basic science and clinical expertise in the pathogenesis and treatment of acne, and have assembled an outstanding group of contributors for this latest addition to our series. We trust that this volume will be of broad interest to scientists and clinicians alike.

Alan R. Shalita, MD
Distinguished Teaching Professor and Chairman
Department of Dermatology
SUNY Downstate Medical Center
Brooklyn, New York, U.S.A.

Preface

The intention of this book is to review the latest developments in the understanding of acne and its treatment. The contents cover the molecular and cell biological aspects of sebocytes, sebaceous glands, and the pilosebaceous unit through to the pathogenesis of acne, its treatment with hormones, antimicrobials, retinoids, and laser. Novel actives are reviewed, such as the effect of octadecenedioic acid, sphingolipids, and enzyme inhibitors. Formulation principles and the importance of follicular delivery through sebum are overviewed and, finally, in vitro testing methods. This book is an invaluable resource for dermatologists as well as scientists working in the pharmaceutical and skin care industries. Each chapter reviews the most relevant literature and gives personal insight into tackling the problems associated with the treatment of acne, its underlying pathophysiology, and its therapy.

The book is a result of the contributions of experts in their own areas and is the work of an international team representing scientists from many disciplines. Dermatologists, cosmetic scientists, and researchers will find *Acne and Its Therapy* an invaluable and in-depth analysis of the pathogenesis of acne and its treatment.

Guy F. Webster
Anthony V. Rawlings

Contents

Contributors

John Bajor   Department of Research and Development, Home and Personal Care Division, Unilever PLC, Trumbull, Connecticut, U.S.A.

Steve Boothroyd   Department of Research and Development, Reckitt Benckiser PLC, Hull, U.K.

William J. Cunliffe   Department of Dermatology, Leeds Foundation for Dermatological Research, Leeds General Infirmary, Leeds, U.K.

Michaela M. T. Downie   Sequenom GmbH, Hamburg, Germany

Peter Elsner   Department of Dermatology and Allergology, Friedrich-Schiller-University Jena, Jena, Germany

Mike Farwick   Degussa, Goldschmidt Personal Care, Essen, Germany

Gabi Gross   Department of Research and Development, Reckitt Benckiser PLC, Hull, U.K.

Terence Kealey   The Clore Laboratories, University of Buckingham, Buckingham, U.K.

Saskia K. Klee   Degussa, Goldschmidt Personal Care, Essen, Germany

Helen Knaggs   Department of Research and Development, Nu Skin Enterprises, Provo, Utah, U.S.A.

Daniela Kroshinsky   Department of Dermatology, SUNY Downstate Medical Center, Brooklyn, New York, U.S.A.

Peter Lersch   Degussa, Goldschmidt Personal Care, Essen, Germany

Nigel Lindner   Department of Research and Development, Uniqema, Gouda, The Netherlands

Monica R. Motwani   College of Pharmacy, Rutgers University, Piscataway, New Jersey, U.S.A.

Michael P. Philpott   Centre for Cutaneous Research, Institute of Cell and Molecular Science, Barts and the London, Queen Mary's School of Medicine and Dentistry, University of London, London, U.K.

Anthony V. Rawlings   AVR Consulting Ltd., Northwich, Cheshire, U.K.

Linda D. Rhein   School of Natural Sciences, Fairleigh Dickinson University, Teaneck, New Jersey, U.S.A.

Thomas Schreier Department of Research and Development, Pentapharm Ltd., Basel, Switzerland

Alan R. Shalita Department of Dermatology, SUNY Downstate Medical Center, Brooklyn, New York, U.S.A.

Diane Thiboutot Department of Dermatology, Pennsylvania State University College of Medicine, Hershey, Pennsylvania, U.S.A.

Rainer Voegeli Department of Research and Development, Pentapharm Ltd., Basel, Switzerland

Guy F. Webster Jefferson Medical College of Thomas Jefferson University, Philadelphia, Pennsylvania, U.S.A.

Philip W. Wertz Dows Institute, University of Iowa, Iowa City, Iowa, U.S.A.

Johann W. Wiechers JW Solutions, Gouda, The Netherlands

Joel L. Zatz College of Pharmacy, Rutgers University, Piscataway, New Jersey, U.S.A.

Christos C. Zouboulis Departments of Dermatology and Immunology, Dessau Medical Center, Dessau, Germany

Part I: The Biology of the Sebaceous Gland and Pathophysiology of Acne

---

1	# Overview of the Pathogenesis of Acne

Guy F. Webster

Jefferson Medical College of Thomas Jefferson University, Philadelphia, Pennsylvania, U.S.A.

INTRODUCTION

Acne is an extremely complex disease with elements of pathogenesis involving defects in epidermal keratinization, androgen secretion, sebaceous function, bacterial growth, inflammation, and immunity. In the past 30 years, much has been worked out, and we now have a fairly detailed understanding of the events that result in an acne pimple, although there is also much left to be discovered.

COMEDO FORMATION

The initial event in acne is the formation of comedo, a plug in the follicle, which is termed "open" if a black tip is visible in the follicular orifice and "closed" if the opening has not distended enough to be visible without magnification. Patients (and their mothers) erroneously conclude that this black tip is due to dirt in the follicle. Rather, it represents oxidized melanin and perhaps certain sebaceous lipids (1,2). The earliest lesion is termed microcomedo and is clinically inapparent, but is the lesion that gives rise to inflammatory acne. Microcomedones are best visualized by harvesting them using cyanoacrylate glue (3). By this method, microcomedones are seen to be numerous on the skin of acne patients, and much less prevalent and less robust on the skin of normal individuals.

Comedo formation begins with faulty desquamation of the follicular lining. Instead of shedding as fine particles, the epithelium comes off in sheets that are incapable of exiting through the follicular orifice, and hence a plug results. Concentric laminae of keratinous material fill and distend the follicle. This process is first detectable at the junction of the sebaceous duct and the follicular epithelium and involves in distal cells later. The granular layer becomes prominent, tonofilaments increase, and lipid inclusions form the desquamated keratin (1,4).

Most comedones contain hairs, usually small vellus hairs, and the age of a comedo may be reflected by the number of hairs that it contains (5). Terminal hairs are almost never seen in comedones. It may be that the presence of a stout hair in the follicle provides a mechanical opening that prevents comedo distention. Is it possible that the conversion of vellus to terminal hairs as acne patients mature is the explanation for the decrease in acne in the late teens and early 20s?

The cause of the faulty desquamation that leads to comedo formation is not known. Comedones have been demonstrated before puberty, so activation of sebaceous secretion cannot be the key event (1). Many compounds have been shown to induce comedones in experimental systems (e.g., coal tar, sulfur, squalene, halogenated biphenyls, and cutting oils), but none are obviously relevant to the natural course of acne formation (6–8). Two experimental systems exist for studying comedo formation: the rabbit ear model and the backs of human volunteers.

In general, the rabbit ear is more sensitive and forms plugs easily, but there is generally good agreement between the two systems for most compounds (6–8).

Physical agents may also enhance comedogenesis. Favre–Racouchaut syndrome consists of severe photodamage accompanied by open comedones on the face (9). Mills et al. (10,11) have demonstrated that UV irradiation will enhance the comedo formation in the rabbit ear engendered by squalene, cocoa butter, sebum, and some sunscreens.

Inflammation may also play a role in the formation of comedones. A ring of comedones may be occasionally seen around a large inflammatory nodule on the back of patients with severe acne. In vitro studies have shown that *Propionibacterium acnes* cell walls will induce follicular plugging in proportion to the degree of inflammation triggered by bacteria in the skin of rats (12). More recent studies in an in vitro model of the acne follicle show that cytokines such as interleukin (IL)1-a modulate the cornification of the epidermis and may be involved in the inflammatory induction of comedones (13,14).

Another potential cause of comedo formation is the lipid contents of the follicle itself. Bacterial lipolysis will liberate fatty acids from sebaceous triglycerides that are comedogenic, but the presence of microcomedones in the skin of prepubertal children (who have no follicular microflora and no sebum) argues against a major role of bacterial action in early comedogenesis (15). Strauss et al. (16) have shown that the sebum of acne patients is relatively deficient in linoleic acid, perhaps reflective of high sebum secretion rates and have suggested that local linoleic acid deficiency may be involved in comedo formation. Further study of this possibility is warranted.

BACTERIAL FACTORS

The skin microflora is greatly influenced by the onset of puberty. Before this hormonal flood, the sebaceous gland is inactive and bacterial populations are low. The arrival of a lipid product with about 50% triglyceride on the skin greatly stimulates bacterial growth and selects bacteria that can effectively metabolize triglycerides. A once sterile follicle becomes the residence of *P. acnes*, an anaerobe, it metabolizes the glycerol fraction of triglycerides, which sterile follicle liberates with an extracellular lipase (17). Lipase cleaves triglycerides into fatty acids and glycerol, and the fatty acids remain in sebum in proportion to the *P. acnes* population (18). It was once thought that these fatty acids were the primary stimulants for inflammation in acne, but now they are believed to be a relatively minor contributor to the process.

Although tens of millions of *P. acnes* present in a square centimeter area on the face (19,20), yet infection with the organism is rare and is typically postsurgical. It is truly a commensal, incapable of surviving in skin without unusual conditions. We may derive some benefits from *P. acnes* colonization. Group A streptococci are inhibited by fatty acids produced by *P. acnes* (21), which may account for the rarity of facial streptococcal impetigo after puberty.

P. acnes populations are proportional to the amount of sebum produced but there is variation amongst the cutaneous microenvironments. Sebum-rich areas such as the face and upper trunk carry mean log populations between 4.8 and $5.5 \, \text{cm}^{-2}$, whereas the lipid deficient legs harbor only $0.5 \, \text{cm}^{-2}$ (20). Animal skin does not support the growth of *P. acnes*, because animal sebum does not contain triglyceride (22), a major reason why there is no satisfactory animal model available for inflammatory acne. The distribution of active sebaceous glands and high

P. acnes populations are reason for the distribution of inflammatory acne lesions. The largest and most active sebaceous glands are located on the face, upper trunk, and arms, regions where acne is common (23). The lower trunk and distal extremities have negligible sebaceous activity, trivial *P. acnes* populations, and no acne (19).

The severity of acne is also somewhat linked to sebaceous secretion and *P. acnes* populations. Teenage acne patients have higher levels of bacteria in their follicles than do age-matched controls (24). Although there is a good degree of overlap between acne and nonacne groups, in general, teenage acne patients have higher sebum production than their normal counterparts, accounting for their greater bacterial populations (25). Interestingly, this difference is less pronounced in older individuals with the disease.

INFLAMMATION IN ACNE

Formation of acne pimples and pustules typically begins at the microcomedones formation. Kligman (1) has observed that visible comedones only, rarely, become inflamed and microcomedones have been shown to contain evidence of neutrophil activity, even though they came from areas of the skin with no acne lesions (26). The trigger for the inflammation of the microcomedo is the comedonal resident *P. acnes* that has many characteristics that incite the inflammatory and immune responses.

The organism *P. acnes* is a potent activator of many facets of the innate immune system, and under the archaic name of *Corynebacterium parvum*, *P. acnes* has been found to be a potent macrophage activator similar to BCG (27). *P. acnes* makes chemotactic substances that attract neutrophils and monocytes. Low molecular weight peptides are produced as a consequence of postsynthetic protein processing by the organism. Neutrophils recognize these peptides by the same receptor as other bacterial chemotactic peptides (28,29) (Tables 1 and 2). These peptides are <2 kDa in mass and accumulate as the organism grows. Presumably small enough to leach out from an intact follicle, these compounds may be part of the initial stimulus for inflammation. *P. acnes* produces at least one other chemotaxin; the lipase that cleaves triglycerides in sebum is also attractive to leukocytes (30).

P. acnes is a potent activator of the classic and complement pathways. It is the major and perhaps sole activator in the comedo (31) and complement deposition around the inflamed acne lesions is great (32). The alternative pathway activator is a mannose-containing cell-wall polysaccharide that shares characteristics with the macrophage-activating factor in *P. acnes* cell wall (33–35). In the classical pathway, the activation is through the formation of immune complexes with anti-*P. acnes* antibody. The more the antibody present, the more the activation occurs (36). Thus, complement activation and the subsequent generation of C5-derived chemotactic factors are greatest in patients with high levels of anti-*P. acnes* immunity.

TABLE 1 Factors Involved in the Development of Acne

Dystrophic keratinization
  Comedo formation
Androgen secretion
     ↓
Bacterial proliferation
     ↓
Immune/inflammatory response

TABLE 2 Inflammatory Factors Involved in Acne

Propionibacterium acnes-derived
Peptide chemoattractants
Large MW molecules, e.g., lipase
Innate immune activators of
Complement
TLR
Leukocyte-derived
IL1-b
TNF-a
IL-8

Abbreviations: IL, interleukin; MW, molecular weight; TLR, toll-like receptors; TNF, tumor necrosis factor.

Toll-like receptors (TLRs) are more recently discovered components of innate immunity, which involve cell-mediated defenses in response to the pathogens in the absence of an immune response. Vowels et al. (37) have demonstrated that *P. acnes* stimulates proinflammatory cytokines such as IL-8, tumor necrosis factor (TNF)-a, and IL1-b in monocytes. Lee et al. (38) have shown that *P. acnes* cell-wall components activate TLR-2 in monocytes, resulting in the production of TNF-a, IL1-b, and IL-8 that attract both neutrophils and lymphocytes to the follicle. This process that is involved in acne is supported by the identification of monocytes in inflamed acne lesions, expressing TLR2 on their surfaces. Activation of TLRs by *P. acnes* also accounts for the observation that CD4-bearing lymphocytes appear at the comedo, early in the initiation of acne inflammation (39).

RESOLUTION OF ACNE LESIONS

Surprisingly, little is known about the processes involved in the healing of acne lesions, which often takes weeks to occur. Kligman (1) observed the evolution and healing of acne lesions and noted a late influx of lymphocytes and the formation of granulomas. Electron microscopy has shown these cells to be synthetically and metabolically active (40). The stimulus for the inflammation is probably persistence of *P. acnes*. The organism is unusually difficult for leukocytes to degrade. Injected *P. acnes* will remain in tissue for weeks, inciting ongoing inflammation (41,42). In vitro studies find that the organism is far more resistant to degradative enzymes from neutrophils and monocytes than a genuine pathogen such as *Staphylococcus aureus* (43) that is degraded within hours. In contrast, *P. acnes* degradation procedes at a glacial pace, requiring 24 hours for the release of only 10% of cell-wall mass supporting the observation of persistence of injected organisms after many weeks.

THE ROLE OF *PROPIONIBACTERIUM ACNES*–SPECIFIC IMMUNITY IN ACNE

The presence of elevated immunity to *P. acnes* may be the factor that determines the severity of a patient's acne. Other potential explanations such as elevated androgens and subsequent increased sebum secretion clearly may play a role in determining acne severity, but their influence is probably not the primary issue.

It is known that virilized women may have more severe acne (44), but not all hyperandrogenic women fit this stereotype. In fact, many hirsuite, hyperandrogenic women have no acne at all, and among those who do have acne, it tends not to be particularly severe (45,46). Moreover, correction of the hyperandrogenicity typically results in an improvement, but not a complete resolution of the acne (47). Thus, virilization is permissive for severe acne, but not the prime factor that causes it.

There is substantial evidence that a patient's anti-*P. acnes* immunity may be the factor that determines acne severity. Agglutinating and complement-fixing antibodies to *P. acnes* are elevated in proportion to the severity of acne inflammation (48–51). Lymphocyte proliferation in response to *P. acnes* antigens is likewise elevated (52,53). Skin test reactivity to comedonal contents and to *P. acnes* fractions is proportional to acne severity as well (54).

There is substantial evidence that elevated immunity makes *P. acnes* a more potent inflammatory stimulus. Complement activation by comedonal contents is increased by the addition of anti-*P. acnes* antibody (31). Complement activation by *P. acnes* organisms in vitro is intensified by increasing amounts of anti-*P. acnes* antibody (33) and results in the generation of increased amounts of neutrophil chemoattractants. When neutrophils encounter the organism, they release destructive hydrolases into tissue in proportion to the amount of anti-*P. acnes* antibody present in the system (55). Thus, humoral immunity to the organism is proinflammatory, rather than protective of infection, and most likely serves to intensify inflammation and tissue damage. Which then comes first, immunity or acne? In the absence of direct experimental data, the author would contend that the hypersensitivity to *P. acnes* is an inherited tendency and is the factor that accounts for many cases of severe acne in unfortunate families.

What is the future of acne research? Much is left to be understood regarding the role of endogenous antimicrobial peptides and TLRs in controlling the inflammatory response in acne, and methods to decrease severe scarring are lacking.

REFERENCES

1. Kligman AM. An overview of acne. J Invest Dermatol 1974; 62:268–287.
2. Blair C, Lewis CA. The pigment of comedones. Br J Dermatol 1970; 82:572–583.
3. Marks R, Dawber RPR. Skin surface biopsy: an improved technique for examination of the horny layer. Br J Dermatol 1971; 84:117–123.
4. Knutson DD. Ultrastructural observations in acne vulgaris: the normal sebaceous follicle and acne lesions. J Invest Dermatol 1974; 62:288–307.
5. Leyden JJ, Kligman AM. Hairs in acne comedones. Arch Dermatol 1972; 106:851–853.
6. Kaidbey KH, Kligman AM. A human model for coal tar acne. Arch Dermatol 1974; 109:212–215.
7. Morris WE, Kwan SC. Use of the rabbit ear model in evaluating the comedogenic potential of cosmetic ingredients. J Soc Cosmet Chem 1983; 34:215–225.
8. Kligman AM, Kowng T. An improved rabbit ear model for assessing comedogenic substances. Br J Dermatol 1979; 100:699–702.
9. Izumi A, Marples RR, Kligman AM. Senile comedones. J Invest Dermatol 1973; 61:46–50.
10. Mills OH, Kligman AM. Comedogenicity of sunscreens. Arch Dermatol 1982; 118:417–419.
11. Mills OH, Porte M, Kligman AM. Enhancement of comedogenic substances by ultraviolet readiation. Br J Dermatol 1978; 98:145–150.
12. Deyoung LM, Spires DA, Ballaron SJ. Acne like chronic inflammatory activity of *Propionibacterium acnes* preparations in an animal model. J Invest dermatol 1985; 85:255–258.

13. Guy R, Kealey T. The effects of inflammatory cytokines on the isolated human sebaceous epithelium. J Invest Dermatol 1998; 110:410–415.

14. Guy R, Green MR, Kealey T. Modeling acne invitro. J Invest Dermatol 1996; 106: 176–182.

15. Lavker RM, Leyden JJ, McGinley KJ. The relationship between bacteria and the abnormal follicular keratinization in acne vulgaris. J Invest Dermatol 1981; 77:325–330.

16. Morello AM, Downing DT, Strauss JS. Octadecaenoic acids in the skin surface lipids of acne patients and normal controls. J Invest Dermatol 1976; 66:319–332.

17. Leyden JJ, McGinley KJ, Webster GF. Cutaneous bacteriology. In: Goldsmith L, ed. The Physiology and Biochemistry of the Skin. London: Oxford Press, 1983:1153–1165.

18. Marples RR, Downing DT, Kligman AM. Control of free fatty acids in skin surface lipid by *Corynebacterium acnes.* J Invest Dermatol 1971; 56:127–131.

19. McGinley KJ, Webster GF, Leyden JJ. Regional variations of cutaneous propionibacteria. Appl Environ Microbiol 1978; 35:62–66.

20. McGinley KJ, Webster GF, Ruggieri MR, Leyden JJ. Regional variations of cutaneous propionibacteria, correlation of *Propionibacterium acnes* populations with sebaceous secretion. J Clin Microbiol 1980; 12:672–675.

21. Speert DP, Wannamaker LW, Gray ED, Clawson CC. Related articles, Bactericidal effect of oleic acid on group A streptococci: mechanism of action. Infect Immun 1979; 26(3):1202–1210.

22. Webster GF, Ruggieri MR, McGinley KJ. Correlation of *Propionibacterium acnes* populations with the presence of triglycerides on non-human skin. Appl Environ Microbiol 1981; 41:1269–1270.

23. Cunliffe WJ, Perera WDH, Thackray P. Pilosebaceous duct physiology III. Observations on the number and size of pilosebaceous ducts in acne vulgaris. Br J Dermatol 1970; 82:572–583.

24. Leyden JJ, McGinley KJ, Mills OH, Kligman AM. Propionibacterium levels in patients with and without acne vulgaris. J Invest Dermatol 1975; 65:382–384.

25. Pochi P, Strauss JS, Rao RS. Plasma testosterone and sebum production in males with acne vulgaris. J Clin Endocrinol Metab 1965; 51:287–291.

26. Webster GF, Kligman AM. A method for the assay of inflammatory mediators in follicular casts. J Invest Dermatol 1979; 73:266–268.

27. Cummins CS, Johnson JL. *Corynebacterium parvum*: a synonym for *Propionibacterium acnes*? J Gen Microbiol 1974; 80(2):433–442.

28. Webster GF, Leyden JJ, Tsai C-C. Characterization of serum independent polymorphonuclear leukocyte chemotactic factors produced by *Propionibacterium acnes*. Inflammation 1980; 4:261–271.

29. Puhvel SM, Sakamoto M. Cytotoxin production by comedonal bacteria. J Invest Dermatol 1978; 71:324–329.

30. Lee WL, Shalita AR, Sunthralingam K. Neutrophil chemotaxis to *P. acnes* lipase and its inhibition. Infect Immun 1982; 35:71–78.

31. Webster GF, Leyden JJ, Nilsson UR. Complement activation by in acne vulgaris, consumption of complement by comedones. Infect Immun 1979; 26:186–188.

32. Leeming JP, Ingham E, Cunliffe WJ. Microbial contents and complement C3 cleaving activity of comedones in acne vulgaris. Acta Derm Venereol 1988; 68:469–473.

33. Webster GF, Nilsson UR, McArthur WR. Activation of the alternative pathway of complement by *Propionibacterium acnes* cell fractions. Inflammation 1981; 5:165–176.

34. Webster GF, McArthur WR. Activation of components of the alternative pathway of complement by *Propionibacterium acnes* cell wall carbohydrate. J Invest Dermatol 1982; 79:137–140.

35. Cummins CS, Linn DM. Related articles. Reticulostimulating properties of killed vaccines of anaerobic coryneforms and other organisms. J Natl Cancer Inst 1977; 59(6):1697–1708.

36. Webster GF, Leyden JJ, Norman ME, Nilsson UR. Complement activation in acne vulgaris: in vitro studies with *Propionibacterium acnes and Propionibacterium granulosum.* Infect Immun 1978; 22:523–529.

37. Vowels BR, Yang S, Leyden JJ. Induction of proinflammatory cytokines by a soluble factor of *Propionibacterium acnes* implications for chronic inflammatory acne. Infect Immun 2000; 63:3158–3165.
38. Kim J, Ochoa M-T, Krutzik SR, et al. Activation of toll-like receptor 2 in acne tiggers inflammatory cytokine responses. J Immunol 2002; 169:1535–1541.
39. Norris JFB, Cunliffe WJ. A histological and immunocytochemical study of early acne lesions. Br J Dermatol 1988; 118:651–659.
40. Lavker RM, Leyden JJ, Kligman AM. The anti-inflammatory activity of isotretinoin is a major factor in the clearing of acne conglobata. In Marks R, Plewig G, eds. Acne and Related Disorders. London: Dunitz, 1989:207–216.
41. Sadler TE, Crump WA, Castro JE. Radiolabelling of Corynebacterium parvum and its distribution in mice. Br J Cancer 1977; 35:357–368.
42. Dimitrov NV, Greenberg CS, Denny T. Organ distribution of Corynebacterium parvum labeled with I-125. J Nat Canc Inst 1977; 58:287–294.
43. Webster GF, Leyden JJ, Musson RA, Douglas SD. Susceptibility of Propionibacterium acnes to killing and degradation by human monocytes and neutrophils in vitro. Infect Immun 1985; 49:116–121.
44. Marynick SP, Chakmakjian ZH, McCaffree DL, Herndon JH. Androgen excess in cystic acne. N Engl J Med 1983; 308:981–986.
45. Vexiau P, Husson C, Chivot M. Androgen excess in women with acne alone compared to women with acne and or hirsuitism. J Invest Derm 1990; 94:279–283.
46. Steinberger E, Smith KD, Rodrigues-Ridau LJ. Testosterone, dehydroepiandrosterone and dehydroepiandrosterone sulfate in hyperandrogenic women. J Clin Endocrinol Metab 1984; 59:47–477.
47. Nader S, Rodriguez-Rigau LJ, Smith KD, Sternberger E. Acne and hyperandrogenism. Impact of lowering androgen levels with glucocorticoid treatment. J Am Acad Derm 1984; 11:256–259.
48. Puhvel SM, Barfatani M, Warnick M. Study of antibody levels to Corynebacterium acnes. Arch Derm 1964; 90:421–427.
49. Puhvel SM, Hoffamn CK, Sternberg TH. Presence of complement fixing antibodies to Corynebacterium acnes in the sera of acne patients. Arch Derm 1966; 93:364–368.
50. Webster GF, Indrisano JP, Leyden JJ. Antibody titers to Propionibacterium acnes cell wall carbohydrate in nodulocystic acne patients. J Invest Derm 1985; 84:496–500.
51. Holland KT, Holland DB, Cunliffe WJ, Cutcliffe AG. Detection of Propionibacterium acnes polypeptides which have stimulated an immune response in acne patients but not in normal individuals. Exp Derm 1993; 2:12–16.
52. Puhvel SM, Amirian DA, Weintraub J. Lymphocyte transformation in subjects with nodulocystic acne. Br J Derm 1977; 97:205–210.
53. Gowland G, Ward RM, Holland KT, Cunliffe WJ. Cellular immunity to P. acnes in the normal population and in patients with acne. Br J Derm 1978; 99:43–48.
54. Kersey P, Sussman M, Dabl M. Delayed skin test reactivity to P. acnes correlates with the severity of inflammation in acne vulgaris. Br J Derm 1980; 103:651–655.
55. Webster GF, Leyden JJ, Tsai CC, McArthur WP. Polymorphonuclear leukocyte lysosomal enzyme release in response to Propionibacterium acnes in vitro and its enhancement by sera from patients with inflammatory acne. J Invest Der 1980; 74:398–401.

2 Cell Biology of the Pilosebaceous Unit

Helen Knaggs

Department of Research and Development, Nu Skin Enterprises, Provo, Utah, U.S.A.

INTRODUCTION

This chapter reviews the structure and function of the pilosebaceous unit and the controlling influences on the pilosebaceous unit and sebum secretion. The chapter is divided into three sections. Section I gives an account of the structure and function of the normal pilosebaceous unit; Section II describes the biochemistry and regulation of pilosebaceous unit biology; and finally, Section III deals briefly with the biochemical changes occurring in the pilosebaceous duct in acne.

SECTION ONE: ANATOMY
Structure of the Pilosebaceous Unit

In humans, pilosebaceous units or pilosebaceous follicles are found on all skin surfaces, apart from the palms of the hands and soles of the feet. Essentially, they are invaginations of the epidermis into the dermis. Each comprises a duct, which ends in the dermal papilla, a hair fiber (or pilus) produced by the dermal papilla, a sebaceous gland and its associated sebaceous duct. The duct supports and protects the hair fiber and also drains sebum produced by the sebaceous gland and carries it to the skin surface. In addition, in split thickness wounds, the cells of the ductal epithelium are a source of proliferating keratinocytes, which migrate to re-epithelialize the wound (1). A specialized population of epithelial cells called stem cells, located in the bulge region situated below the sebaceous gland, are believed to be crucial for this (2). These cells are pluripotent and can also differentiate in some circumstances to produce ductal keratinocytes and sebocytes (3,4). Both the hair and sebum are products of pilosebaceous follicles, emerging onto the skin surface. Sebum is a holocrine secretion from the sebaceous gland cells or sebocytes, which means that the cells are destroyed when sebum is released. The function of sebum in humans is unclear, but as will be discussed later it may play a role in several skin functions (5,6).

According to Kligman (7), three types of pilosebaceous units may be distinguished histologically based on the relative proportions of duct, gland, and hair in each: the terminal follicle, the vellus follicle, and the sebaceous follicle. Terminal follicles produce long hairs and are found, for example, on the scalp (Fig. 1). These pilosebaceous ducts are long, relative to those of other follicles, penetrating deep into the dermis, and the associated sebaceous glands are relatively small. The hair acts as a wick facilitating the passage of sebum and possibly also desquamating ductal cells to the surface of the skin. In contrast, vellus and sebaceous follicles have small, vestigial hairs and relatively large sebaceous glands. Sebaceous follicles are distinguished from vellus follicles by their large sebaceous gland and large follicular orifices (pores), which are visible clinically to the naked eye. However, based on

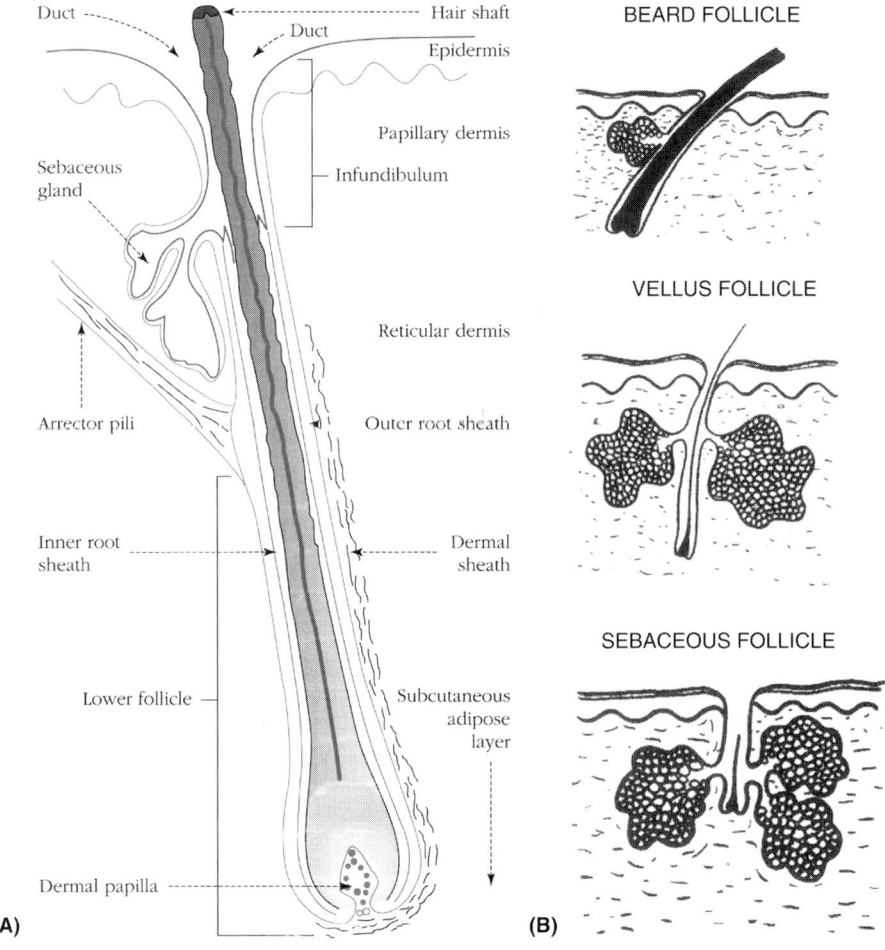

FIGURE 1   (**A**) Basic structure of a terminal pilosebaceous unit in anagen (growth phase). The hair penetrates deep into the scalp and the associated sebaceous gland is relatively small. (**B**) Structures of the different types of pilosebaceous units. The hair, sebaceous gland, and duct vary in size relative to each other.

microdissection of skin, studies (8,9) appear to show that there is a spectrum of different sized follicles as compared to the three types described by Kligman.

Neonatal pilosebaceous units begin as clusters of basal epidermal cells (pregerms) that bud down into the dermis during the third and fourth months following conception (10). Budding is believed to be controlled by inductive messages, transmitted from the mesenchyme to the pregerms (11) and proper hair follicle development is dependent on a series of several inductive factors travelling between epithelial and mesenchymal follicle progenitors (12). Regulation of Wnt, β-catenin, and hedgehog signaling pathways directs proper follicle morphogenesis, along with many growth factors including epidermal growth factors (EGFs), transforming growth factors (TGFs), bone morphogenic proteins, fibroblast growth factors (FGFs), and neurotrophins (13). Specialized mesenchymal cells accumulate beneath and around the pregerms and direct the elongation of the cells to form oblique hair pegs in the dermis. By approximately the fifth month, the pilosebaceous units are clearly visible and the keratinization of the duct begins. At this stage there are no follicular orifices. As cells in the center of what is to be the duct senesce, a central canal forms allowing the development of the hair fiber. The growth of the hair upwards removes the cellular debris from the canal and produces the follicular pore. It is believed that no new pilosebaceous units are formed after birth (14). However, recent work indicates that the epidermis can still maintain its capacity to produce follicles, if it is combined with embryonic trichogenic dermis by transplantation (15).

Sebaceous glands form from the outgrowths of the outer root sheaths of hair follicles and are clearly visible by the 15th week of fetal life (16). The factors surrounding the development of sebaceous glands are complex, although there are data supporting a critical role for the hedgehog-signaling pathway. Thus, inhibition of hedgehog signaling blocked the development of sebocytes, while activation led to a striking increase in size and number of sebaceous glands in transgenic mice (17,18). In the embryo, sebum secretion contributes to the vernix caseosa and the amniotic fluid. During the neonatal period, sebaceous gland function is regulated by both fetal steroid synthesis and maternal androgens. At parturition, the sebaceous glands are well developed, largely due to the influence of the maternal androgens. However, during the first six months of life they become small and atrophic, remaining so until puberty, when they mature and become active under the influence of pubertal androgens.

Distribution

As mentioned earlier, all skin areas excluding the glabrous skin, that is, the palmar (palms) and plantar (soles), possess pilosebaceous units. Although the number of secreting follicles, and consequently sebum output, varies greatly between individuals, the distribution and shape of follicles tend to follow the same pattern over the human body (19). The highest density of sebaceous and vellus follicles is found on the face, especially on the forehead, where there may be as many as 900 glands/cm^2 in some areas (20), but the number varies according to the study: Blume et al. (21) determined a density of 423 follicles/cm^2, Pagnoni et al. (22) found 455 follicles/cm^2 on the lateral forehead and up to 1220 follicles/cm^2 in the nose area, and most recently, Otberg et al. (23) determined a number of 292 follicles/cm^2 on the forehead. Nevertheless, there is agreement that sebum output is maximal on the forehead, nose, and chin, the so-called "t-zone" and decreases toward the outer edges of the face (22). Elsewhere on the body, there may be fewer than 100 pilosebaceous units/cm^2 (23). The face contains the largest sebaceous glands, but despite this the ducts serving these glands are smallest on the face, particularly, on the forehead and have a significantly smaller pore compared to those found on the back. It has been calculated that the smaller duct creates a five times greater resistance to sebum output on the forehead compared to the back (24). This greater resistance exerted by the small duct on sebum flow, may, in part, explain the prevalence of pilosebaceous diseases on the face, involving high sebum secretion, such as acne.

Other types of sebaceous glands are found in humans distributed over epithelial surfaces and open directly onto the surfaces upon which they secrete. These so-called free sebaceous glands are particularly prevalent in transitional areas between skin and mucosal membranes for example, anogenital region, lips, and meibomian glands in the eyelids. Sebaceous glands are also located in oral mucosa (called Fordyce spots), the digestive and respiratory tract, and the areoles of the nipples.

Structure of the Pilosebaceous Duct

The pilosebaceous duct is lined by a stratified, squamous epithelium consisting of keratinocytes. The duct lumen is frequently colonized by bacteria that rely on the keratinocytes and sebum as a source of nutrients.

Several distinct anatomical parts of the duct can be recognized. The opening of the duct onto the surface of the skin is the orifice or ostium. The sebaceous follicles on the back frequently group together and emerge through one orifice (25), while those on the face and chest show no such "grouping" (26). Grouped follicles may be more prone to bacterial colonization, which may, in turn, have important implications for follicular diseases. The size of the duct orifice can decrease by as much as 50% in conditions of high humidity due to hydration of keratin in the pilosebaceous duct (27). During this time, sebum excretion is significantly reduced, but then increases above its original level when the duct reverts to its original size.

The region of duct from the orifice to the point of insertion of the sebaceous duct is called the infundibulum. The hair shaft lies unprotected in the infundibulum, while in the lower duct (i.e., below the insertion of the sebaceous gland) it is surrounded by the inner and outer root sheaths (Fig. 1).

In terminal follicles, the whole of the infundibular lining closely resembles the interfollicular epidermis, the cells of which undergo the same basic pattern of terminal differentiation, as do those of the epidermis. However, in sebaceous and vellus follicles only the upper fifth resembles the contiguous epidermis. This region is termed the acroinfundibulum. The lower four-fifths of the duct, down to the insertion of the sebaceous duct, the infrainfundibulum, display distinct structural and functional differences when compared with the epidermis. The granular layer is thin and inconspicuous and the keratinocytes often contain glycogen granules in contrast to those of the acroinfundibulum. The cornified layer that develops from this is thin, being composed of only two to three layers, and the corneocytes have been described as fragile (28), as opposed to the interfollicular epidermis, where the stratum corneum is well defined. Based upon histological observations, there appears to be little adherence between the ductal cells or corneocytes (28), and as a consequence it is thought that they slough off and disintegrate to form a loose disorganized mass within the lumen which is normally eliminated along with sebum and shed vellus hairs (7). Desmosomes are present between the cells of the follicular epithelium and there is no difference in their expression in acroinfundibulum versus infrainfundibulum (29). The ductal stratum corneum is observed to be relatively thick near the orifice, but it thins as it extends down the follicular canal until it is almost absent at the junction with the sebaceous duct. At these sites, it is thought that the stratum corneum may present an incomplete barrier, allowing the entry of microorganisms and drugs.

The sebaceous duct is lined by a thin epithelium consisting mainly of a basal and granular layer. These cells contain small lipid droplets, whose origin is unclear, but they are thought to be derived from the secretion of the sebaceous glands (7), keratin filaments, and sparse keratohyalin granules. The horny cells here are fragile and are sloughed off in the stream of sebum (7).

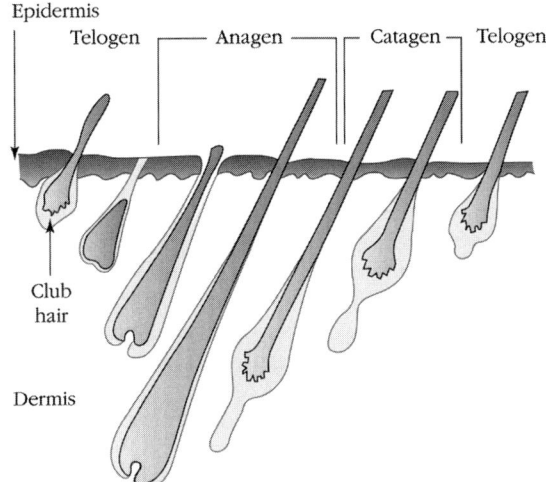

Epidermis

Telogen —— Anagen —— Catagen — Telogen

Club hair

Dermis

FIGURE 2 All follicles produce a hair from the dermal papilla, and hair growth is cyclical, comprising anagen (growth), catagen (breakdown), and telogen (resting) phases successively.

All follicles produce a hair from the dermal papilla and the hair growth is cyclical, comprising of anagen (growth), catagen (breakdown), and telogen (resting) phases, successively (Fig. 2). The amount of hair growth in any area of the body, therefore, depends on several factors, including the duration of anagen, the proportion of time spent in anagen, and the growth rate of the hair (Table 1). The length of a hair shaft is directly proportional to the time the follicle grows (anagen). At the end of an anagen, the follicle stops growing and regresses, transiting in terminal follicles from a deep lower follicle portion in the reticular dermis to a shallow structure in the papillary dermis. Both FGF5 and EGF are believed to play a role in the anagen–catagen switch; transgenic mice lacking FGF5 have an extended anagen phase and have an angora phenotype (30), while topical addition of EGF to sheep can cause spontaneous induction of catagen (31). In the catagen phase, hair growth is arrested by a sudden shrinkage of the lower follicle and papilla. The dermal papilla is released from the hair bulb, accompanied with degradation of the lower follicle followed by apoptosis (32). In order to achieve this, the lower portion from which the hair has been growing begins to break down aided by a perifollicular mast cell infiltrate that may function to remove some of the excess components and end products of apoptosis. During this process, the lower follicle is destroyed and the dermis is remodeled appropriately. In telogen, the follicle is quiescent and no hair growth occurs and finally the hair is shed. The Wnt/β catenin pathway plays an important role in telogen–anagen transition and reactivation of follicle growth during postnatal hair cycling hair follicle (33). More is known about hair follicle cycling in terminal follicles and the influence of steroid hormones

TABLE 1 Characteristics of the Hair Cycle in Vellus and Terminal Follicles

	Vellus	Terminal
Anagen	Short—30–60 days	Long—up to 12 yr
Catagen	Long	Short
Telogen	Fine hair—<30 μm	Large; occupies most of the infundibulum

and receptor expression, compared to sebaceous and vellus follicles. Terminal hair follicle cycling is well reviewed by Stenn and Paus (34).

The Cells of the Pilosebaceous Duct

The duct is lined with keratinocytes, which undergo the same basic pattern of terminal differentiation as do those of the epidermis. This process of terminal differentiation of keratinocytes has been well characterized for the epidermis, but is less well understood for the pilosebaceous duct, largely due to the small amounts of material available for experimentation. Most of the information comes from immunohistochemical studies. Our present understanding of keratinocyte biochemistry within the infundibulum of terminal, vellus, and sebaceous follicles is outlined briefly in the next paragraph.

In the epidermis, cytokeratins form the major structural proteins of keratinocytes, forming the cytoskeleton. Reports on the expression of keratins in the ducts of terminal follicles vary according to the antisera used (35–37). Moll et al. (36) reported that the expression of keratins in the infundibulum of terminal follicles resembled that of the interfollicular epidermis. However, other researchers made very specific antibodies to the highly variable C-terminal region of keratins and reported finding the hyperproliferative keratin 16 suprabasally in the infundibulum, indicating that follicular epithelium may naturally have a higher cell turnover compared to interfollicular epithelium.

Keratins 1 and 10, normally found suprabasally in epidermis, are expressed throughout the infundibulum of sebaceous and vellus follicles, except for the area around the point of insertion of the sebaceous duct, where expression of K16 and K17 was noted, suprabasally (9). It is surprising that no gross differences were reported between the acroinfundibulum and the infrainfundibulum despite the fact that the latter is reported to produce only a thin stratum granulosum and stratum corneum in the sebaceous follicle (38). In comparison with terminal follicles, sebaceous follicles were found to have less extensive expression of keratins 16 and 19 in the outer root sheath of the lower duct (39,40), suggesting that the follicular epithelia of lower ducts in terminal follicles are more hyperproliferative than in other follicles. The keratin pairs 1 and 10, 5 and 14, and 16 and 17 were expressed in the sebaceous duct cells.

Histological observations made by Plewig and Kligman (28) led them to describe the cornified envelopes formed in the infrainfundibulum as fragile, since they disintegrated more readily than did those of the acroinfundibulum. These purely histological observations have never been followed up by isolating and examining the shapes of cornified envelopes from ducts. In fact, ductal cornified envelopes were shown to be antigenically identical throughout the infundibulum, but different from interfollicular cornified envelopes (41). Rupniak et al. (42) also showed that psoriatic keratinocytes express epitopes similar to those expressed by the cornified envelopes of keratinocytes in the follicular duct.

Immunohistochemical staining for transglutaminase demonstrated that this enzyme is expressed throughout the follicular epithelium of sebaceous follicles (H. Knaggs, unpublished observations). A hair follicle specific transglutaminase, which is structurally distinct from the other types of transglutaminase, exists in the inner root sheath and in the medulla of the terminal hair follicles (43,44). Transglutaminase catalyzes the crosslinking of various precursor proteins via

γ-glutamyl-ε-lysine bonds in a calcium-dependent acyl transfer reaction. Proteins that can be incorporated into the cornified envelope include desmosomal components, compounds obtained following organelle destruction, and involucrin. Staining for involucrin in the duct is restricted to the upper spinous and granular layers at the cell boundaries (45). Other transglutaminase substrates such as loricrin, keratolinin, pancornulins (46), and sciellin (47) may be more important than involucrin in cornified envelope formation, although the location of these proteins within the sebaceous follicle has not been reported. In terminal follicles of rats, loricrin is found predominantly in the upper duct (48).

The lumen of the duct provides a suitable environment for bacterial colonization, but recently it has been demonstrated that the keratinocytes of follicles are a source of antimicrobial peptides called defensins (49).

Structure of the Pilosebaceous Gland

All sebaceous glands are similar in structure. They consist of either a single lobule (acinus) or a collection of acini. The glands are separated from the dermis by a connective tissue capsule, consisting of fine collagen fibers, fibroblasts, and a capillary plexus. The ultrastructure of human sebaceous cells does not vary significantly from one skin site to another nor does the ultrastructure of sebocytes of prepubertal children differ significantly from that of adults, implying that increased levels of androgens at puberty do not induce gross ultrastructural changes (50).

In human skin, the cells of sebaceous glands, called sebocytes, which are modified keratinocytes, can be divided into three major cell types determined by structure: undifferentiated or dividing, differentiated, and mature. The undifferentiated cells are attached to the basement membrane by hemidesmosomes. These cells tend to be cuboidal and are characterized by the possession of large nuclei, numerous mitochondria, tonofilaments, small golgi bodies, a high free ribosome, and glycogen granule content. No sebum is apparent in these cells. A second pool of dividing cells has been described to occur near the insertion of the sebaceous duct. These cells have a higher labeling index with tritiated thymidine (19–24%) compared to the germinative cells at the periphery of the gland (8–10%), implying that these cells have a higher turnover rate. Langerhans cells, which participate in the immune function of skin, are also found among the undifferentiated layer.

The sebocytes differentiate centripetally, that is, toward the center of the lobule. They take on a rounded appearance and the volume of cytoplasm decreases as the cells become filled with lipid containing vacuoles. The cells develop an extensive golgi apparatus, smooth endoplasmic reticulum, numerous mitochondria, free ribosomes, and glycogen. As differentiation progresses, lysosomes become apparent, which are thought to originate from the golgi apparatus. These are enriched with acid phosphatase activity. The mature cells in the center of the gland, near the insertion of the sebaceous duct, are approximately 100 to 150 times larger in volume than the basal cells. At this point, cytoplasmic organelles and nuclei degenerate and the mature cells disintegrate to produce the oily liquid sebum, a so-called holocrine secretion.

In sebaceous glands, the release of sebum from the mature cells into the sebaceous duct is thought to be a consequence of physical displacement of mature cells by new cells from the basal layer. Acid esterases and phosphatases have been demonstrated histochemically in the central portion of sebaceous glands (51), where they may be involved in holocrine secretion (52).

It was generally accepted that sebaceous glands were not innervated (53) until a very specific silver staining procedure was used on sections of sebaceous glands. This showed that nerve fibers do, in fact, penetrate the connective tissue capsule of the gland and enter between the lobules, reaching the inner part of the sebaceous lobule (54). These fibers may play a role in the holocrine secretion of sebum or they may secrete neuropeptides into sebum before the sebum exits from the gland. Certainly in acne, there is evidence of increased innervation of the sebaceous gland with increased expression of nerve growth factor (NGF) (55).

SECTION TWO: SEBUM
Sebum Production

Sebum is an oily liquid containing triglycerides, free fatty acids, wax esters, squalene, and a little cholesterol produced by the gland. It is modified by bacteria that hydrolyze triglycerides to produce free fatty acids, thus a sample of skin surface lipids has a different composition compared to sebum produced by the gland (Table 2).

The delay between sebum synthesis, as measured by the incorporation of injected 14-C acetate into forehead skin of four healthy male subjects, and the subsequent excretion of radiolabeled sebum was determined to be eight days (56). This was similar to the five days reported for the delay between the onset of fasting and initial change in composition of skin surface lipids reported by Pochi et al. in 1970 (57). However, the overall process from sebocyte cell division to cell rupture is longer, about 14 days (58). In the beard and scalp follicles, it is believed that the hairs act as a wick to facilitate the passage of sebum to the surface of the skin. In follicles, which possess a vellus hair, the sebum may pool and form a follicular reservoir (59). Thus, the rate of sebum excretion onto the skin surface is a function of the rate of sebocyte proliferation, lipid synthesis, cell lysis, and the rate of flow through the follicular reservoir.

Sebum secretion is increased around puberty under the influence of androgens, concomitant with sebaceous gland enlargement. In human males, sebum secretion continues until the age of 80, but in females it drops significantly in the decade after menopause (60). In elderly individuals, sebaceous glands may undergo hyperplasia, but this does not seem to result in an increase in sebum output (61).

TABLE 2 Composition of Sebum

	Sebum produced by gland (%)	Sebum obtained from skin surface (%)
Triglycerides	60	40
Free fatty acids	40	20
Wax esters	25	25
Squalene	15	15
Cholesterol + cholesterol esters	1−2	1−2

Function of Sebum

In animals, sebum may provide odor: it contains pheromones and may also condition the hair. However, in humans, the function of sebum is unclear (5) and it has been speculated that the sebaceous glands are vestigial (20). There is now an increasing body of evidence indicating that the sebaceous gland and the components of sebum play a crucial role in the homeostasis of skin (6). Sebum transports vitamin E, a lipophilic antioxidant, to the skin surface where it may play a key role in protecting skin surface lipids from peroxidation (62). Glycerol, a major component of sebaceous triglycerides, may play a role in maintaining epidermal barrier function, since asebic mice lacking sebum and, therefore, glycerol have a poorly functioning epidermal barrier (63). Other proposed functions include antibacterial, lubrication, and/or to provide precursor substrates for epidermal metabolism and synthesis of lipids and/or vitamin D (5). In equine follicles, the sebaceous gland and sebum are required to regulate growth of the hair sheath (64) and an intact sebaceous gland in sheep and human terminal follicles was shown to be required for the inner root sheath breakdown (65,66). Whether this holds true for human sebaceous and vellus follicles, remains to be determined. Alopecia is present in asebic mice with hypoplastic sebaceous glands, that may also indicate a role of the sebaceous gland in hair follicle growth (67).

It seems unlikely that lack of sebum is a causative factor in the production of dry skin. The distribution of sebaceous glands and amount of sebum produced does not correlate with dry skin. Dry skin in the elderly is, apparently, not related to sebum output (68), nor does a low sebum output in prepubertal children lead to dry skin (69). In addition, subjective self-assessment of skin type as dry, normal, or oily does not always correlate with the amount of sebum as measured using a sebumeter (70).

Lipogenesis

Human sebum is quite distinct in composition and biological complexity compared to that of other animals, and also compared to epidermal lipids synthesized by keratinocytes. It is unique in containing high levels of squalene and characteristic free fatty acids, for which the rate-limiting enzymes of the biosynthetic pathways are 3-hydroxy-3-methylglutaryl (HMG) CoA reductase and acetyl CoA carboxylase, respectively. Both enzymes are inactivated by phosphorylation through a cAMP-activated protein kinase. Comparison of the kinetic parameters for these enzymes with those previously described in the literature found in other organs, indicates that the sebaceous gland enzymes have similar affinities for substrates and similar responses to allosteric effectors such as citrate. However, there are key points of differences and these will be discussed in turn.

Squalene Biosynthesis

Human sebum contains a high percentage of squalene, in contrast to the epidermal lipids, which contain a higher proportion of cholesterol. In the sebaceous glands, therefore, the cholesterol biosynthetic pathway appears to be partly arrested in the steps after the production of squalene. This may be due to low activity of squalene epoxidase, or other enzyme of cholesterol biosynthesis, or the availability of substrates. For example, a ready supply of acetate appears to direct lipogenesis toward squalene biosynthesis, while glucose, glutamine, and isoleucine preferentially result in more triacylglyceride production in vitro (71). Limiting levels of

NADPH had previously been suggested, but this is not believed to be responsible for the low levels of cholesterol produced. Since squalene is unique to sebum, it is often used as a marker to differentiate sebaceous lipids from epidermal lipids.

The activity of HMG CoA reductase in sebocytes regulates the amount of squalene produced. This can be reduced by 200 µg/mL of low-density lipoproteins (LDL) in isolated glands (72), similar to LDL downregulation of cholesterol production in fibroblasts, which may work via HMG CoA reductase suppression. Cholesterol itself is a weak repressor of HMG CoA reductase, with the oxygenated cholesterol derivatives mediating suppression of the enzyme. Thus, low concentrations of 25-hydroxycholesterol (2 µg/mL) did not have an effect on squalene synthesis in sebocytes. However, synthesis was reduced by 65% by a 10-fold higher concentration of 25-hydroxycholesterol (73). Mevalonate, the end product of the reaction catalyzed by HMG CoA reductase, can downregulate the reaction and a structurally related compound, mevinolin (lovastatin), inhibits the synthesis of squalene and cholesterol in isolated sebaceous glands (74).

Other compounds that inhibit cholesterol synthesis such as oral aluminum nicotinate and clofibrate had no effect on sebum production (75). Eicosa-5:8:11:14-tetraynoic acid, given orally, suppressed squalene synthesis by 13% to 64% between subjects (76), but its site of action has never been determined.

Free Fatty Acids

Sebum contains numerous fatty acids and many are quite unique in structure, including a wide variety of straight, branched, saturated, and unsaturated fatty acids (77). In human sebum, about 27% of fatty acids chains are saturated, with the greatest proportion being unsaturated (68%). The vast majority of these are monounsaturated (64%) and about 4% are diunsaturated, with the remainder being composed of fatty acid chains longer than 22 carbons (78). Monounsaturated fatty acids of sebum have a double bond usually inserted at position $\Delta 9$. However, in human sebum there is an unusual placing of the double bond at $\Delta 6$ to produce sapienic acid. Sapienic acid is a very abundant and important monounsaturated fatty acid with 16-carbons and a *cis* double bond located at the sixth carbon from the carboxyl terminal. This fatty acid has been implicated in acne and is produced by an enzyme unique to sebaceous glands, the $\Delta 6$ desaturase, which has recently been isolated from human skin, and its expression is demonstrated in human sebaceous glands (79). This is the first time that a sebaceous gland-specific functional marker has been demonstrated.

In mice, a similar enzyme has been located in sebaceous glands producing unsaturation between carbons 9 and 10, in other words, a $\Delta 9$ desaturase. Loss of expression of this enzyme in mice results in profound effects with hypoplastic sebaceous glands and an asebic phenotype (80). Although the reason for the presence of these unique fatty acids is not understood, it is speculated that they may impart fluidity on the sebum allowing it to reach the skin surface. An area of active interest is, whether subtle changes in these lipids occur causing blockage in the duct leading to skin diseases such as acne (81) or not. The ratio of $\Delta 6:\Delta 9$ fatty acids depends on the rate of sebum secretion—in prepubertal children, and in sebum from the vernix caeosa, as well as elderly individuals the $\Delta 9$ fatty acid predominates. The $\Delta 6$ form is found most commonly in sebum from adults and increases concomitantly with sebum excretion rate. This is thought to be due to a higher level of the $\Delta 6$ desaturase enzyme located in differentiating sebocytes, compared to the enzyme responsible for producing the $\Delta 9$ unsaturated fatty acids, which predominates in undifferentiated sebocytes (82). Thus, as sebum secretion increases, the $\Delta 6$ fatty acid increases and dilutes the $\Delta 9$ fraction. Since high levels of sebum production are implicated in acne, the increased content of sapienate may be relevant to the pathogenesis of this disease.

Diunsaturated fatty acids in sebum have double bonds at positions $\Delta 5$ and $\Delta 8$ or at positions $\Delta 7$ and $\Delta 10$. The major form of dienoic acid was identified as 18:2 $\Delta 5$:8 and named sebaleic acid. This is presumably synthesized by action of the $\Delta 6$ desaturase on palmitic acid (16:0) to produce 16:1 $\Delta 6$, which then undergoes further desaturation at the 5,6 position following chain elongation to 18 carbons (83). Sebaleic acid is thought to be a major component of sebaceous membrane phospholipids and this may explain the increased levels associated with increased rates of sebum excretion and acne. Another important dienoic acid of sebum is linoleic acid (18:2 $\Delta 9$,12), and the levels are inversely related to sebum excretion, with lower levels being found in subjects with high sebum excretion rates (84). As the cells enlarge during differentiation, they may need additional diunsaturated fatty acids for membrane synthesis and presumably synthesize sebaleic acid as a subsititute for linoleic acid, thus explaining the change in ratio of these fatty acids accompanying high sebum excretion (81). There is evidence that linoleic acid from sebum is incorporated into epidermal acylceramides, but when levels of sebum are low it is replaced by sapienic acid, and this could impair barrier function.

There is evidence to suggest that the types of fatty acids synthesized by individuals is controlled by genotype (85) and is unchanged by fluctuations in diet or metabolism. Site to site variations in free fatty acids in skin surface lipids have also been reported (86). It is important to note that the types of fatty acids synthesized seem to vary significantly during the life of an individual: there are several reported examples of this. In addition to those mentioned earlier, a similar effect is seen with some branched chain fatty acids (82). Although human fatty acids are predominantly straight chain, branched chain components were detected with gas chromatography, and saturated fatty acids of human sebum were found to contain methyl branches on one or more of the even numbered carbon atoms throughout the chain (87). The terminally isobranched 15 and 17 carbon species, often comprising wax esters, occur in higher proportions in the sebum of young children, when sebum secretion is low, and in lower quantities in adult sebum (88).

Another enzyme involved in fatty acid synthesis is acetyl CoA carboxylase and this controls the rate-limiting step of this biosynthetic pathway. It exists in different isoforms, but it is not known whether any of these forms predominates in sebocytes. These cells incorporate fatty acids into triglycerides and wax esters. Palmitate, palmitoleate, stearate, and oleate seem to be the main fatty acids used for further esterification in the gland (89). Of all the fatty acids investigated, linoleic acid was unique, since it was preferentially broken down to 2-carbon units to fuel further fatty acid synthesis, such as palmitic and oleic acids, and squalene synthesis.

The processes of lipid biosynthesis and terminal differentiation in human sebocytes are quite well understood, but the pathways that control holocrine secretion are still unknown. Immortalized humans (SZ95) sebocytes were found to exhibit DNA fragmentation after a six-hours culture followed by increased lactate dehydrogenase release after 24 hours, indicating cell damage, indicating at least in culture this cell line that lipid release is accompanied by apoptosis (90).

Regulation of Pilosebaceous Unit Activity

There are many controlling influences on the pilosebaceous unit (Fig. 3). The development of model systems for the sebaceous gland and duct has made it easier to study these pathways in vitro.

Androgens

Perhaps the most profound and well-known effect of hormones on the pilosebaceous unit is the one caused by androgens, more specifically in causing sebaceous gland enlargement, sebocyte proliferation, and lipid metabolism (91,92). It is well established that the increase in lipid production and enlargement of the sebaceous glands at puberty is attributable to an increase in circulating androgens from the testes in males, the ovaries in females, and the adrenal glands of both sexes. Androgen-insensitive subjects do not produce sebum (93). Furthermore, the local application of testosterone to skin resulted in a 15-fold increase in sebum excretion rate, although admittedly this was a small study in which 2% testosterone cream was applied to the foreheads of prepubertal boys. In fact, three subjects failed to respond, but this study does demonstrate that skin can respond to local androgens (94).

Androgen sensitivity of pilosebaceous units has been confirmed by the positive detection of androgen receptors in pilosebaceous units by immunohistochemistry (Fig. 4) (95–97) and by their isolation from sebaceous gland cells (98). However, it has not been possible to demonstrate differences in receptor levels that explain androgen dependent dermatoses, such as acne or the different rates of sebum production in different individuals. There is a strong correlation between sebum excretion rate and acne grade (99,100), but it has not been possible

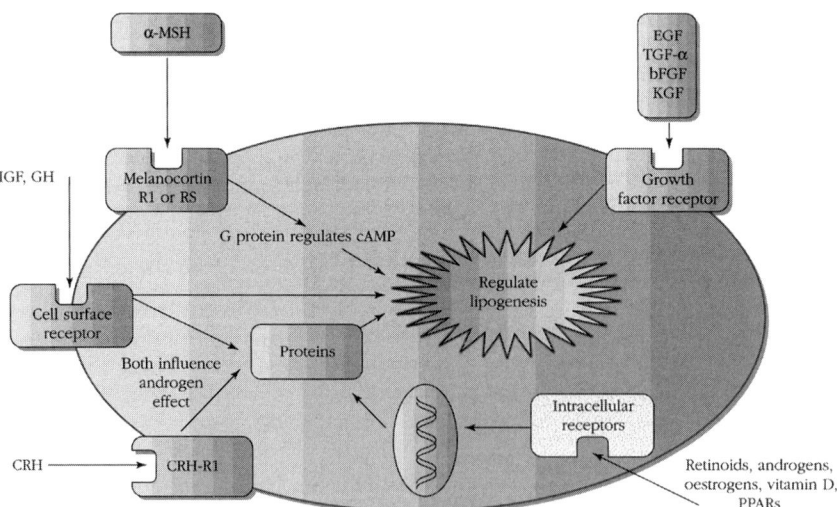

FIGURE 3 A schematic representation of potential pathways in sebocytes that can regulate lipogenesis. *Abbreviations*: CAMP, cyclic adenosine monophosphate; CRH, corticotrophic releasing hormone; EGF, epidermal growth factor; FGF, fibroblast growth factor; GH, growth hormone; IGF, insulin-like growth factors; KGF, keratinocyte growth factor; MSH, melanocyte stimulating hormone; PPARs, peroxisome proliferator-activated receptors; TGF, transforming growth factor.

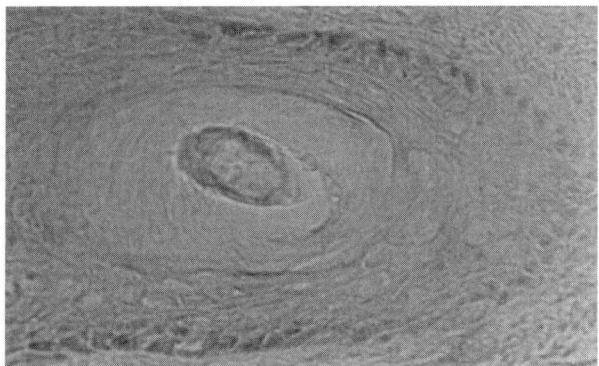

FIGURE 4 Immunohistochemical labeling of a cross-section through the infundibulum of a sebaceous follicle stained with a monoclonal antibody for androgen receptors. Positively stained nuclei are dark gray.

to relate the rate of sebum production to differences in androgen receptor levels in different acne patients.

Androgen receptor antagonists, such as oral cyproterone acetate and spironolactone compete with androgens for the androgen receptor-binding site (101), and while both compounds effectively decrease sebum production, they also have feminizing side-effects. Since their effect is not specific for skin, their use is restricted to women. Antiandrogens also decrease follicular impactions (see later) (102), but this may be secondary to a reduction in sebum flow or a change in sebaceous lipid composition.

An important feature of the effect of androgens on pilosebaceous unit metabolism is the metabolic conversion of the androgens themselves, and much work has been done in the last decade to define the pathways of androgen metabolism. It is now clear that pilosebaceous units possess all the steroid metabolizing enzymes needed to convert dehydroepiandrosterone to the most potent androgen, dihydrotestosterone (DHT), including 3-β-hydroxsteroid dehydrogenase (103–105), and 5-α-reductase (5-α-R) (106). These latter two enzymes exist in several isoforms: type 2 isozyme of 17 β-hydroxy steroid dehydrogenase (β-HSD) is predominant in sebaceous glands and type 1 5α-R is highest in sebaceous glands (107,108), isolated and cultured infundibular keratinocytes, and in epidermis (109). This would explain why 5α-R II inhibitors such as finasteride, do not produce a significant reduction in sebum output (93).

Furthermore, sebocytes have the biosynthetic capacity to produce their own androgens from cholesterol through the cytochrome P450 side-chain cleavage system (P450scc) (110). Along with its cofactors, adrenodoxin, adrenodoxin reductase, and the transcription factor, steroidogenic factor 1, P450scc converts cholesterol to pregnenolone, which is also the precursor for estrogen synthesis. Positive staining using antibodies to these proteins was demonstrated in hair follicles in human facial skin, and biochemical activity was demonstrated in vitro confirming that sebaceous glands are locally steroidogenic with the capacity to produce the highly potent DHT from cholesterol. The conclusion from this body of work is that the skin has its own capacity to metabolize androgens suggesting that the skin exercises local control over the ultimate effects of circulating androgens on the target tissue.

Genes for lipid biosynthesis are regulated in sebaceous glands by androgen-dependent transcription (111). Topical application of 0.005% DHT to hamster ear activated the steroid regulating element (SRE) binding proteins in sebaceous glands, with an upregulation of the mRNA expression for enzymes involved in lipid production, including HMG CoA reductase and synthase, glycerol 3-phosphate acyltransferase, and stearoyl CoA desaturase. SREs are present in the promoter regions of the genes for these enzymes (112).

Estrogens
In contrast to the stimulatory effect of androgens on the sebaceous glands, estrogens and compounds that have estrogenic activity, such as phenol red (113), reduce lipogenesis in vitro. In vivo, the effect of estrogens is contradictory, although at pharmacological doses estrogens are sebosuppressive in rat preputial gland (114) and in humans also producing feminizing side effects (115). This action of estrogens is indirect and occurs by inhibiting the adrenals and gonads via the pituitary, thereby reducing the production of androgens. During hormonal treatments, such as hormone replacement therapy (HRT), the effect on skin surface lipids depends on the predominant hormone given. Skin surface lipids are increased during combined HRT, possibly reflecting stimulatory effects of the progestogen component on sebaceous gland activity, while estrogen alone has a sebum-suppressive action (116).

Local effects of estrogens have been demonstrated (115). Thus, ethinyl estradiol is capable of reducing sebum secretion when applied to the forehead. In addition, sebum secretion was reduced at sites on the forehead distal to the site of application. In agreement with a local effect, both α and β receptor subtypes for estrogens are detected in sebaceous glands of human terminal follicles in both basal and partially differentiated sebocytes (117). There was also widespread expression of estrogen receptor β in the terminal hair follicle, where it was localized to the nuclei of the outer root sheath, epithelial matrix, dermal papilla cells, and in the cells of the bulge (118).

Retinoids
Retinoids exert dramatic, dose-dependent effects on sebocytes in vitro and in vivo. The effect of retinoids is mediated through nuclear receptors [retinoic acid receptor (RAR), retinoid X receptor (RXR)] expressed in sebocytes (119), and in vitro, sebocytes respond differently to retinoids depending upon whether RAR or RXR agonists are given. Activation of RAR by all-*trans*-retinoic acid (all-*trans*-RA) mediated the antiproliferative and antidifferentiation effects, while RXR agonists caused differentiation and only weak proliferation in rat preputial cells (120).

Vitamin A was essential for the proliferation, lipogenesis, and differentiation of immortalized human sebocytes in vitro (121), but these cells showed different responses to other retinoids and the effects were dose dependent. In delipidized serum (i.e., in the absence of vitamin A), isotretinoin [13-*cis*-retinoic acid (13-*cis*-RA)] and acitretin at concentrations $\leq 10^{-7}$M enhanced sebocyte proliferation and lipid synthesis, whereas at concentrations $> 10^{-7}$M–sebocyte proliferation was inhibited (121). In contrast, with cells cultured in media containing vitamin A, further addition of either isotretinoin or to a lesser extent, all-*trans*-RA at concentrations ranging from 10^{-8}M to 10^{-5}M inhibited cell proliferation and lipid synthesis, and altered keratin expression (122). For 13-*cis*-RA to affect sebocyte proliferation, differentiation, and lipogenesis, it must apparently be first isomerized to all-*trans*-RA (123), so it is perhaps not surprising that these retinoids show similar effects.

Other culture systems support the inhibitory role for retinoids in sebaceous glands. Retinoids significantly inhibited proliferation in the rank order 13-*cis*-RA > all-*trans*-RA ≫ acitretin in immortalized sebocytes (124) and in sebaceous gland organ culture, 13-*cis*-RA caused a significant decrease in lipogenesis over seven days (113,125), and reduced thymidine uptake in pilosebaceous duct organ culture (126).

Clinically, 13-*cis*-RA is given orally for severe acne at doses of 1 mg/kg/day for four months and produces a rapid reduction in sebum excretion, for example, down to 20% of its former level within four weeks (127). This is due to sebaceous gland atrophy as demonstrated by histological methods (128) but the mechanism involved is unknown. 13-*cis*-RA and the derivatives, 3,4-didehydroretinoic acid, and 3,4-didehydroretinol are potent competitive inhibitors of the oxidative 3 α-HSD, potentially downregulating the production of potent androgens, DHT, and androstandione, in vitro (129). 13-*cis*-RA does not however have any effect on 5-α-R responsible for the production of DHT (107). There is also a strong increase in cellular retinoic acid binding protein II expression in the sebaceous gland, and to some extent, in the infundibular structures compared with the level of expression in the epidermis in biopsies obtained from patients treated with 13-*cis*-RA. Strongest staining was always found in layers of suprabasal sebocytes lacking lipid droplets, and staining was absent in the basal layers (130).

Vitamin D
The effect of topical vitamin D on human sebocytes and sebum secretion has not been documented, although receptors for vitamin D have been demonstrated in the nuclei of basal sebocytes (131,132). In a culture system of hamster auricular sebocytes, 1-α,25-dihydroxyvitamin D_3, decreased the triglyceride level by 34.3%, but augmented the accumulation of wax esters by 30%, with no difference in the level of cholesterol produced (133).

Peroxisome Proliferator-Activated Receptors
Peroxisome proliferator-activated receptors (PPARs) are a subfamily of so-called orphan receptors belonging to the nonsteroid receptor family of nuclear hormone receptors. Several major types of PPARs have been identified. Activation of PPARs regulates many of the lipid metabolic genes contained in peroxisomes, mitochondria, and microsomes, with the net effect of stimulating lipogenesis. Adipocytes, for example, are induced to differentiate and accumulate lipid through PPARγ2. Therefore, there is interest in PPARs functioning as regulators of lipogenesis in sebocytes (134,135). Certainly in rat preputial sebocytes, PPARγ is selectively expressed and has been implicated in the regulation of sebocyte differentiation (136). Fatty acids are PPAR ligands and act as regulators of lipogenesis (137). For example, linoleic acid incubation for 48 hours in immortalized sebocytes induced abundant lipid synthesis. Furthermore, the effect of androgens appears to be additive with the PPAR pathways: androgens appear to upregulate downstream PPAR expression, which in turn influences terminal differentiation of sebocytes (137,138). PPARs can also form heterodimers with RXRs and there is some evidence that there is cooperation between RXR agonists and PPAR agonists in sebocyte growth and development (139). This is a complex area and the role of these receptors in lipid

production in sebocytes is just beginning to be understood with the help of model systems.

Thyroid Hormones

Thyroid hormones exert an effect on sebum secretion since thyroidectomy decreases the rate of sebum secretion in rats and administration of thyroxine reverses this effect (140). Increases in sebum secretion rate were observed when thyroxine was given to hypothyroid patients (141), and immunohistochemical localization of thyroid hormone nuclear receptors has been demonstrated in human scalp follicles in the nuclei of the outer root sheath cells, dermal papilla cells, sheath cells, and sebaceous gland cells (142). Other than this, little attention has been paid to the effect of thyroid hormones on sebum secretion.

Melanocortins

Melanocortins are small peptides, including α-melanocyte stimulating hormone (αMSH) and adrenocorticotrophic hormone (ACTH), known to regulate immune functions, lipid metabolism, and pigmentation pathways. These small peptides are derived from a larger precursor, proopiomelanocortin (POMC), a 241 amino acid peptide secreted by the pituitary, which is cleaved to liberate the melanocortins. Evidence has existed since the 1970s demonstrating that the sebaceous gland is influenced by pituitary secretions. For example, removal of the posterior pituitary in rats significantly reduced lipid secretion from rat preputial glands, addition of αMSH stimulated a dose-dependent increase in sebum secretion in rats (143), and patients with hypopituitarism show reduced sebum secretion (141). The expression of POMC-derived peptides in hair follicles in mice varies during the hair cycle, with high levels of β-endorphin expressed during anagen and catagen (144).

The biological effects of melanocortins are mediated through specific transmembrane receptors, known as melanocortin receptors, which are coupled to G-proteins to modulate intracellular levels of cAMP. To date, five receptor subtypes (MCR1–5) have been cloned (145) and, of these, MCR-1 was detected in human sebaceous glands using immunostaining (146), and in an immortalized human sebocyte cell line (147). MCR-5 expression was demonstrated in microdissected human sebaceous glands (148), but could not be detected using immunostaining of sections. Specific transcripts for MCR-1, but not for MCR-5, were present in an immortalized sebocyte cell line and these sebocytes responded to αMSH by modulating interleukin-8 (IL-8) secretion (147). In rat preputial cells, MCR-5 was detected perhaps explaining the earlier observations of the effect of melanocortin on these cells (143); and in transgenic mice, targeted disruption of MCR-5 gave marked reduction of sebum secretion (149). Other investigators showed that sebocytes derived from normal human facial skin were stimulated to differentiate and produce prominent lipid droplets when POMC-derived peptides, αMSH, and ACTH were added, and this correlated with an increase in expression of MCR-5 (150). Together, these data support the regulation of human sebum production by melanocortins and may offer an explanation for the link between stress and acne, with high circulating levels of ACTH acting directly on the sebaceous gland to mediate sebum production (148).

Growth Factors and Neuropeptides

EGF, TGF-α, basic FGF, and keratinocyte growth factor (KGF) all inhibit lipogenesis and with the exception of KGF are mitogenic in cultured hamster sebocytes (133,151). In organ culture of human sebaceous glands, EGF produced a dose-dependent inhibition of lipid synthesis and inhibited DNA synthesis (152), and removal of EGF from the medium caused an increase in the rate of lipogenesis without affecting cell turnover (113). In vivo, the presence of EGF inhibited the sebaceous gland differentiation in sheep (153), and in hamster ears, it stimulated the sebaceous glands to proliferate (154). Receptors for EGF are found in sebaceous glands (155). Based on this evidence, Kealey and colleagues proposed that EGF may be, in part, responsible for sebaceous gland atrophy observed during acne lesion formation (7,152). EGF can also induce changes in sebum composition. Ridden (156), reported that there was a fall in the amount of squalene and a corresponding rise in cholesterol, although this was not corroborated by other researchers (157).

Sebocyte proliferation is stimulated by insulin, thyroid-stimulating hormone, and hydrocortisone (158). In rat preputial cells, growth hormone (GH) increased sebocyte differentiation and was more potent than either insulin-like growth factors (IGFs) or insulin. Furthermore, GH enhanced the effect of DHT on sebocyte differentiation perhaps complementing the effect of androgens in increasing sebum during puberty. IGFs, in contrast, had a greater effect on increasing DNA synthesis compared to GH, and had no effect on the response of the cell to DHT (159), although a role for IGF in causing the observed increase in sebum production at puberty has not been ruled out. This suggests that antagonists of IGF may offer a way of decreasing sebum synthesis.

Corticotrophic-releasing hormone (CRH), a key regulator in the central nervous system, has been implicated in sebum production (160). CRH and its receptor are expressed in cultured sebocytes, where the hormone appears to upregulate expression of 3 β-HSD—a key enzyme in the androgen biosynthetic pathways. Therefore, CRH could indirectly influence lipid synthesis by modifying the local production of androgens.

Incubation of sebaceous glands in organ culture with neuropeptides (e.g., calcitonin gene-related peptide, substance P, vasoactive intestinal polypeptide, or neuropeptide Y), or NGF up to a final concentration of 10^{-7}M showed that only substance P had any effect on sebaceous gland ultrastructure as observed in the electron microscope, and this effect was dose dependent (161). Skin samples cultured with substance P showed sebaceous glands with an increased gland area (in sections) compared with control samples. The sebocytes were engorged with numerous lipid droplets.

Cytokines

Expression of IL-1α and β was demonstrated in sebaceous glands by immunohistochemistry (162), and mRNA for IL-1α was detected in cultured sebocytes (163). No change in staining pattern was observed when sebum was extracted from the samples, indicating that IL-1 is not associated with sebum. The function of IL-1 in normal sebaceous glands is unclear, although in vitro IL-1α and tumor necrosis factor α, inhibited sebaceous lipogenesis in sebaceous gland organ culture and induced de-differentiation of human sebocytes into a keratinocyte-like phenotype (152). In organ culture, IL-1α at 1 ng/mL promoted ductal cornification (164) and upregulated mRNA and protein synthesis of vascular endothelial growth factor (VEGF) (165). Thus in follicular diseases, liberation of IL-1 into the dermis may contribute toward inflammation and increased levels of VEGF by follicular keratinocytes can stimulate angiogenesis. In acne, high levels of IL-1α bioactivity existed in comedonal contents (166).

SECTION THREE: DISEASES
Disorders Affecting Pilosebaceous Unit Biology
Various disorders affect pilosebaceous units, although these diseases are rarely life threatening. Three types of skin cysts exist: epidermoid cysts result from squamous metaplasia of a damaged sebaceous gland, while trichilemmal cysts and steatocystoma are both genetically determined structural aberrations of the pilosebaceous duct. Accumulation of material in the follicular lumen results in distension of the follicle, leading to the formation of noninflamed lesions that are typical of acne, which is the most common follicular disease. In terminal follicles, plugging of the pilosebaceous duct may occur and result in keratosis pilaris. Inflammation around follicles is often seen at the skin surface, for example in folliculitis or acne. In folliculitis, there is extensive colonization of the follicular lumen by microflora.

Acne
Acne is the most common follicular disorder and accounts for the majority of dermatological visits by patients between the ages of 15 to 45 years, with treatment costs likely to exceed $1 billion in the United States (167). Problems associated with follicles often occur on the face and thus can cause great psychological problems for the sufferer. Four main factors contribute to acne: increased sebum production, ductal hypercornification, increased bacterial activity in the duct, and inflammation. The changes that occur in the pilosebaceous biology will be reviewed briefly.

Changes in the Pilosebaceous Unit in Acne
There is no doubt that sebum plays an important etiological role in acne (99,168–170). Patients with acne secrete more sebum than unaffected individuals and sebosuppressive treatments alleviate acne: the greater the inhibition the more profound the clinical response. In addition to elevated sebum excretion, it is well-established that acne is associated histologically and clinically with hypercornification of the duct epithelium (7,38,171). Ductal hypercornification results initially in the formation of microcomedones and eventually comedones, a process termed comedogenesis. On the basis of a detailed histological study Kligman (7) concluded that comedogenesis began in the infrainfundibulum and was closely followed by hyperkeratosis of the sebaceous duct. This is now generally accepted to a reasonable description of what is likely to happen.

Essentially, microcomedones are those follicles containing "impactions," "follicular casts," or "sebaceous filaments" of corneocytes, bacteria, sebum, and vellus hairs within the follicular lumen. There are no clinical signs of these changes occurring, although they are more common in patients with acne (7,172). Microcomedones may develop either into noninflamed, or inflamed lesions, or even resolve (173). The contents of the normal infundibulum from nonacne

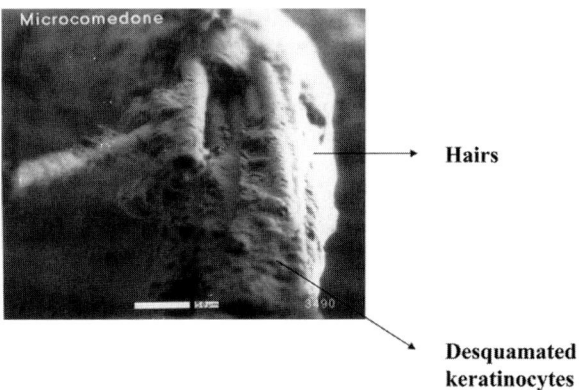

Hairs

Desquamated
keratinocytes

FIGURE 5 Environmental scanning electron micrograph of a microcomedone removed from a pilosebaceous duct. Keratinocytes are seen covering multiple hairs.

control patients were easy to extrude and contained numerous empty spaces in the cells which appeared to have lost their contents and had no clear cytoskeleton. In contrast, the contents of follicles from acne patients were hard to extrude and the cells were firm and compact (7).

An extensive ultrastructural study on the cornified material in follicular impactions was carried out by Al Baghdadi (174). He showed that corneocytes are arranged into three layers in the follicular impaction: a loosely attached outer layer; a densely packed middle layer; and a further loosely attached layer in the middle of the cast. Lipid droplets occur inside the cornified cells (38,175) and as a result the corneocytes become balloon-like in appearance. Abnormal lamellar inclusions of lipid have been described as a marker for abnormal keratinization (176). Scanning electron microscopy of comedonal contents revealed a complex system of numerous internal channels or "canaliculi" composed of concentric lamellae of corneocytes enclosing bacteria and sebum (177) (Fig. 5).

The overall composition of follicular casts was reported to be water (20–60%), lipids (20%), proteins (15%), and microorganisms (178). Bladon et al. (179) analyzed the protein content of comedones and found both epidermal keratins and degraded keratins to be present in the comedones.

Biochemical Changes in the Infundibulum During Comedogenesis
The process of comedogenesis is thought to be due to hyperproliferation of ductal keratinocytes, inadequate separation of the ductal corneocytes, or a combination of both factors, resulting in microcomedones. Hyperproliferation of basal keratinocytes in acne has been demonstrated (180,181) and correlates with keratin 16 expression, a marker for hyperproliferation suprabasally (182). Aldana et al. (183) proposed a cycling of normal follicles through different levels of expression of Ki-67 (a proliferation marker) and keratin 16 and that these represent different stages of development of the microcomedone. The point at which both Ki-67 and keratin 16 are coexpressed by the follicle is when the follicle is susceptible to comedogenic changes (184).

A more extensive investigation of adhesion in follicles is required. In epidermis, intercellular adhesion is mediated by lipids, cellular adhesion molecules, and desmosomes. At the present time, the relative importance of follicular intercellular lipids in normal and acne follicles is unclear due to the experimental difficulties encountered obtaining sufficient material for analysis. Hypercornification from the retention of desmosomes was described to be a contributory factor to the formation of acne lesions. However, no differences were detected between staining for these epitopes in the wall of normal and comedonal follicles (29).

CONCLUSION

Although it is clear that we now know a great deal about the pilosebaceous unit at the structural, biochemical, and physiological levels, there are still considerable gaps in our understanding. Much of the early work was descriptive biology of the structure obtained using immunohistochemical studies. Over the last decade, several in vitro models systems (isolated organ culture, cultured sebocytes) have made it easier to study the cellular processes in the follicle, including sebum production and the effect of inhibitors and stimulators. There is also now a good deal of information about the chemistry and biosynthesis of sebum components, and we also have a much better understanding of the cell biology of the pilosebaceous duct. Even so, we are still unable to precisely define the cause of one of the most common skin diseases, namely acne, which affects a very large proportion of the population globally.

ACKNOWLEDGMENTS

The author wishes to acknowledge and thank Professor W Cunliffe for kindly allowing the use of Figure 1B, and the journal "Retinoids and Lipid Soluble Vitamins in Clinical Practice" for kindly allowing the use of Figures 1A, 2, and 3.

REFERENCES

1. Eisen AZ, Holyoke JB, Lobitz WC. Responses of the superficial portion of the human pilosebaceous apparatus to controlled injury. J Invest Dermatol 1955; 25:145–156.
2. Alonso L, Fuchs E. Stem cells of the skin epithelium. Proc Natl Acad Sci USA 2003; 30(suppl 1):11830–11835.
3. Cotsarelis G, Sun TT, Lavker R. Label-retaining cells reside in the bulge area of pilosebaceous unit: implications for follicular stem cells, hair cycle and skin carcinogenesis. Cell 1990; 61:1329–1337.
4. Oshima H, Rochat A, Kedzia C, Kobayashi K, Barrandon Y. Morphogenesis and renewal of hair follicles from adult multipotent stem cells. Cell 2001; 104:233–245.
5. Shuster S. Biological purpose of acne. Lancet 1976; 1:1328–1329.
6. Zouboulis C. Sebaceous gland in human skin—the fantastic future of a skin appendage. J Invest Dermatol 2003; 120(6):xiv-xv.
7. Kligman AM. An overview of acne. J Invest Dermatol 1974; 62:268–287.
8. Leeming JP, Holland KT, Cunliffe WJ. The microbiological ecology of pilosebaceous units from human skin. J Gen Microbiol 1984; 130:803–807.
9. Hughes BR. The Structure and Function of the Pilosebaceous Duct in Health and Disease—with Special Reference to Acne Vulgaris. MD thesis, University of Leeds, UK, 1992.

10. Holbrook KA. Structure and function of the developing human skin. In: Goldsmith LA, ed. Physiology, Biochemistry and Molecular Biology of the Skin. Vol. 1. Oxford: Oxford University Press, 1991:83–89.
11. Westgate GE, Shaw DA, Harrap GJ, Couchman JR. Immunohistochemical localisation of basement membrane components during hair follicle morphogenesis. J Invest Dermatol 1984; 82:259–264.
12. Millar SE. Molecular mechanisms regulating hair follicle development. J Invest Dermatol 2002; 118:216–225.
13. McElwee KJ, Hoffman R. Growth factors in early hair follicle morphogenesis. Eur J Dermatol 2000; 10:341–350.
14. Ebling FJG. Embryology. In: Rook A, Wilkinson DS, Ebling FJG, eds. Textbook of Dermatology. Oxford: Blackwell Scientific, 1968:16–22.
15. Ferraris C, Bernard BA, Dhouailly D. Adult epidermal keratinocytes are endowed with pilosebaceous forming abilities. Int J Dev Biol 1997; 41:491–498.
16. Serri F, Huber WM. In Advances in Biology of Skin. Vol. 4. Oxford: Pergamon Press, 1963:1–18.
17. Allen M, Grachtchouk M, Sheng H, et al. Hedgehog signaling regulates sebaceous gland development. Am J Path 2003; 163:2173–2178.
18. Niemann C, Unden AB, Lyle S, Zouboulis ChC, Toftgard R, Watt FM. Indian hedgehog and beta-catenin signaling: role in the sebaceous lineage of normal and neoplastic mammalian epidermis. Proc Natl Acad Sci USA 2003; 100(suppl 1): 11873–11880.
19. Piérard GE. Follicle to follicle heterogeneity of sebum excretion. Dermatologica 1986; 173:61–65.
20. Montagna W. Advances in Biology of the Skin. Vol. 4. Oxford, U.K.: Pergamon Press, 1963.
21. Blume U, Ferracin J, Verschoore M, Czernielewski JM, Schaefer H. Physiology of the vellus hair follicle: hair growth and sebum excretion. Br J Dermatol 1991; 124: 21–28.
22. Pagnoni A, Kligman AM, el Gammal S, Stoudemayer T. Determination of density of follicles on various regions of the face by cyanoacrylate biopsy: correlation with sebum output. Br J Dermatol 1994; 131:862–865.
23. Otberg N, Richter H, Schaefer H, Blume-Peytavi U, Sterry W, Lademann J. Variations of hair follicle size and distribution in different body sites. J Invest Dermatol 2004; 122:14–19.
24. Cunliffe WJ, Perera WDH, Thackray P, Williams M, Forster RA, Williams SM. Pilosebaceous duct physiology III. Observations on the number and size of pilo-sebaceous ducts in acne vulgaris. Br J Dermatol 1976; 95:153–156.
25. Price VH, Cappas A, Uno H. Compound follicles presenting as folliculitis and scarring alopecia [abstr]. J Invest Dermatol 1992; 98:582.
26. Cunliffe WJ, Cotterill JA. The Acnes-Clinical Features, Pathogenesis and Treatment. London: WB Saunders, 1975.
27. Williams M, Cunliffe WJ, Gould D. Pilosebaceous duct physiology I. Effect of hydration on pilosebaceous duct orifice. Br J Dermatol 1974; 90:631–635.
28. Plewig G, Kligman AM. Acne, Morphogenesis and Treatment. Berlin: Springer-Verlag, 1975.
29. Knaggs HE, Hughes BR, Morris C, Holland DB, Wood EJ, Cunliffe WJ. Immunohistochemical study of desmosomes in acne vulgaris. Br J Dermatol 1994; 130:731–737.
30. Rosenquist TA, Martin GA. Fibroblast growth factor signalling in the hair growth cycle: expression of the fibroblast growth factor receptor and ligand genes in the murine hair follicle. Dev Dyn 1996; 205:379–386.
31. Danilenko DM, Ring BD, Pierce GF. Growth factors and cytokines in hair follicle development and cycling: recent insights from animal models and the potential for clinical therapy. Mol Med Today 1996; 2:460–467.
32. Paus R, Cotsarelis G. The biology of hair follicles. N Engl J Med 1999; 341:491–497.
33. Van Mater D, Kolligs FT, Dlugosz AA, Fearon ER. Transient activation of β-catenin signalling in cutaneous keratinocytes is sufficient to trigger the active growth phase of the hair cycle in mice. Genes Dev 2003; 17:1219–1224.

34. Stenn K, Paus R. Controls of hair follicle cycling. Physiol Rev 2003; 81:449–494.
35. Heid HW, Moll I, Franke WW. Patterns of expression of trichocytic and epithelial cytokeratins in mammalian tissues I. Human and bovine hair follicle. Differentiation 1988; 91:553–559.
36. Moll R, Franke WW, Volk Platzer B, Koepler R. Different keratin polypeptides in epidermis and other epithelia of human skin: a specific cytokeratin of molecular weight 46000 in epithelia of the pilosebaceous tract and basal cell epitheliomas. J Cell Biol 1982; 95:285–295.
37. Wilson CL, Deane D, Wojnarowska F, Lane EB, Leigh IM. Follicular keratin expression in normal and psoriatic scalp [abstr]. J Invest Dermatol 1990; 95:495.
38. Knutson DD. Ultrastructural observations in acne vulgaris. The normal sebaceous follicle and acne lesions. J Invest Dermatol 1974; 62:288–307.
39. Kluznik AR, Cunliffe WJ. Keratin biosynthesis in the pilosebaceous ducts in acne vulgaris. Biochem Soc Trans 1988; 220:330–331.
40. Stark H-J, Breitkreutz, Limat A, Bowden PE, Fusenig NE. Keratins of the human hair follicle: "Hyperproliferative" keratins consistently expressed in outer root sheath cells in vivo and in vitro. Differentiation 1987; 35.236–248.
41. Rupniak HT, Turner DM, Cunliffe WJ, Dhuna R, West MR. Cell envelope production in acne. In: Marks R, Plewig G, eds. Acne and Related Disorders. London: Martin Dunitz, 1989:87–93.
42. Rupniak HT, Turner DM, Wood EJ, Cunliffe WJ. Characteristics of the cell envelope system in normal and psoriatic epidermis [abstr]. J Invest Dermatol 1986; 87:164.
43. Peterson LL, Wuepper KD. Epidermal and hair follicle transglutaminases and cross-linking in skin. Mol Cell Biochem 1984; 58:99–111.
44. Rothnagel JA, Rogers GE. Transglutaminase-mediated cross-linking in mammalian epidermis. Mol Cell Biochem 1984; 58:113–119.
45. Murphy GF, Flynn TC, Rice RH, Pinkus G. Involucrin expression in normal and neoplastic skin: a marker for keratinocyte differentiation. J Invest Dermatol 1984; 82:453–457.
46. Greco MA, Ladas D, Rudolph S, Baden H. Modulation of pancornulin expression by calcium and relative confluence [abstr]. J Invest Dermatol 1992; 98:640.
47. Kvedar JC, Manabe M, Phillips SB, Ross BS, Baden HP. Characterisation of sciellin, a precursor to the cornified envelope of human keratinocytes. Differentiation 1992; 49:195–204.
48. Hohl D, Olana BR, Schnyder UW, Roop DR. Loricrin is a marker of squamous differentiation in rodents and a marker of epidermal differentiation in higher mammals [abstr]. J Invest Dermatol 1991; 96:1030.
49. Philpott MP. Defensins and acne. Mol Immunol 2003; 40:457–462.
50. Bell M. A comparative study of the ultrastructure of the sebaceous glands of man and other primates. J Invest Dermatol 1974; 62:132–143.
51. Brandes D, Bertini F. Role of lysosomes in cellular lytic processes II. Cell death during holocrine secretion in sebaceous glands. Exp Mol Pathol 1965; 11:245–265.
52. Im MJC, Hoopes JE. Enzymes of carbohydrate metabolism in normal human sebaceous glands. J Invest Dermatol 1974; 62:153–160.
53. Hurley HJ, Shelley WB, Koelle GB. The distribution cholinesterases in human skin, with special reference to eccrine and apocrine sweat glands. J Invest Dermatol 1953; 21:139–147.
54. Pawlowski A, Weddell G. The lability of cutaneous neural elements. Br J Dermatol 1967; 79:14–19.
55. Toyoda M, Nakamura M, Morohashi M. Neuropeptides and sebaceous glands. Eur J Dermatol 2002; 12:422–427.
56. Downing DT, Strauss JS, Ramasastry P, Abel M, Lees CW, Pochi PE. Measurement of the time between synthesis and surface excretion of sebaceous lipids in sheep and man. J Invest Dermatol 1975; 64:215–219.
57. Pochi PE, Downing DT, Strauss JS. Sebaceous gland response in man to prolonged total caloric deprivation. J Invest Dermatol 1970; 55:303–309.

58. Downing DT, Strauss JS. On the mechanism of sebum secretion. Arch Dermatol Res 1982; 272:343–349.
59. Downing DT, Straniesi AM, Strauss JS. The effect of accumulated lipids on measurements of sebum secretion in human skin. J Invest Dermatol 1982; 79:226–228.
60. Pierard-Franchimont C, Pierard GE. Postmenopausal aging of the sebaceous follicle: a comparison between women receiving hormone replacement therapy or not. Dermatology 2003; 204(1):17–22.
61. Zouboulis CC, Boschnakow A. Chronological ageing and photoageing of the human sebaceous gland. Clin Exp Dermatol 2001; 26(7):600–607.
62. Thiele JJ, Weber SU, Packer L. Sebaceous gland secretion is a major physiologic route of vitamin E delivery to skin. J Invest Dermatol 1998; 113:390–395.
63. Fluhr JW, Man M-Q, Brown BE, et al. Glycerol regulates stratum corneum hydration in sebaceous gland deficient (asebia) mice. J Invest Dermatol 2003; 120: 728–737.
64. Williams D, Siock P, Stenn K. 13-cis-Retinoic acid affects sheath-shaft interaction of equine hair follicles in vitro. J Invest Dermatol 1996; 106(2):356–361.
65. Williams D, Stenn K. Transection level dictates the pattern of hair follicle sheath growth in vitro. Dev Biol 1994; 165:469–479.
66. Philpott MP, Sanders DA, Kealey T. Is the sebaceous gland important for inner root sheath breakdown? In: Van Neste D, Randall VA, eds. Hair Research for the Next Milennium. Amsterdam: Elsevier, 1996:393–395.
67. Gates AH, Karasek M. Hereditary absence of sebaceous glands in mouse. Science 1965; 148:1471–1473.
68. Downing DT, Stewart ME, Strauss JS. Changes in sebum secretion and the sebaceous gland. Clin Geriatr Med 1989; 5(1):109–114.
69. Kligman AM. The uses of sebum. Br J Dermatol 1963; 75:307–319.
70. Youn SW, Kim SJ, Hwang IA, Park KC. Evaluation of facial skin type by sebum secretion: discrepancies between subjective descriptions and sebum secretion. Skin Res Technol 2002; 8(3):168–172.
71. Downie MMT, Kealey T. Lipogenesis in the human sebaceous gland: glycogen and glycerophosphate are substrates for the synthesis of sebum lipids. J Invest Dermatol 1998; 1111:199–205.
72. Marsden JR, Middleton B. Lipogenesis in isolated human sebacoues glands: effects of different precursors and inhibitors of cholesterol synthesis. In: Marks R, Plewig G, eds. Acne and Related Disorders. London, U.K.: Martin Dunitz, 1989:35–38.
73. Smythe CDW, Greenall M, Kealey T. The activity of HMG-CoA reductase and actyl-CoA carboxylase in human apocrine sweat glands, sebaceous glands and hair follicles is regulated by phosphorylation and by exogenous cholesterol. J Invest Dermatol 1998; 111:139–148.
74. Marsden JR, Middleton B, Cox J. Lipogenesis in isolated human sebaceous glands: effect of inhibitors. Br J Dermatol 1986; 116:448.
75. Cunliffe WJ, Burton JL, Shuster S. Effect of aluminium nicotinate on sebum excretion. Br J Dermatol 1969; 81:867–868.
76. Strauss JS, Pochi PE, Whitman EN. Suppression of sebaceous gland activity with eicosa-5:8:11:14-tetraynoic acid. J Invest Dermatol 1967; 48(5):492–493.
77. Nicolaides N, Kellum RE, Woolley PV. The structures of the free unsaturated fatty acids of human skin surface fat. Arch Biochem Biophys 1964; 105:634–639.
78. Nicolaides N, Fu HC, Ansari MN, Rice GR. The fatty acids of wax esters and sterol esters from vernix caesosa and from human skin surface. Lipids 1972; 7:506–517.
79. Ge L, Gordon JS, Hsuan C, Stenn K, Prouty SM. Identification of the Δ-6 desaturase of human sebaceous glands expression and enzyme activity. J Invest Dermatol 2003; 120:707–714.
80. Zheng Y, Eilertsen KJ, Ge L, et al. Scd1 is expressed in sebaceous glands and is disrupted in the asebia mouse. Nat Genet 1999; 23(3):268–270.
81. Downing DT, Stewart ME, Wertz PW, Strauss JS. Essential fatty acids and acne. J Am Acad Dermatol 1986; 14:221–225.
82. Stewart ME, Quinn MA, Downing DT. Variability in the fatty acid composition of wax esters from vernix caseosa and its possible relation to sebaceous gland activity. J Invest Dermatol 1982; 78:291–295.

83. Thody A, Shuster S. Control and function of sebaceous glands. Physiol Rev 1989; 69:383416.
84. Stewart ME, Grahek MO, Cambier LS, Wertz PW, Downing DT. Dilutional effect of increased sebaceous gland activity on the proportion of linoleic acid in sebaceous wax esters and in epidermal acylceramides. J Invest Dermatol 1986; 87:733–736.
85. Stewart ME, Greenwood R, Cunliffe WJ, Strauss JS, Downing DT. Effect of cyproterone acetate-ethinyl estradiol treatment on the proportions of linoleic and sebaleic acids in various skin surface lipid classes. Arch Dermatol Res 1986; 278:481–485.
86. Kotani A, Kusu F. HPLC with electrochemical detection for determining the distribution of free fatty acids in skin surface lipids from the human face and scalp. Arch Dermatol Res 2002; 294(4):172–177.
87. Nicolaides N, Apon JM. The saturated methyl branched fatty acids of adult human skin surface lipid. Biomed Mass Spectrom 1977; 4:337–347.
88. Stewart ME, Downing DT. Proportions of various straight and branched fatty acid chain types in the sebaceous wax esters of young children. J Invest Dermatol 1985; 84:501–503.
89. Pappas A, Anthonavage M, Gordon JS. Metabolic fate and selective utilisation of major fatty acids in human sebaceous gland. J Invest Dermatol 2002; 118:164–171.
90. Wrobel A, Seltmann H, Fimmel S, et al. Differentiation and apoptosis in human immortalized sebocytes. J Invest Dermatol 2003; 120(2):175–181.
91. Hamilton JB. Male hormone substance: a prime factor in acne. J Clin Endocrinol 1941; 1:570–592.
92. Rosenfield RL, Deplewski D. Role of androgens in the developmental biology of the pilosebaceous unit. Am J Med 1995; 16(suppl):80–88.
93. Imperato-McGinley J, Gautier T, Cai LQ, Yee B, Epstein J, Pochi P. The androgen control of sebum production. Studies of subjects with dihydrotestosterone deficiency and complete androgen insensitivity. J Clin Endocrinol Metab 1993; 76:524–528.
94. Holland DB, Cunliffe WJ, Norris JFB. Differential response if sebaceous glands to exogenous testosterone. Br J Dermatol 1998; 139:102–103.
95. Henderson CA, Knaggs H, Clark A, Highet AS, Cunliffe WJ. Apert's syndrome and androgen receptor staining of the basal cells of sebaceous glands. Br J Dermatol 1995; 132(1):139–143.
96. Whitaker SB, Vigneswaran N, Singh BB. Androgen receptor status of the oral sebaceous glands. Am J Dermatopathol 1997; 19(4):415–418.
97. Choudhry R, Hodgins MB, Van der Kwast TH, Brinkmann AO, Boersma WJ. Localization of androgen receptors in human skin by immunohistochemistry: implications for the hormonal regulation of hair growth, sebaceous glands and sweat glands. J Endocrinol 1992; 133(3):467–475.
98. Sawaya M. Purification of androgen receptors in human sebocytes and hair. J Invest Dermatol 1992; 98(suppl):92–96.
99. Cunliffe WJ, Shuster S. Pathogenesis of acne. Lancet 1969; 1:685–687.
100. Cunliffe WJ. In: Marks R, ed. Androgen abnormalities in acne subjects. Acne. London: Martin Dunitz, 1989:158–160.
101. Akamatsu H, Zouboulis CC, Orfanos CE. Spironolactone directly inhibits proliferation of cultured human facial sebocytes and acts antagonistically to testosterone and 5 alpha-dihydrotestosterone in vitro. J Invest Dermatol 1993; 100:660–662.
102. Cunliffe WJ, Forster RA. Androgen control of the pilosebaceous duct. [abstr]. Br J Dermatol 1986; 116:449.
103. Sawaya ME, Penneys NS. Immunohistochemical distribution of aromatase and 3β-hydroxysteroid dehydrogenase in human hair follicle and sebaceous gland. J Cutan Pathol 1992; 19(4):309–314.
104. Thiboutot D, Martin P, Volikos L, Gilliland K. Oxidative activity of the type 2 isozyme of 17beta-hydroxysteroid dehydrogenase (17beta-HSD) predominates in human sebaceous glands. J Invest Dermatol 1998; 111(3):390–395.
105. Thiboutot D, Knaggs H, Gilliland K, Lin G. Activity of 5-alpha-reductase and 17-beta-hydroxysteroid dehydrogenase in the infrainfundibulum of subjects with and without acne vulgaris. Dermatology 1998; 196(1):38–42.

106. Luu-The V, Sugimoto Y, Puy L, et al. Characterization, expression, and immunohisto-chemical localization of 5 alpha-reductase in human skin. J Invest Dermatol 1994; 102(2):221–226.
107. Thiboutot D, Harris G, Iles V, Cimis G, Gilliland K, Hagari S. Activity of the type 1 5-alpha-reductase exhibits regional differences in isolated sebaceous glands and whole skin. J Invest Dermatol 1995; 105:209–214.
108. Bayne EK, Flanagan J, Einstein M, et al. Immunohistochemical localization of types 1 and 2 5-alpha-reductase in human scalp. Br J Dermatol 1999; 141(3):481–491.
109. Thiboutot DM, Knaggs H, Gilliland K, Hagari S. Activity of type 1 5 alpha-reductase is greater in the follicular infrainfundibulum compared with the epidermis. Br J Dermatol 1997; 136(2):166–171.
110. Thiboutot D, Jabara S, McAllister JM, et al. Human skin is a steroidogenic tissue: ster-oidogenic enymes and cofactors are expressed in epidermis, normal sebocytes and an immortalised sebocyte cell line (SEB-1). J Invest Dermatol 2003; 120:905–914.
111. Ideta R, Seki T, Adachi K, Nakayama Y. The isolation and characterization of androgen-dependent genes in the flank organs of golden Syrian hamsters. Dermatology 1998; 196(1):47–50.
112. Rosignoli C, Nicolas JC, Jomard A, Michel S. Involvement of the SREBP pathway in the mode of action of androgens in sebaceous glands in vivo. Exp Dermatol 2003; 12:480–489.
113. Guy R, Ridden C, Kealey T. The improved organ maintenance of the human sebaceous gland: modeling in vitro the effects of epidermal growth factor, androgens, estrogens, 13-cis retinoic acid, and phenol red. J Invest Dermatol 1996; 106(3):454–460.
114. Ebling FJ, Skinner J. The local effects of topically applied estradiol, cyproterone acetate and ethanol on sebaceous secretion in intact male rats. J Invest Dermatol 1983; 81:448–451.
115. Strauss JS, Kligman AM, Pochi PE. Effects of androgens and estrogens on human sebac-eous glands. J Invest Dermatol 1962; 39:139–155.
116. Sator PG, Schmidt JB, Sator MO, Huber JC, Honigsmann H. The influence of hormone replacement therapy on skin ageing: a pilot study. Maturitas 2001; 25:43–55.
117. Thornton MJ, Taylor AH, Mulligan K, et al. The distribution of estrogen receptor beta is distinct to that of the estrogen receptor a and the androgen receptor in human skin and the pilosebaceous unit. J Invest Dermatol Sym Proc 2003; 8:100–103.
118. Thornton MJ, Taylor AH, Mulligan K, et al. Oestrogen receptor beta is the predominant oestrogen receptor in human scalp skin. Exp Dermatol 2003; 12(2):181–190.
119. Doran TI, Lucas DA, Levin AA, et al. Biochemical and retinoid receptor activities in human sebaceous cells. In: Saurat J-H, ed. Retinoids: 10 Years On. Basel: Karger, 1991:243–253.
120. Kim MJ, Ciletti N, Michel S, Reichert U, Rosenfield RL. The role of specific retinoid receptors in sebocyte growth and differentiation in culture. J Invest Dermatol 2000; 114:349–353.
121. Zouboulis CC, Korge BP, Miscke D, Orfanos CE. Altered proliferation, synthetic activity, and differentiation of cultured human sebocytes in the absence of vitamin A and their modulation by synthetic retinoids. J Invest Dermatol 1993; 101:628–633.
122. Zouboulis CC, Korge B, Akamatsu H, et al. Effects of 13-cis-retinoic acid, all trans-retinoic acid and acitretin on the proliferation, lipid synthesis and keratin expression of cultured human sebocytes in vitro. J Invest Dermatol 1991; 96:792–797.
123. Tsukada M, Schroder M, Roos TC. 13 cis-retinoic acid exerts its specific activity on human sebocytes through selective intracellular isomerisation to all trans-retinoic acid and binding to retinoid acid receptors. J Invest Dermatol 2000; 115:321–327.
124. Zouboulis CC, Seltmann H, Neitzel H, Orfanos CE. Establishment and characterization of an immortalized human sebaceous gland cell line (SZ95). J Invest Dermatol 1999; 113(6):1011–1020.
125. Ridden J, Ferguson D, Kealey T. Organ maintenance of human sebaceous glands: in vitro effects of 13-cis retinoic acid and testosterone. J Cell Sci 1990; 95:125–136.
126. Guy R, Ridden C, Barth J, Kealey T. Isolation and maintenance of the human pilosebac-eous duct: 13-cis retinoic acid acts directly on the duct in vitro. Br J Dermatol 1993; 128(3):242–248.

127. Stewart ME, Benoit AM, Stranieri AM, Rapini RP, Strauss JS, Downing DT. Effect of oral 13-cis-retinoic acid at three dose levels on sustainable rates of sebum secretion and on acne. J Am Acad Dermatol 1983; 8:532–538.

128. Dalziel K, Barton S, Marks R. The effects of isotretinoin on follicular and sebaceous gland differentiation. Br J Dermatol 1987; 117:317–323.

129. Karlsson T, Vahlquist A, Kedishvili N, Torma H. 13-cis-retinoic acid competitively inhibits 3 alpha-hydroxysteroid oxidation by retinol dehydrogenase RoDH-4: a mechanism for its anti-androgenic effects in sebaceous glands? Biochem Biophys Res Commun 2003; 303(1):273–278.

130. Sitzmann JH, Bauer FW, Cunliffe WJ, Holland DB, Lemotte PK. In situ hybridization analysis of CRABP II expression in sebaceous follicles from 13-cis retinoic acid-treated acne patients. Br J Dermatol 1995; 133(2):241–248.

131. Stumpf WE, Koike N, Hayakawa N, et al. Distribution of 1,25-dihydroxyvitamin D3[22-oxa] in vivo receptor binding in adult and developing skin. Arch Dermatol Res 1995; 287:294–303.

132. Stumpf WE, Perez-Delgado MM, Li L, Bidmon HJ, Tuohimaa P. Vitamin D_3 (soltriol) nuclear receptors in abdominal scent gland and skin of Siberian hamster (Phodopus sungorus) localised by autoradiography and immunohistochemistry. Histochemistry 1993; 100:115–119.

133. Sato T, Imai N, Akimoto N, Sakiguchi T, Kitamura K, Ito A. Epidermal growth factor and 1-25-dihydroxy-vitamin D_3 suppress lipogenesis in hamster sebaceous gland cells in vitro. J Invest Dermatol 2001; 117:965–970.

134. Tontonoz P, Hu E, Spigelman B. Stimulation of adipogenesis in fibroblasts by PPARγ2, a lipid-activated transcription factor. Cell 1994; 79:1147–1156.

135. Tontonoz P, Hu E, Spigelman BM. Regulation of adipocyte gene expression and differentiation by peroxisome proliferators activated receptor. Curr Opin Genet Dev 1995; 5:571–576.

136. Rosenfield RL, Kentsis A, Deplewski D, Ciletti N. Rat preputial sebocyte differentiation involves peroxisome proliferator-activated receptors. J Invest Dermatol 1999; 112:226–232.

137. Chen W, Yang CC, Sheu HM, Seltmann H, Zouboulis CC. Expression of peroxisome proliferator-activated receptor and CCAAT/enhancer binding protein transcription factors in cultured human sebocytes. J Invest Dermatol 2003; 121(3):441–447.

138. Rosenfield RL, Deplewski D, Kentsis, Ciletti N. Mechanisms of androgen induction of sebocyte differentiation. Dermatology 1998; 196:43–46.

139. Kim MJ, Deplewski D, Ciletti N, Michel S, Reichert U, Rosenfield RL. Limited cooperation between peroxisome proliferator-activated receptors and retinoid X receptor agonists in sebocyte growth and differentiation. Mol Genet Metab 2001; 74:362–369.

140. Thody AJ, Shuster S. A study of the relationship between the thyroid gland and sebum secretion in the rat. J Endocrinol 1972; 54:239–244.

141. Goolamali SK, Evered D, Shuster S. Thyroid disease and sebaceous function. Br Med J 1973; 1:432–433.

142. Ahsan MK, Urano Y, Kato S, Oura H, Arase S. Immunohistochemical localisation of thyroid hormone nuclear receptors in human hair follicles and in vitro effect of L-triiodothyronine on cultured cells of hair follicles and skin. Lab Med Invest 1998; 44:179–184.

143. Thody AJ, Shuster S. Control of sebum secretion by the posterior pituitary. Nature 1972; 237:346–347.

144. Slominski A, Paus R, Mazurkiewicz JE. Proopiomelanocortin expression in the skin during induced hair growth in mice. Experientia 1992; 48:50–54.

145. Cone RD, Lu D, Koppula S, et al. The melanocortin receptors, agonists, antagonists and the hormonal control of pigmentation. Recent Prog Horm Res 1996; 51:287–318.

146. Stander S, Bohm M, Brzoska T, Zimmer KP, Luger T, Metze D. Expression of melanocortin-1 receptor in normal, malformed and neoplastic skin glands and hair follicles. Exp Dermatol 2002; 11(1):42–51.

147. Bohm M, Schiller M, Stander S, et al. Evidence for expression of melanocortin-1 receptor in human sebocytes in vitro and in situ. J Invest Dermatol 2002; 118:533–539.

148. Thiboutot D, Sivarajah A, Gilliland K, Cong Z, Clawson G. The melanocortin-5-receptor is expressed in human sebaceous glands and rat preputial cells. J Invest Dermatol 2000; 115:614–619.
149. Chen W, Kelly MA, Opitz-Araya X, Thomas RE, Low MJ, Cone RD. Exocrine gland dysfunction in MC5-R-deficient mice: evidence for coordinated regulation of exocrine gland function by melanocortin peptides. Cell 1997; 91:789–798.
150. Zhang L, Anthonavage M, Huang Q, Li WH, Eisinger M. Proopiomelanocortin peptides and sebogenesis. Ann NY Acad Sci 2003; 994:154–161.
151. Akimoto N, Sato T, Sakiguchi T, Kitamura K, Kohno Y, Ito A. Cell proliferation and lipid formation in hamster sebaceous gland cells. Dermatology 2002; 204:118–123.
152. Downie MMT, Sandera DA, Kealey T. Modelling remission of individual acne lesions in vitro. Br J Dermatol 2002; 147:869–878.
153. Moore GPM, Panaretto BA, Carter NB. Epidermal hyperplasia and wool follicle regression in sheep infused with epidermal growth factor. J Invest Dermatol 1985; 84:172–175.
154. Matias JR, Orentriech N. Stimulation of hamster sebaceous glands by epidermal growth factors. J Invest Dermatol 1983; 80:516–519.
155. Green MR, Basketter DA, Couchman JR, Rees DA. Distribution and number of epidermal growth factor receptors in skin related to epithelial cell growth. Dev Biol 1983; 100:506–512.
156. Ridden J. Ph.D. thesis, University of Cambridge, U.K., 1990.
157. Guy R. Ph.D. thesis, University of Cambridge, U.K., 1994.
158. Zouboulis CC, Xia L, Akamatsu H, et al. The human sebocyte culture model provides new insights into development and management of seborrhoea and acne. Dermatology 1998; 196:21–31.
159. Deplewski D, Rosenfield RL. Growth hormone and insulin-like growth factors have different effects on sebaceous cell growth and differentiation. Endocrinology 1999; 140:4089–4094.
160. Zouboulis CC, Seltmann H, Hiroi N, et al. Corticotrophin-releasing hormone: an autocrine hormone that promotes lipogenesis in human sebocytes. Proc Natl Acad Sci 2002; 99:7148–7153.
161. Toyoda M, Morohashi M. Pathogenesis of acne. Med Electron Microsc 2001; 34:29–40.
162. Anttila HSI, Reitamo S, Saurat JH. Interleukin 1 immunoreactivity in sebaceous glands. Br J Dermatol 1992; 127:585–588.
163. Horneman S, Seltmann H, Kodelija V, Orfanos CE, Zouboulis C. Interleukin-1α mRNA and protein are expressed in cultured human sebocytes at a steady state and their levels are barely influenced by lipopolysaccharides [abstr]. J Invest Dermatol 1997; 108:382.
164. Guy R, Kealey T. Modelling the infundibulum in acne. Dermatology 1998; 196:32–37.
165. Kozlowska U, Blume-Peytavi U, Kodelja V, et al. Vascular endothelial growth factor expression induced proinflammatory cytokines (Interleukin 1α,β) in cells of the human pilosebaceous unit. Dermatology 1998; 196:89–92.
166. Ingham E, Eady EA, Goodwin CE, Cove JH, Cunliffe WJ. Pro-inflammatory levels of interleukin-1α – like bioactivity are present in the majority of open comedones in acne vulgaris. J Invest Dermatol 1992; 98:895–901.
167. Stern RS. Medication and medical service utilization for acne 1995-1198. J Am Acad Dermatol 2000; 43:1042–1048.
168. Strauss JS, Pochi PE. The quantitative gravimetric determination of sebum production. J Invest Dermatol 1961; 36:293–298.
169. Burton JL, Shuster S. The relationship between seborrhoea and acne vulgaris. Br J Dermatol 1971; 85:197–198 (letter).
170. Cotterill JA, Cunliffe WJ, Williamson B. Severity of acne and sebum excretion rate. Br J Dermatol 1971; 85:93–94.
171. Van Scott EJ, MacCardle RC. Keratinisation of the duct of the sebaceous gland and the growth cycle of the hair follicle in the histogenesis of acne in human skin. J Invest Dermatol 1956; 27:405–429.
172. Holmes RL, Williams M, Cunliffe WJ. Pilosebaceous duct obstruction and acne. Br J Dermatol 1972; 87:327–332.

173. Blake J, Cunliffe WJ, Holland KT. The development and regression of individual acne lesions [abstr]. J Invest Dermatol 1986; 87:130.
174. Al Baghdadi H. The Structure and Function of the Skin in Relation to Acne Vulgaris. A Clinical and Functional Study Using Non-Intrusive Dermatological Sampling Techniques. Ph.D. thesis, University of Leeds, U.K., 1984.
175. Wolff HH, Plewig G, Braun-Falco O Ultrastructure of human sebaceous follicles and comedones following treatment with vitamin A acid. Acta Derm Venereol 1975; 74(suppl):99–110.
176. Lavker RM, Leyden JJ. Lamellar inclusions in follicular horny cells: a new aspect of abnormal follicular keratinisation. J Ultra Res 1979; 69:362–370.
177. Hoyberg K, Knaggs HE. Environmental scanning electron microscopy of microcomedones. Proc Ann Microsc Soc Am 1994; 52:370–371.
178. Lees CW, Strauss JS, Downing DT, Pochi PE, Bachta M. Analysis of soluble proteins in comedones. Acta Derm Venereol (Stockh) 1977; 57:117–120.
179. Bladon PT, Cooper NF, Cunliffe WJ, Wood EJ. Protein content of comedones from patients with acne vulgaris. Acta Derm Venereol (Stockh) 1985; 65:413–418.
180. Plewig G, Fulton JE, Kligman AM. Cellular dynamics of comedo formation in acne vulgaris. Arch Dermatol Forsch 1971; 242:12–29.
181. Knaggs HE, Holland DB, Morris C, Wood EJ, Cunliffe WJ. Quantification of cellular proliferation in acne using the monoclonal antibody, Ki-67. J Invest Dermatol 1994; 102:89–92.
182. Hughes BR, Cunliffe WJ, Morris C, Leigh IM, Lane EB. Keratin profiles of the pilosebaceous unit in sites prone to acne vulgaris—an in situ study [abstr]. J Invest Dermatol 1990; 95:473.
183. Aldana OL, Holland DB, Cunliffe WJ. Variation in pilosebaceous duct keratinocyte proliferation in acne patients. Dermatology 1998; 196:98–99.
184. Cunliffe WJ, Holland DB, Clark SM, Stables GI. Comedogenesis: some new aetiological, clinical and therapeutic strategies. BJD 2000; 142:1084–1091.

3 Sebum Secretion and Acne

Philip W. Wertz
Dows Institute, University of Iowa, Iowa City, Iowa, U.S.A.

COMPOSITION OF HUMAN SEBUM

Sebum is synthesized in sebaceous glands, which are part of the pilosebaceous units of the skin (1). Sebaceous glands are epidermal appendages found in all regions of the skin, except the palmar and plantar surfaces; however, the greatest density of glands is found in the scalp and facial areas.

As sebocytes move from the basal layer at the periphery of the gland toward the lumen, they synthesize neutral lipids, which accumulate as lipid droplets, and eventually all of the carbon-based components of the cell are converted into lipid. The composition of sebum is species-specific. Human sebum, as it is synthesized in the gland (2), consists of squalene (15%), wax esters (25%), cholesterol esters (2%), triglycerides (57%), and cholesterol (1%). The small proportion of free cholesterol and cholesterol esters are thought to be derived from cholesterol in the basal sebocyte plasma membrane. Differentiating sebocytes do not express the enzymes of the cholesterol biosynthetic pathway beyond those leading to the production of squalene (3). This mixture of sebaceous lipids is liquid phase at skin temperature.

As it flows out through the follicle and over the skin surface, the triglycerides undergo at least partial hydrolysis to liberate free fatty acids (4). The first investigation of the free fatty acids derived from human sebum was conducted by Weitkamp et al. in 1947 (5). Using fractional distillation, fatty acids ranging from 7 through 22 carbons in length were detected. Shorter chains may have been present, but the 7-carbon entity was the shortest that could be detected. In addition, series of $\Delta6$- and $\Delta9$-monoenes were identified, with the $\Delta6$ series dominating. The 16- and 18-carbon species were the most abundant. Small proportions of 1,2-diglycerides and 1,3-diglycerides are also produced through lipase action (4). The esterases responsible for sebaceous triglyceride hydrolysis are bacterial (6) and probably also of epidermal origin (7).

Of the fatty acids released from sebaceous triglycerides lauric acid (C12:0) and sapienic acid (C16:1$\Delta6$) are the most potent antimicrobials (8; Drake DR and Wertz PW, unpublished observations). Sapienic acid is the single most abundant fatty acid in human sebum and is not found in abundance in any other known source, whereas lauric acid is a relatively minor sebaceous fatty acid. These two fatty acids both have potent antimicrobial properties, especially against gram-positive bacteria.

Frequently, alkanes are found in lipid samples collected from the human skin surface. Carbon dating has proven this material to be derived from petroleum (9), although it is not certain if it is simply surface contamination, as opposed to an internalized contaminant that is delivered to the skin surface through the sebaceous secretions.

In addition to the sebaceous lipids synthesized in the gland, hydrophobic materials from the circulation may partition into the sebaceous glands. This includes the antioxidants vitamin E (10,11) and coenzyme Q10 (11). Sebum secretion appears to be the major route for delivery of these antioxidant vitamins to the skin surface. This may be of particular significance for defense against reactive oxygen species and protection of the linoleate containing acylceramides in the stratum corneum (12).

The major fatty acids in human sebum range in length from 12 carbons through 20 carbons, with the 16- and 18-carbon species predominating (13,14). In prepubertal children, some longer fatty chains are found (15). As noted, C16:1Δ6 is the most abundant fatty acid in human sebum. C18:1Δ8 is produced from C16:1Δ6 by chain extension. An unusual characteristic of human sebum is the presence of various methyl branched fatty acids (13,14). These include saturated iso- and anteisomethyl branched chains, but also various other internal and multi-methyl branched chains. The methyl branching pattern of saturated fatty acids varies among individuals, but is invariant with time for a given individual (14). This indicates genetic control.

Saturated and monounsaturated fatty acids predominate in the sebaceous esters with only small proportions of dienes being present (4). Among the wax ester fatty acids, the saturated-to-monounsaturated fatty acid ratio is approximately 40 to 60; whereas in the cholesterol ester and triglyceride fractions this ratio is 65:35 and 70:30, respectively (13,16). The dienoic fatty acids include linoleic acid (C18:2 Δ9,12), derived from the diet, and an isomer thereof (C18:2 Δ5,8), which is synthesized in the gland (17). The proportion of C18:2 Δ9,12 relative to C18:2 Δ5,8 is decreased in acne. This is consistent with the suggestion that comedogenesis is initiated by a localized essential fatty acid deficiency (18).

MEASUREMENT OF SEBUM SECRETION
Cigarette Paper Method
One of the most widely used methods for measurement of sebum secretion rates is the cigarette paper method of Strauss and Pochi (19). In this method, the forehead was first cleansed to remove surface lipid. A previously extracted cigarette paper was then placed against the skin of the forehead and held in place with an ace bandage. After a three-hour collection period, the cigarette paper was removed. Lipids were extracted from the paper using ethyl ether and quantitated either by weighing (19) or by quantitative thin-layer chromatographic analysis (4,20).

Bentonite Method
Subsequently, bentonite has been used to adsorb sebum on the forehead (21). After washing the forehead with soap and water and swabbing with an ethanol-soaked gauze pad, a thin layer of bentonite gel was applied to the forehead. In initial studies, two 1.8-mm diameter circular disks of Dacron mesh were pressed into the bentonite, and these were covered with additional bentonite. At three hours interval thereafter, the Dacron disks and adhering bentonite were replaced and sampling continued to 24 hours. The amount of sebum adsorbed per disk over three hours decreased steadily for about the first 12 hours, after which the rate of sebum secretion became constant. The excess sebum secreted during the initial 12 hours of collection was interpreted as a reflection of a follicular reservoir. Only after this reservoir was depleted was the sustainable sebum secretion rate

measurable. This sustainable secretion rate is equal to the rate of synthesis in the glands. In later studies, bentonite was applied to the forehead, and a rectangular piece of Dacron mesh large enough to cover most of the forehead was pressed into the gel and covered with additional bentonite. After seven hours, the Dacron mesh on the forehead was replaced, and after another seven hours to deplete the reservoir, the rectangular Dacron was replaced with two circular disks of Dacron for a final three-hour collection period, reflecting the sustainable rate of sebum secretion. The lipids were extracted from the bentonite into ethyl ether and analyzed by quantitative thin-layer chromatography. In a variant on this method, the final collection period after depletion of the follicular reservoir was extended to nine hours, and the extracted sebum was quantitated gravimetrically.

Sebutape
More recently, Sebutape (Cuderm Corporation, Dallas, Texas, U.S.A.) has been introduced for assessment of pore patterns and sebum secretion (22,23). This adsorbant polymeric tape is white but turns transparent at the points where sebum is adsorbed. This tape is used after clearing sebum from the surface, but not depletion of the follicular reservoir, although there is no fundamental reason why this could not be done. Typically, the Sebutape is removed from the forehead after three hours, although it has been suggested that one hour would be adequate (24), and placed on a black background. The pore pattern then appears as black dots on a white background, and the total black area determined by image analysis is proportional to the amount of sebum secreted (25). One can qualitatively assign the pore pattern to one of five categories, referring to images provided by the manufacturer: prepubertal, pubertal, acne, mature, or senescent (26). It is also possible to extract lipids from the Sebutape and to analyze them by thin-layer chromatography (23).

Instrumental Methods
In 1970, Schaefer and Kuhn-Bussius (27) demonstrated that sebum secretion could be measured by collecting it on a frosted glass plate and measuring the transparency. As sebum is adsorbed on the rough surface, it spreads and fills the microscopic pockets within the glass. This smooths the surface and will result in less light scattering when the plate is illuminated with a beam of light. The relationship between the amount of adsorbed lipid and light transmission was quantitated and shown to be nonlinear. Subsequently, several instruments based on this principle have become commercially available. The first of this is the Lipometre introduced by L'Oreal (Aulnay's Bois, France). More recently, the Sebumeter has been introduced by Courage & Khazaka (Koln, Germany). These instruments allow measurements of the amount of sebum on the skin surface or the sebum secretion rate, which can be made easily within a few minutes. However, calibration can be difficult, and unless the sebaceous reservoir has been depleted, this will be the least accurate means for measuring sebum secretion rates.

Proposed Hybrid Method
The biggest obstacle to accurate measurement of sebum secretion rates is the need to deplete the sebaceous follicles. This can be overcome by 12 to 14 hours of adsorption onto bentonite prior to measurement. Once the reservoir is depleted, the

Sebutape method is appealing for the actual sebum secretion measurement. The collection time could be shortened to one hour, and a digitized image of the Sebutape on its black backing should be captured immediately. Subsequently, this image can be analyzed to estimate the sebum secretion rate from the total black area. In addition, information on the number, the pattern and the activity of individual glands can be obtained. The Sebutape can be removed from the backing and the lipids can be extracted and examined by thin-layer chromatography in conjunction with photodensitometry. In this way, one could obtain two measures of the sebum secretion rate, the overall lipid class composition and information on the pore density and variation in the activity of individual glands.

HORMONAL CONTROL

At the time of birth, sebaceous glands are large and active, probably as a result of androgenic stimulation in utero (28). Shortly after birth, the sebaceous glands undergo atrophy and remain relatively small until the onset of puberty. The rate of sebum secretion in prepubertal children is generally low, but there is a measurable increase in sebum secretion beginning at about an age of seven (29). This is thought to reflect increasing secretion of dehydroepiandrosterone and its sulfated form from the adrenal glands. At the onset of puberty in males, the testes produce increased levels of testosterone. In the skin, this is metabolized to dihydrotestosterone, which binds to a cytoplasmic receptor protein. This complex translocates to the cell nucleus and modulates gene expression (30). In females, the ovaries do produce testosterone, androstenedione, and dehydroepiandrosterone; however, adrenal hormones are the major circulating androgens in women (31). In general, sebum secretion rates reach a maximum in the mid-teen years and slowly decline thereafter as circulating androgen levels decline.

Hormonal control of sebaceous gland activity (Thiboutot) and the etiology of acne (Strauss) are discussed at length in later chapters of this book.

SEBUM SECRETION AND AGE

As noted earlier, sebaceous glands are active in utero under the influence of maternal hormones, and sebaceous lipids are major components of the vernix caseosa (13). Vernix caseosa also contains exfoliated corneocytes. In the later stages of development, lung surfactant is produced and can be detected in the amniotic fluid. This surfactant at least partially dislodges vernix caseosa, and this material is ingested (32). Whether this has significance beyond possible provision of nutrients is unknown.

The mean rate of sebaceous wax ester secretion in six-year old boys and girls was $5 \mu g/10 \text{ cm}^2/3$ hr. This increased to about $25 \mu g/10 \text{ cm}^2/3$ hr in seven-year olds and $50 \mu g/10 \text{ cm}^2/3$ hr in eight-year olds (29). There is a major, age-dependent increase in the mean sebum secretion rate for both genders from ages 10 to 15 (33). After age 10, the mean sebum secretion rate at any given age was always greater for males. At age 15, the mean wax ester secretion rates were $0.75 \text{ mg}/10 \text{ cm}^2/3$ hr for boys and $0.55 \text{ mg}/10 \text{ cm}^2/3$ hr for girls (31,33). Sebum secretion rates appear to decline exponentially thereafter, reaching rates approximately half of secretion rates of 15-year olds at about age 50 (33). In individuals older than about 65 years, sebum secretion rates are in the same range as prepubertal children.

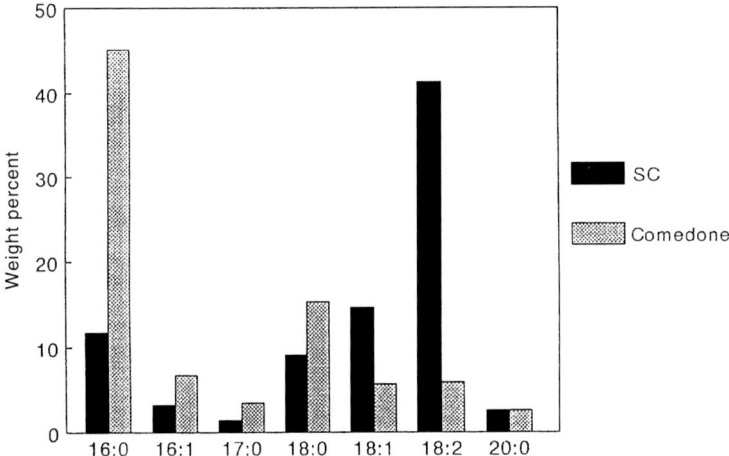

FIGURE 1 Relative proportions of ester-linked fatty acids from acylceramide of comedones compared with acylceramide from the skin surface of normal control subjects. *Abbreviation*: SC, stratum corneum. *Source*: From Ref. 37.

SEBUM SECRETION AND ACNE

It has long been established that elevated rates of sebum secretion are associated with acne, and treatments that lower sebaceous gland activity are therapeutic (34). It should be noted that with the bentonite method for measurement of sebum secretion, the mean sebum secretion rates for nonacne control subjects, mild-to-moderate acne, and severe acne are significantly different with higher secretion rates, occurring with more severe disease (35). The role of sebum in comedogenesis and initiation of acne and the available therapies are discussed in later chapters of this book. In general, any treatment that significantly reduces sebum secretion is therapeutic for acne.

INTERACTION OF SEBACEOUS LIPIDS WITH THE EPIDERMIS

It has been demonstrated that sebaceous lipids can increase the permeability of the skin (36). This was first demonstrated after application of human sebum to neonatal rat skin in vivo. The follicles have not penetrated to the surface of the neonatal rodent skin, so there is no endogenous sebum. It was found that the application of human sebum to this skin surface resulted in a two-fold increase in permeability. In addition, in accord with the localized essential fatty acid hypothesis, it has been shown that in comedones, sebaceous fatty acids can replace linoleate in the acylceramide (37). This is illustrated in Figure 1. More recently, it has been reported that barrier function is impaired in acne patients compared to normal controls (38).

REFERENCES

1. Montagna W. The sebaceous gland in man. In: Montagna W, Ellis RA, Silver AS, eds. Advances in Biology of Skin. Oxford: Pergamon Press, 1963:19–31.
2. Stewart ME, Downing DT, Pochi PE, et al. The fatty acids of human sebaceous gland phosphatidylcholine. Biochim Biophys Acta 1978; 529(3):380–386.

3. Bloch K. The biological synthesis of cholesterol. Science 1965; 150(692):19–28.
4. Downing DT, Strauss JS, Pochi PE. Variability in the chemical composition of human skin surface lipids. J Invest Dermatol 1969; 53(5):322–327.
5. Weitkamp AW, Smiljanic AM, Rothman S. The free fatty acids of human hair fat. J Am Chem Soc 1947; 69(8):1936–1939.
6. Marples RR, Kligman AM, Lantis LR, et al. The role of the aerobic microflora in the genesis of fatty acids in human surface lipids. J Invest Dermatol 1970; 55(3): 173–178.
7. Gilbert D, Madison KC, Sando GN, et al. Acid lipase in lamellar granules. J Dent Res 2000; 79(special issue):322.
8. Bergsson G, Arnfinnsson J, Steingrimsson O, et al. Killing of gram-positive cocci by fatty acids and monoglycerides. APMIS 2001; 109(10):670–678.
9. Bortz JT, Wertz PW, Downing DT. On the origin of alkanes found in human skin surface lipids. J Invest Dermatol 1989; 93(6):723–727.
10. Thiele JJ, Schroeter C, Hsieh SN, et al. The antioxidant network of the stratum corneum. Curr Probl Dermatol 2001; 29:26–42.
11. Passi S, De Pita O, Puddu P, et al. Lipophilic antioxidants in human sebum and aging. Free Radic Res 2002; 36(4):471–477.
12. Ponec M, Weerheim A, Lankhorst P, et al. New acylceramide in native and reconstructed epidermis. J Invest Dermatol 2003; 120(4):581–588.
13. Nicolaides N, Fu HC, Ansari MNA, et al. The fatty acids of wax esters and sterol esters of vernix caseosa and from human skin surface. Lipids 1972; 7(8):506–517.
14. Green SC, Stewart ME, Downing DT. Variation in sebum fatty acid composition among adult humans. J Invest Dermatol 1984; 83(2):114–117.
15. Stewart ME, Downing DT. Unusual cholesterol esters in the sebum of young children. J Invest Dermatol 1990; 95(5):603–606.
16. Downing DT, Pochi PE, Strauss JS. Synthesis and composition of surface lipids of human skin. J Invest Dermatol 1974; 62(3):228–244.
17. Krakow R, Downing DT, Strauss JS, et al. Identification of a fatty acid in human skin surface lipids apparently associated with acne vulgaris. J Invest Dermatol 1973; 61(5):286–289.
18. Downing DT, Stewart ME, Wertz PW, et al. Essential fatty acids and acne. J Am Acad Dermatol 1986; 14(2 Pt 1):221–225.
19. Strauss JS, Pochi PE. The quantitative gravimetric determination of sebum production. J Invest Dermatol 1961; 36(4):293–298.
20. Downing DT. Photodensitometry in the thin-layer chromatographic analysis of neutral lipids. J Chromatogr 1968; 38(1):91–99.
21. Downing DT, Stranieri AM, Strauss JS. The effect of accumulated lipids on measurement of sebum secretion in human skin. J Invest Dermatol 1982; 79(4):226–228.
22. Pierard GE. Follicle to follicle heterogeneity of sebum excretion. Dermatologica 1986; 173(2):61–65.
23. Nordstrom KM, Schmus HG, McGinley KJ, et al. Measurement of sebum output using a lipid adsorbent tape. J Invest Dermatol 1986; 87(2):260–263.
24. Kligman AM, Miller DL, McGinley K. Sebutape: a device for visualizing and measuring human sebaceous secretion. J Soc Cosmet Chem 1986; 37(4):369–374.
25. Pierard-Franchimont C, Pierard GE, Saint-Leger D, et al. Comparison of the kinetics of sebum secretion in young women with and without acne. Dermatologica 1991; 183(6):120–122.
26. Clarys P, Barel A. Quantitative evaluation of skin surface lipids. Clin Dermatol 1995; 13(4):307–321.
27. Schaefer H, Kuhn-Bussius H. A method for the quantitative determination of human sebum secretion. Arch Klin Exp Dermatol 1970; 238(4):429–435.
28. Agache P, Blanc D, Barrand C, et al. Sebum levels during the first year of life. Br J Dermatol 1980; 103(6):643–649.
29. Stewart ME, Downing DT. Measurement of sebum secretion rates in young children. J Invest Dermatol 1985; 84(1):59–61.

30. Leyden JJ. New understandings of the pathogenesis of acne. J Am Acad Dermatol 1995; 32(5 Pt 3):S15–S25.
31. Downing DT, Stewart ME, Strauss JS. Changes in sebum secretion and the sebaceous gland. Dermatol Clin 1986; 4(3):419–423.
32. Narendran V, Wickett RR, Pickens WL, et al. Interaction between pulmonary surfactant and vernix: a potential mechanism for induction of amniotic fluid turbidity. Pediatr Res 2000; 48(1):120–124.
33. Jacobsen E, Billings JK, Frantz RA, et al. Age-related changes in sebaceous wax ester secretion rates in men and women. J Invest Dermatol 1985; 85(5):483–485.
34. Strauss JS. Sebaceous gland, acne and related disorders—an epilogue. Dermatology 1998; 196(1):182–184.
35. Harris HH, Downing DT, Stewart ME, et al. Sustainable rates of sebum secretion. J Am Acad Dermatol 1983; 8(2):200–203.
36. Squier CA, Wertz PW, Williams DM, Cruchley AT. Permeability of oral mucosa and skin with age. In: Squier CA, Hill MH, eds. The Effect of Aging in Oral Mucosa and Skin. Boca Raton: CRC Press, 1994:91–98.
37. Wertz PW, Miethke MC, Long SA, et al. The composition of ceramides from human stratum corneum and from comedones. J Invest Dermatol 1985; 84(5):410–412.
38. Yamamoto A, Takenouchi K, Ito M. Impaired water barrier function in acne vulgaris. Arch Dermatol Res 1995; 287(2):214–218.

4 The Molecular Biology of Retinoids and Their Receptors

Anthony V. Rawlings

AVR Consulting Ltd., Northwich, Cheshire, U.K.

INTRODUCTION

Acne vulgaris is a multifactorial disease of the skin in areas rich in sebaceous follicles. It is characterized by seborrhea, hypercornification of the infundibulum (the neck of the sebaceous gland), and the presence of comedones and inflammatory lesions such as papules and pustules. The inflammatory pathway is mediated by antigenic and inflammatory products of *Propionibacterium acnes* (1). Although acne is mostly associated with puberty, persistent or late onset acne may be similar in physiology to pubertal acne, with hyperandrogenicity and increased sebogenesis, being the key factors (2). The hyperproliferation of the infundibulum keratinocytes, characterized by the expression of the hyperproliferative marker proteins, Ki67 and K6/16, and the resulting immature stratum corneum does not desquamate efficiently, leading to clumps of squames that attach to the hair follicle causing a blockage to sebum flow. Hypercornification of the infrainfundibulum is an early feature of the microcomedones, preceding the clinically observable inflammatory process (3).

Hypovitaminosis A has been proposed as an inducer of sebogenesis, as retinoids suppress sebogenesis. Follicles with a high sebum output are thought to become deficient in vitamin A, which will disturb the keratinization process of the infundibulum of the gland, culminating in the initial formation of microcomedones in these glands (4).

Recently, comedogenesis has been related to a subclinical microinflammatory state in the sebaceous gland (3). The increased interleukin-1 levels may influence the production of other growth factors by fibroblasts that then cause the ductal hyperproliferation and faulty differentiation (5). Increased transcription factor signaling occurs following binding of the cytokines to their receptors, activator protein-1 (AP-1) and nuclear factor kappa-b, thereby activating the signaling pathways. As a result, suppression of these signaling pathways will be beneficial for acne. Retinoids can improve epidermal differentiation, reduce sebogenesis, and decrease AP-1 driven inflammatory pathways. It is not too surprising, therefore, that this class of agents improve the acne status. This chapter reviews the molecular biology and biochemistry of this important class of molecules.

NUCLEAR HORMONE RECEPTORS AND THE RETINOID RECEPTORS

In the last several years, the structure and function of nuclear receptors have been determined (6). Based on the similarities among the sequences, it has been possible to classify the receptor superfamilies. The endocrine receptors include the retinoic acid receptors (RARs) and the thyroid hormone receptors, and the adopted orphan

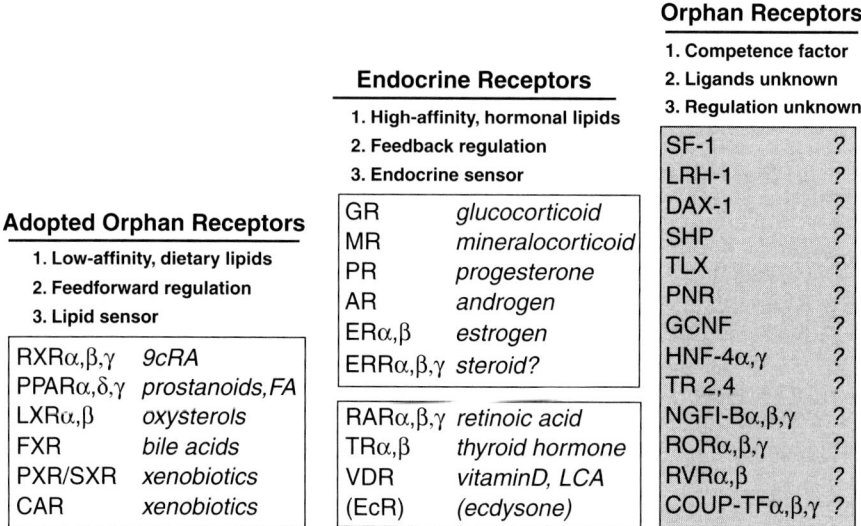

FIGURE 1 Classification of nuclear and orphan receptors. *Abbreviations*: LXR, liver-X-activated receptor; PPAR, peroxisomal proliferators activated receptor; RXR, retinoid X receptor; TR, thyroid hormone receptors, 9cRA, 9-*cis*-retinoic acid.

receptors include the retinoid X receptors (RXRs). These retinoid receptors are active as heterodimers (typical receptors are illustrated in Fig. 1).

The two classes of nuclear receptors mediate the action of endogenous retinoids (7). Both types of receptors are composed of three subtypes (alpha, beta, and gamma) (8). Each subtype consists of six distinct domains referred to as A to F based on homology with other members of the nuclear receptor superfamily (Fig. 2). Domains A and B are at the amino terminal and contain isoform-specific ligand-independent transactivation function-1 (AF-1). The DNA-binding domain (C or DBD) is highly conserved and contains two zinc-binding motifs responsible for the recognition of the retinoic acid response element (RARE), located in the promoter region of target genes. The E domain is the ligand-binding domain (LBD) and is responsible for the dimerization of the receptors, ligand-dependent transcriptional AF-2, and translocation to the nucleus (Fig. 2) (9).

The DNA response element of nuclear receptors comprises of two hexameric motifs with the nucleotide structure AGGTCA. The organization of these repeat palindromes and the length of the nucleotide spacing between the two hexamers determine the binding specificity of a particular receptor. The simplest is the direct repeat-1 of the RXR–RXR homodimer, RARE. However, the polarity of binding to the response element is reversed in these receptors with the RXRs occupying the 5′ half-site when coupled to the RAR (9).

The pleotropic effects of retinoids are due to the existence of multiple RAR isoforms and as a result of the different combinations of RAR–RXR heterodimers. RARs and RXRs mainly act as heterodimers on binding to the RAREs. The RARs can be activated by binding all-*trans*-retinoic acid (all-*trans*-RA) or 9-*cis*-RA; however, of the different retinoids, RXRs can only be activated by 9-*cis*-RA. The RXRs predominate in human skin, especially RXR alpha. Of the RARs, 87%

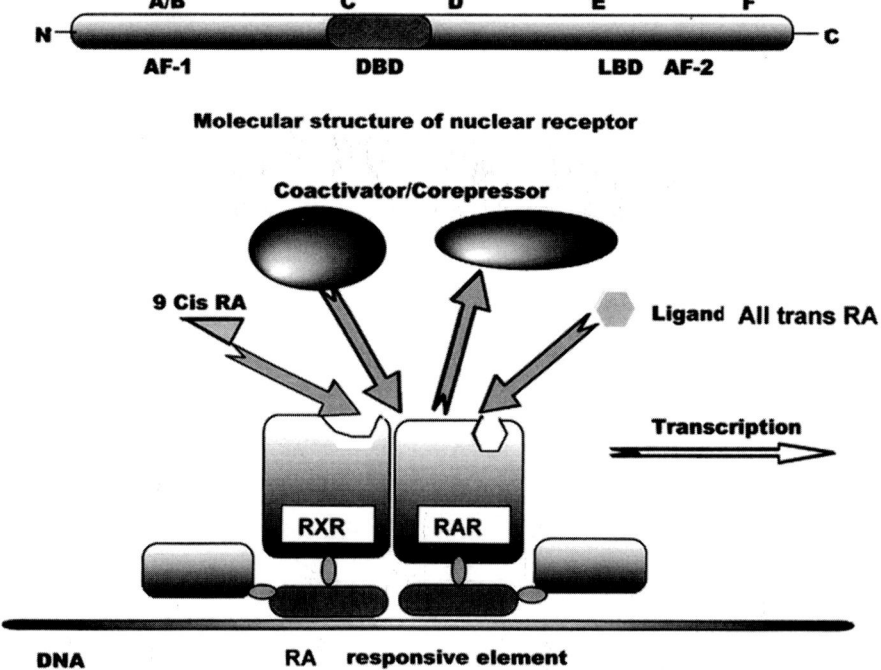

FIGURE 2 Schematic overview of the retinoic acid receptor/retinoid X receptor, receptor dimerization, and binding to the retinoic acid response element in the promoter region of a gene. *Abbreviations*: AF, activation function; DBD, DNA-binding domain; LBD, ligand binding domain; RA, retinoic acid; RAR, retinoic acid receptor RXR, retinoid X receptor.

is gamma and 13% alpha. Only small amounts of RAR beta are found in dermal cells and melanocytes. Human sebocytes in vitro also express mRNA or RAR alpha and gamma together with RXR alpha. Although both all-*trans*-RA and 9-*cis*-RA bind RAR in vivo, RAR gamma preferentially binds all-*trans*-RA. Both 9-*cis*-RA and 13-*cis*-RA can be isomerized to all-*trans*-RA. The isomerization of 9-*cis*-RA has been reported to occur in keratinocytes (8).

The ligand-binding pockets of nuclear receptors have been determined by X ray crystallography (10). This domain consists of a series of alpha helices that give rise to a novel antiparallel alpha-helical sandwich. Side chains of the amino acid, which constitute this structure, also include the homo- and heterodimeric interfaces and the surfaces that provide binding sites for the nuclear corepressor and coactivator molecules (Fig. 2). Binding of ligands to the LBD induces conformational changes in the receptors (11). Although this is true of all the ligand activated nuclear receptors, it is particularly true of the RXRs. The ligand-binding pocket is a deep hydrophobic pocket within the LBD, and it is different in its architecture, which plays a significant role in contributing to the different ligand-binding properties. For instance, in the peroxisomal proliferators activated receptor, the ligand-binding pocket is relatively large (1200–1500 nm^3) and when ligands bind to these receptors they occupy only a small fraction of the available volume usually 15% to 25%, the rest being occupied by water molecules (12). The large binding pocket and the limited number of ligand-receptor contact points result in a relatively low affinity of binding of ligands to these receptors and because of the large pocket, the receptor is promiscuous and binds a diverse range of molecules. In contrast to these low affinity receptors, the other nuclear receptors have a much higher affinity for their ligands. In general, the ligand-binding pocket is much smaller ($400–500$ nm^3), and the ligand occupies a high fraction of the available volume; for example, 9-*cis*-RA occupies 75% of the ligand-binding pocket of RXR alpha while all-*trans*-RA occupies 60% (13). The ligand-binding pocket of the RARs can accommodate both the all-*trans*-RA and 9-*cis*-RA, but due to the bulkier side chains of the aminoacid residues of the RXRs, it only permits binding of 9-*cis*-RA.

One important region of the LBD is the dimerization interface (14). For the RARs, symmetric assembly of the dimerization interface to form homodimers is energetically unfavorable. Asymmetric interactions between the interfaces of the RXR give rise to an extended area of intermolecular contact that stabilizes heterodimer formation. The RXR is unique among the nuclear receptors, having a dimerization interface that is stable in both the symmetrical configuration (RXR/RXR homodimers) and the asymmetrical confirmation (RXR/RAR heterodimers). The RXR homodimer (but not the heterodimer) generates a new dimerization interface that allows tetramer formation, and a large fraction of the unliganded RXRs is also found in this formation. Binding of ligands to the apo-RXR tetramer induces conformational changes that destabilizes the tetramer conformation to form homo- or heterodimers. In the tetramer form, however, even though the homodimers of RXR do not bind all-*trans*-RA, the distorted ligand-binding pocket binds it but does not induce dissociation of the tetramer format. In fact, all-*trans*-RA can act as a competitive antagonist of ligand-induced RXR tetramer dissociation. In this tetramer state, the RXRs cannot bind corepressor or coactivators and are sequestered in a transcriptionally inactive pool called "auto-silencing." Thus, one of the ways that RXR ligands can activate transcription is by increasing the pool of RXRs available for heterodimerization with RARs (10).

Liganded RXRs preferentially form homo- or heterodimers. The interface between the receptors in heterodimers such as RXR/RAR is substantially larger than the dimer interface (550 vs. 500 nm^3), resulting in a preferential formation of hetero- versus homodimers. Binding of 9-*cis*-RA to the RXR also results in conformational changes that generate an agonist confirmation, dependent on the binding of coactivator molecules. The initiation of a "mouse trap-like" configuration induces structural changes in the protein in such a way that it not only closes the lid of the ligand-binding pocket, but also simultaneously generates a high affinity coactivator-binding site. In the presence of partial agonists like oleic acid, the structural changes cause transrepression rather than activation (10–14).

RXR ligands can alter RXR activity both by altering the availability of RXRs for heterodimer formation and by altering the intrinsic transactivation activity of heterodimeric complexes and receptor degradation pathways. Ligands can accelerate the degradation of the receptor, particularly through the 26S proteasome complex. Binding of ligands to the different isoforms could induce degradation of both receptors or the selective degradation of only one receptor. It can also depend on the subisoform in each receptor class.

Like other nuclear receptors, retinoid-induced transactivation of genes is mediated as a result of alterations in chromatin packing and structure (15). The chromatin is tightly packed inside the nucleus and is a complex, consisting of

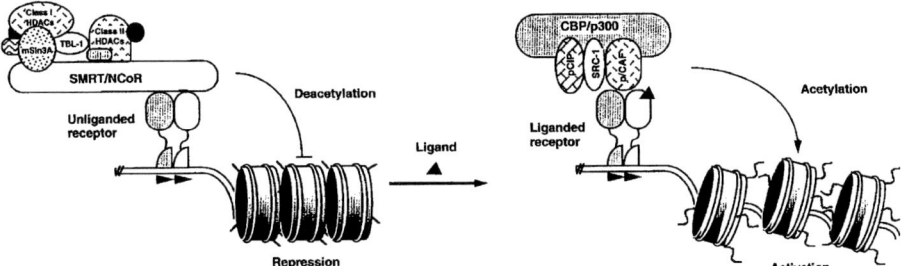

FIGURE 3 Schematic overview of coactivator/corepressor and histone deacetylase proteins and their functions in chromatin condensation and gene activation. *Abbreviations*: HDAC, histone deacetylase; NcoR, nuclear receptor corepressor; SMRT, silencing mediator for retinoid and thyroid; SRC, steroid receptor coactivator.

DNA, histones, and nonhistone proteins. A nucleosome is the basic building block of chromatin, which contains 147 base pairs of DNA wrapped around a core of four histone partners—an H3–H4 tetramer and 2 H2A–H2B dimers. When condensed, this structure represses gene transcription. In the absence of the ligand, the nuclear receptors recruit nuclear corepressor proteins, nuclear receptor corepressor or the silencing mediator for retinoid and thyroid hormone, and Sin 3, which in turn forms a complex with histone deacetylase enzymes (HDAC) resulting in transcriptional silencing of the genes (Fig. 3). This suppression occurs because deacylation of the histone proteins creates conformational changes in the chromatin structure, limiting the access and binding of the nuclear receptors and RNA polymerase to the related genes. At physiological concentrations of RA (10^{-9}–10^{-8} M), the nuclear coreppressors and HDAC are dissociated, which in turn results in recruitment of coactivators with histone acetyltransferase activity such as the steroid receptor coactivator-1. Acetylation of lysine residues in the N-terminal of histones opens up the chromatin structure and allows gene transcription (16). Enhancement of retinoid activity is anticipated by combining HDAC inhibitors with retinoids (see later).

RETINOID METABOLISM AND BINDING PROTEINS

The metabolic fate of retinoids is controlled by two classes of intracellular binding proteins: the cellular retinol binding protein type I (CRBP I) and the cellular retinoic acid binding protein type II (CRABP II) (17,18). These sequester the retinoids, so that it is only available for reaction with specific enzymes. The holo-CRBP retinol complex can serve as a substrate for lecithin retinol acyl transferase (LRAT) (19) when the retinoid status is high, conversely when low, it serves as a substrate for retinol dehydrogenase synthesizing retinal, which ultimately gets converted to all-*trans*-RA (Fig. 4). The transport into the nucleus and further metabolism of all-*trans*-RA is controlled by CRBP I and CRABP II. It is suggested that CRBP I transport all-*trans*-RA into the nucleus, whereas CRABP II sequesters excess all-*trans*-RA in the cytoplasm facilitating its degradation. Metabolic inactivation of all-*trans*-RA to 4-hydroxyretinoic acid occurs via a cytochrome P450 enzyme (CYP26; Fig. 4) (20,21). This hydroxylase activity is actually induced in vivo by RA in human epidermis but can be inhibited by azoles. In the presence of low-dose RA or ROH, azoles amplify the human skin responses to retinoids in a manner characteristic

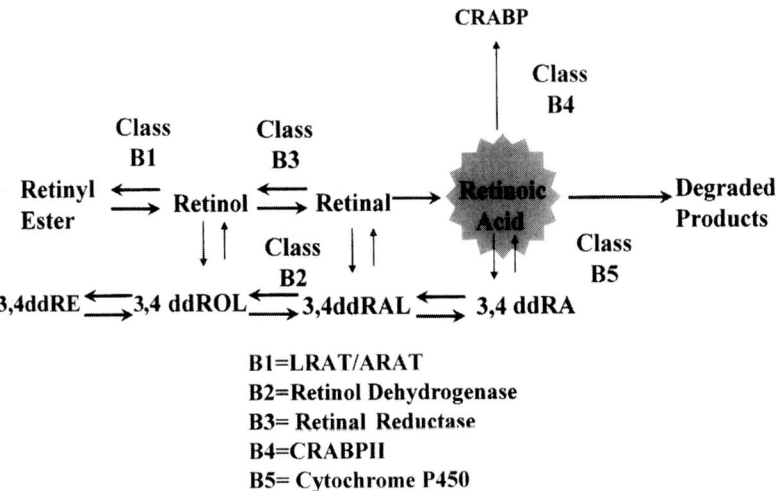

B1=LRAT/ARAT
B2=Retinol Dehydrogenase
B3= Retinal Reductase
B4=CRABPII
B5= Cytochrome P450

FIGURE 4 Schematic representation of retinol metabolism. *Abbreviations*: CRABP, cellular retinoic acid binding protein; LRAT, lecithin retinol acyl transferase; RA, retinoic acid; RAL, retinal; RE, retinyl ester; ROL, retinol.

of the retinoids at a higher dose (22). These agents have been called retinoic acid metabolism breakdown agents (RAMBAs) or retinomimetics. Azoles also inhibit the RA-induced expression of cytochrome 24-hydroxylase, which inactivates 1,25-dihydroxyvitamin D3.

In human keratinocytes, all-*trans*-RA regulates its own biosynthesis from atROH through the regulation of retinol esterification and, as such, RAMBA-type agents are not optimal (23). Treatment with all-*trans*-RA induces retinol-esterifying activity in proliferating keratinocytes. LRAT was induced by all-*trans*-RA and reduces the conversion of ROH to RA, resulting in sequestration of ROH in REs. Acyl retinol acyl transferase activity is also present. Several other enzymatic steps have been identified, which if manipulated can deliver improved retinoid responses (24).

EFFECTS OF RETINOIDS

Hypovitaminosis has been related to the expression of acne (25), and so its addition to skin should alleviate the condition. All-*trans*-RA was the first retinoid used, but it was ineffectual on acne when used systemically. 13-*cis*-RA (isotretinoin), however, is an extremely effective oral anti-acne drug by causing marked sebosuppression (26). 13-*cis*-RA has been shown to inhibit significantly sebocyte proliferation, differentiation, and lipid synthesis in vivo. Despite its potent biological effects, 13-*cis*-RA exhibits only low-binding affinity for CRABP and nuclear receptors (27). This unique antisebotrophic activity results from a selective isomerization to all-*trans*-RA intracellularly in sebocytes, reduces all-*trans*-RA inactivation compared with all-*trans*-RA, and mediates inhibition of sebocyte proliferation (28). The synthesis of CRABP II, which facilitates the degradation of intracellular all-*trans*-RA, was delayed and induced lesser by 13-*cis*-RA when compared with all-*trans*-RA, in vitro. Although all-*trans*-RA in trace amounts promotes sebocyte growth and differentiation, larger doses induce atrophy of the sebaceous gland and decrease sebogenesis. In vitro all-*trans*-RA and selective RAR agonists increase lipid-forming colonies except at higher doses (10^{-6} M), in which only a small number of colonies grew but they were differentiated more greatly. On the other hand, RXR agonists increased the cell growth slightly and lipid-forming colonies dramatically (29–31).

It is important to remember that RA effects in vitro may be completely different to in vivo. Retinoic acid induces sebocyte differentiation in preputial sebocytes, yet in in vivo the opposite occurs. Equally, the effects of RA on the keratinocyte differentiation process are contradictory in vitro and in vivo. Nevertheless, the effects of retinoids on epidermal differentiation will help to improve the acnegenesis state. Increased levels of epidermal transglutaminase and involucrin are observed together with increases in K6, as would be expected for a proliferating epidermis, but the differentiation in keratin markers (K1 and K10) are not inhibited in vivo. A unique keratin, K13 is also induced in vivo. Filaggrin and loricrin are increased in the longer term (four months) application of RA. As it has been recently reported that reduced Langerhans cell (LC) activity decreases in acne, the increases in LC activity by RA will also be beneficial (32).

The mechanism of action of isotretinoin has however remained elusive, as it does not bind itself to the retinoid receptors. Multiple actions have been proposed from inhibition of sebaceous gland activity, inhibition of the growth of *P. acnes*, inhibition of inflammation, and improvements in follicular epithelial differentiation. More recently, it has been shown that isotretinoin competitively inhibits 3 alpha-hydroxysteroid oxidation by retinol dehydrogenase, resulting in reduced formation of dhihydrotestosterone and thereby reduced sebogenesis (33). Retinoids are reported to increase the expression of transforming growth factor (TGF beta 1–3), and these inhibit keratinocyte proliferation. However, TGF beta-2 and 3, but not TGF beta-1, reduce cell proliferation and lipogenesis in human sebaceous glands in organ culture studies, suggesting that these growth factors may also contribute to the effects of retinoids on sebaceous glands (34–37).

At present, Accutane (oral 13-*cis*-RA) is available for the oral treatment of acne, whereas topical treatments include Retin-A (micronized all-*trans*-RA)—Differin (adapalene or CD271). Retinoic acid cannot be used in cosmetic products but retinol can (Fig. 5) (36). This does have some efficacy, but several new routes are being proposed to enhance its activity by inhibiting esterification and degradation enzymes and also manipulation of HDAC activities (37).

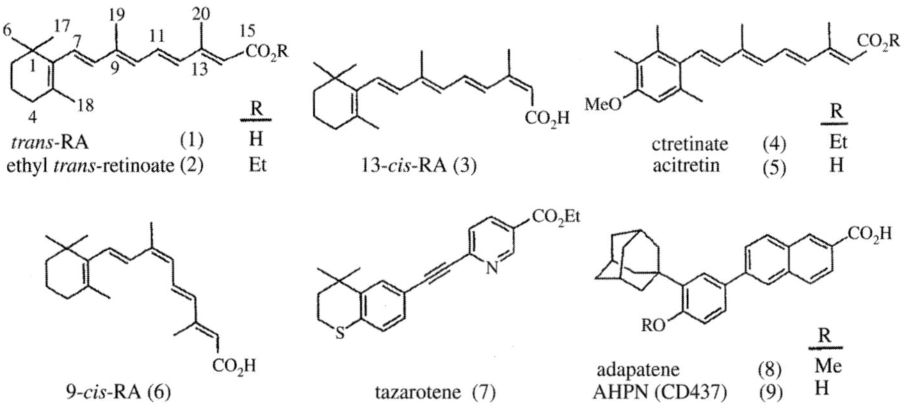

FIGURE 5 Typical structures of retinoids. *Abbreviation*: RA, retinoic acid.

REFERENCES

1. Stern RS. Acne therapy: medication use and sources of care in office-based practice. Arch Dermatol 1996; 132:776–780.
2. Knaggs HE, Wood EJ, Rizer RL, et al. Post-adolescent acne. Int J Cosmet Chem 2004; 26(3):129–138.
3. Jeremy AH, Holland DB, Roberts SG, et al. Inflammatory events are involved in acne lesion initiation. J Invest Dermatol 2003; 121(1):20–27.
4. Macdonald-Hull SM, Cunliffe WJ. Hypovitaminosis A of follicular duct as cause of acne vulgaris. Lancet 1988; 31(2):8626–8627.
5. Angel P, Szabowski A. Function of AP-1 target genes in mesenchymal-epithelial cross-talk in skin. Biochem Pharmacol 2002; 64(5–6):949–956.
6. Aranda A, Pascual A. Nuclear hormone receptors & gene expression. Physiol Rev 2001; 81(3):1269–1304.
7. Mehta K. Retinoids as regulators of gene transcription. J Biol Regul Homeost Agents 2003; 17:1–12.
8. Fisher GJ, Voorhees JJ. Molecular mechanisms of retinoid actions in skin. FASEB J 1996; 10:1002–1013.
9. Rastinejad F. Retinoid X receptor and its partners in the nuclear receptor family. Curr Opin Struct Biol 2001; 11:33–38.
10. Ahuja HS, Szanto A, Nagy L, et al. The retinoid X receptor & its ligands: versatile regulators of metabolic function, cell differentiation & cell death. J Biol Regul Homeost Agents 2003; 17(1):29–45.
11. Wurtz JM, Bourguet W, Renaud JP, et al. A canonical structure for the ligand binding domain of nuclear receptors. Nat Struct Biol 1996; 3:87–94.
12. Gampe RT, Montana VG, Lambert MH, et al. Asymmetry in the PPARgamma/RXRalpha crystal structure reveals the molecular basis of heterodimerization among nuclear receptors. Mol Cell 2000; 5:545–555.
13. Egea PF, Mitschler A, Rochel N, et al. Crystal structure of the human RXRalpha ligand binding domain bound to its natural ligand: 9-cis retinoic acid. EMBO J 2000; 19:2592–2601.
14. Bourguet W, Vivat V, Wurtz JM, et al. Crystal structure of a heterodimeric complex of RAR & RXR ligand-binding domains. Mol Cell 2000; 5:289–298.
15. Khorasanizadeh S. The nucleosome: from genomic organization to genomic regulation. Cell 2004; 53:1003–1009.
16. Jung M. Inhibitors of histone deacetylase as new anticancer agents. Curr Med Chem 2002; 8(12):1505–1511.
17. Roos TC, Jugert FK, Merk HF, et al. Retinoid metabolism in the skin. Pharmacol Rev 1998; 50(2):315–333.
18. Napoli JL. Interactions of retinoid binding proteins & enzymes in retinoid metabolism. BBA 1999; 1440:139–162.
19. Kurlandsky SB, Duell EA, Kang S, et al. Autoregulation of retinoic acid biosynthesis through regulation of retinol esterification in human keratinocytes. J Biol Chem 1996; 271(26):15346–15352.
20. Duell EA, Kang S, Voorhees JJ. Retinoic acid isomers applied to human skin in vivo each induce a 4-hydroxylase that inactivates only trans retinoic acid. J Invest Dermatol 1996; 106(2):316–320.
21. Mirikar Y, Wang Z, Duell EA, et al. Retinoic acid receptors regulate expression of retinoic acid 4-hydroxylase that specifically inactivates all-trans retinoic acid in human keratinocyte HaCaT cells. J Invest Dermatol 1998; 111(3):434–439.
22. Kang S, Duell EA, Kim KJ, et al. Liarozole inhibits human epidermal retinoic acid 4-hydroxylase activity and differentially augments human skin responses to retinoic acid and retinol in vivo. J Invest Dermatol 1996; 107:183–187.
23. Iobst S, Feinberg C, Rawlings AV, et al. Manipulation of retinoid metabolism. J Invest Dermatol 2003; 121:0563.
24. Granger S, Rawlings AV, Scott IR. Compositions to mimic retinoic acid. European Patent WO9813020.

25. Wolbach SB, Howe PR. Tissue changes following deprivation of fat soluble A vitamin. J Exp Med 1925; 42:753–777.
26. Goldstein JS, Socha-Szott A, Thomsen RJ, et al. Comparative effect of isotretinoin and etretinate on acne and sebaceous gland secretion. J Am Acad Dermatol 1982; 6:760–765.
27. Downie MMT, Guy R, Kealey T. Advances in sebaceous gland research: potential new approaches to acne management. Int J Cosmet Chem 2004; 26(6):291–312.
28. Tsukada M, Schroder M, Roos TC, et al. 13-cis retinoic acid exerts its specific activity on human sebocytes through selective intracellular isomerization to all-trans retinoic acid and binding to retinoid receptors. J Invest Dermatol 2000; 115:321–327.
29. Zouboulis CC, Korge B, Akamatsu H, et al. Effects of 13-cis Retnoic acid, all trans retinoic acid and acitretin on the proliferation, lipid synthesis and keratin expression of cultured human sebocytes in vitro. J Invest Dermatol 1991; 96:792–797.
30. Zouboulis CC, Korge B, Mischke D, et al. Altered proliferation, synthetic activity & differentiation of cultured human sebocytes in the absence of vitamin A and their modulation by synthetic retinoids. J Invest Dermatol 1993; 101:628–633.
31. Kim MJ, Ciletti N, Michael S, et al. The role of specific retinoid receptors in sebocyte growth & differentiation in culture. J Invest Dermatol 2000; 114:349–353.
32. Griffiths CEM, Voorhees JJ. Human in vivo pharmacology of topical retinoids. Arch Dermatol Res 1994; 287:53–60.
33. Glick AB, McCune BK, Abdulkarem N, et al. Complex regulation of TGFbeta expression by retinoic acid in the vitamin A deficient rat. Development 1991; 111:1081–1086.
34. Fisher GJ, Tavakkol A, Griffiths CEM, et al. Differential modulation of TGFbeta expression & mucin deposition by retinoic acid & SLS in human skin. J Invest Dermatol 1992; 98:102–108.
35. Han GR, Dohi DF, Lee HY, et al. All trans retinoic acid increases TGFbeta2 & IGFBP-3 expression through a retinoic acid receptor alpha dependent signalling pathway. J Biol Chem 1997; 272:13711–13716.
36. Dawson MI. Synthetic retinoids & their nuclear receptors. Curr Med Chem 2004; 4:199–230.
37. Schehlmann V, Klock J, Maillan P, Vollhardt J, Rawlings AV, Beumer R. Composition comprising an HDAC inhibitor in combination with a retinoid. European Patent WO2005092283, 2005.

5 Molecular Biology of Peroxisome Proliferator-Activated Receptors in Relation to Sebaceous Glands and Acne

Michaela M. T. Downie
Sequenom GmbH, Hamburg, Germany

Terence Kealey
The Clore Laboratories, University of Buckingham, Buckingham, U.K.

INTRODUCTION

Peroxisome proliferators-activated receptors (PPARs) are nuclear hormone receptors belonging to the superfamily of steroid/thyroid receptors. Three types of nuclear PPARs, PPARα, PPARβ/δ, and PPARγ1/γ2, have been identified and cloned, each being encoded by separate genes (1–8). Alternative splicing of one gene product yields two transcripts of PPARγ: PPARγ1 was found to predominate in adipose tissue and large intestines, whereas PPAR γ2 seemed to be a minor isoform (9). These receptors have been named according to their capacity to be activated by many compounds, which share in common the property of inducing peroxisome proliferation, especially in rodent liver (10–12). They are involved in the control of genes encoding lipid metabolism-associated proteins, particularly those of peroxisomal β-oxidation (13–15), and are activated by physiological concentrations of fatty acids (16–18), fibrate hypolipidemic drugs (10,19), and certain plasticizers and herbicides (19,20).

The main response to peroxisomal proliferators is an increase in peroxisome proliferation, stimulation of peroxisomal fatty acidβ-oxidation, and hepatocarcinogenesis. The oxidative degradation is responsible for the formation of hydrogen peroxide, which might lead to DNA damage and tumor initiation (20–22). Besides targeting peroxisomes, PPAR activation has been shown to be important in the regulation of lipid metabolism in fat and liver cells (23,24) and also regulates the expression of target genes involved in many cellular functions, including cell proliferation, differentiation, and immune/inflammatory response (25). The three PPARs (α, β/δ, γ) show the characteristics of ligand binding, and ligand activation can be related to a number of cellular processes: (*i*) fatty acid catabolism and modulation of the inflammatory response for PPARα; (*ii*) embryo implantation, cell proliferation, and apoptosis for PPARβ/δ; and (*iii*) adipocytic differentiation, monocytic differentiation, and cell-cycle withdrawal for PPARγ (18). It has been shown that 3T3 L1 cells can be induced to differentiate into adipocytes, demonstrating that PPARs not only regulate the expression of lipid metabolism-associated proteins but are also directly involved in cell differentiation (26). This suggestion was supported by the finding that PPARγ expression is induced early in the differentiation of 3T3 L1 preadipocytes into adipocytes (27,28). Further, examining the effects of the PPARγ ligands BRL49653, troglitazone, and

15-deoxy-$\Delta^{12,14}$-prostaglandin J_2 on the differentiation of human preadipocytes derived from subcutaneous and omental fat, it could be shown that these ligands enhanced markedly the differentiation of preadipocytes from subcutaneous sites; in contrast, preadipocytes from omental sites in the same individuals were refractory to the PPARγ ligands, although PPARγ was expressed at similar levels in both depots (29,30).

Members of the nuclear hormone receptor family have been implicated in epidermal processes such as differentiation, proliferation, and barrier development (31–34). Activators of PPARα and PPARγ have been shown to regulate differentiation in cultured sebocytes (35–39), the hamster flank organ (40), and human sebaceous gland organ cultures (41), modulating sebum formation. Further, PPARs have been shown to be involved in regulating inflammatory responses, in particular PPARα and PPARγ activation (42–45), and they are able to influence the inflammatory cytokine production and cell recruitment to the inflammatory sites (46).

Acne is a disease of the infundibulum and the sebaceous gland, and is characterized by comedogenesis, inflammation, and increased sebum secretion (47–50). Thus, with their involvement in regulating sebum formation and inflammation, PPARs may open up new avenues in the development of novel acne treatments.

PEROXISOME PROLIFERATOR-ACTIVATED RECEPTOR GENES: STRUCTURE AND LOCALIZATION

The genomic organization of the members of the nuclear hormone receptors, belonging to the superfamily of steroid/thyroid receptors, has provided useful information concerning their degree of relatedness. Their most conserved region contains two zinc fingers that constitute the core of the DNA-binding domain, which specifically recognizes hormone receptor elements. This conservation has been exploited to isolate additional members of the superfamily by sequence analysis, cross-hybridization screening of cDNA libraries, and functional studies. The conserved DNA-binding domain (C-domain) is flanked by a variable N-terminal domain (A/B domain) and a C-terminal ligand-binding domain (E/F domain), whereby the EF domain is linked with a hinge domain (D-domain) to the DNA-binding domain (Fig. 1). The A/B domain contains the activation function 1 (AF-1) that is transcriptionally active in the absence of ligands. The C-domain and

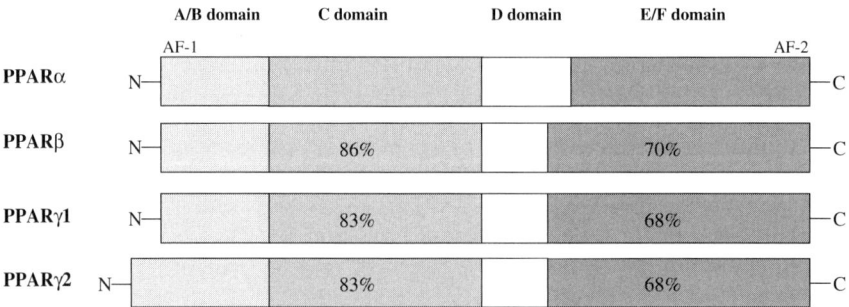

FIGURE 1 Typical structure of a peroxisome proliferator activated receptor gene. *Abbreviations*: AF, activation function; PPAR, peroxisome proliferator activated receptor.

the E/F-domain determine the specificity of promoters in DNA sequence recognition and ligand recognition, respectively. The ligand-binding domain, in addition to determining ligand specificity, contains a ligand-inducible transactivation function and a heptad-repeat motif involved in dimerization of nuclear receptors. This domain contains some regions that are highly conserved between most members of the nuclear receptor superfamily, particularly in the Ti-domain and AF-2 region. The N-terminal domain varies both in length and amino acid composition, and is responsible for the interaction with other transcription factors and transactivation. A distinctive feature of the PPAR subfamily is its great divergence in the ligand-binding domain, allowing researchers to distinguish the different PPAR subtypes pharmacologically (46,51,52).

The chromosomal localization of the human genes encoding PPARα, PPARβ/δ, and PPARγ have been defined. They map on different chromosomes. The PPARγ gene is on chromosome 3 at position 3p25 and has six exons (53). The PPARβ/δ gene is located on chromosome 6 at chromosomal region 6p21.2 and spans approximately 85 kb of DNA consisting of nine exons and eight introns (54). Finally, the PPARα gene has been mapped on chromosome 22 in the general region of 22q12-q13.1 and spans at least 80 kb with eight exons (6).

TRANSCRIPTIONAL ACTIVITY, DIMERIZATION, AND DNA BINDING

The transcriptional activity of the PPARs is regulated by post-translational modifications, such as phosphorylation (55,56) and ubiquitination (57). Phosphorylation of PPARs is controlled by environmental factors, activating different kinase pathways leading to the modulation of their activities (56). PPAR degradation by the ubiquitin–proteasome system modulates the intensity of the ligand response by controlling the level of PPAR proteins in the cells (46,57). It has been shown, moreover, that the novel orphan nuclear hormone receptor, liver-X-activated receptor (LXR)α, which is distinct from retinoic-X-activated receptor (RXR)α, inhibited PPAR signaling by competing with RXRα for PPARα heterodimerization, whereby the LXRα/PPARα heterodimer was unable to form a DNA-binding complex (58).

Dimerization is essential for the function of PPARs (Fig. 2). It has been demonstrated in vitro that PPARs form heterodimers with RXRs and that activation of PPARs can be increased in vitro by the addition of the RXR ligand, 9-*cis*-retinoic acid (59–63). As for other members of the nuclear hormone receptor family, PPARs regulate gene expression by binding to specific peroxisome proliferator response elements (PPRE) in the promoter regions of target genes (64) (Fig. 2). PPARs recognize a hormone response element that comprises a direct repeat (DR) of the hexameric AGGTCA half-site motif, with a one nucleotide spacer between the half elements (DR-1). The complex formed in vitro on such a response element is a PPAR–RXR heterodimer (59–63). The first PPRE characterized was found in the promoter of the acyl-coenzyme A (CoA) oxidase gene and was defined as DR-1 (2). Further, it has been shown that PPARs can achieve gene/tissue specific activity by being selectively bound as heterodimers to PPRE, whereby specific heterodimers such as PPARγ/RXRα or PPARγ/RXRγ bind more strongly to certain PPREs than other heterodimer combinations (65). Binding of PPAR/RXR to certain PPREs mediates transcriptional activation, but this can be negatively controlled by the presence of other heterodimers such as the thyroid hormone receptor/RXR heterodimer, as they can act as competitive inhibitors for PPRE binding that do not activate transcription (66).

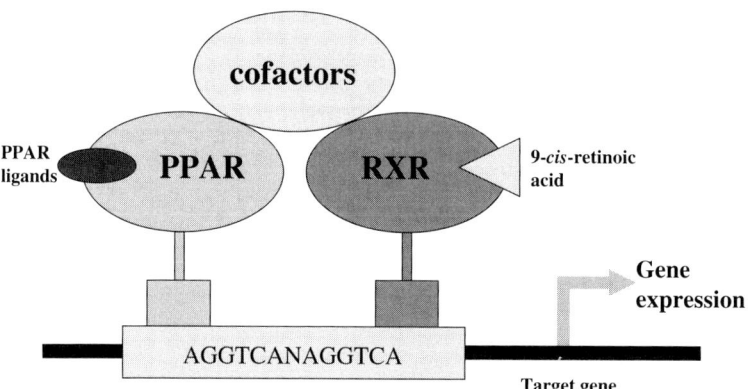

FIGURE 2 Typical peroxisome proliferator activated receptor/retinoic-x-activated receptor heterodimer complex. *Abbreviations*: PPAR, peroxisome proliferator activated receptor; RXR, retinoic-x-activated receptor.

Transcriptional activity is also influenced by cofactors. Using a yeast two-hybrid system, a number of coactivators have been identified, including the steroid receptor coactivator 1, the PPARγ-binding protein, and the PPAR interacting protein (67–69).

DIFFERENTIAL EXPRESSION OF PEROXISOME PROLIFERATOR-ACTIVATED RECEPTORS

The discovery of several subtypes of PPARs has raised the question of the biological significance of PPAR diversity, which can be addressed by looking at their expression patterns. PPARα is expressed preferentially in the liver and in tissues with high fatty acid catabolism, such as the heart, kidneys, muscles, and brown fat (9,70,71), demonstrating lower expression in adrenal, placenta, and lung (71). PPARγ is abundantly expressed in adipose tissue and at much lower levels in colon, spleen, and adrenal tissue (9,72). PPARβ/δ is the most ubiquitously expressed isoform among the three, but relatively little is known about its functions due to the lack of identification of physiological and specific ligands, as well as its remarkably broad tissue distribution (9,73–75).

In the skin, expression of all the three PPAR isoforms has been demonstrated and for recent reviews on PPARs in cutaneous biology, the reader is referred to Kuenzli and Saurat (76) and Wahli (77). PPARβ/δ is the prevalent PPAR subtype in human epidermis, whereas PPARα and PPARγ are expressed at lower levels (34,78,79). In vitro studies have shown that PPARβ/δ expression remains high during keratinocyte differentiation, whereas expression of PPARα and PPARγ increases significantly (34,80,81). In addition, these receptors are also present in rodent keratinocytes where the three isoforms exhibit a specific pattern of expression, suggesting nonredundant functions during development and in the various layers of the epidermis (32,78,79,82,83). PPARα, PPARβ/δ, and PPARγ transcripts are already present in the mouse epidermis at foetal day 13.5 (79). PPAR expression decreases after birth to become undetectable in the interfollicular epidermis of the adult mice. In contrast, all three isoforms remain expressed in

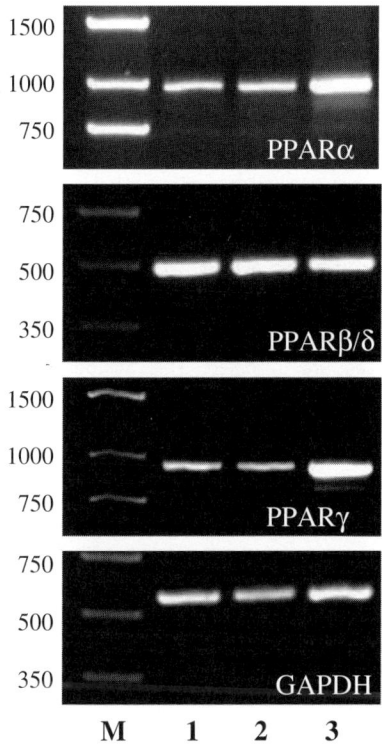

FIGURE 3 Peroxisome proliferator activated receptors are expressed in freshly isolated human sebaceous glands. RNA was extracted and reverse transcription polymerase chain reaction (PCR) performed as previously described. Lanes 1 to 3 show PCRs performed on freshly isolated glands derived from three different subjects. Individual lane numbers in each of the PCR refer to cDNA obtained from the same subject. For example the PCR shown in lane 1 in each gel was performed using an aliquot from the same sample of cDNA. *Abbreviations*: GAPDH, glyceraldehyde-3-phosphate dehydrogenase; PPAR, peroxisome proliferator activated receptors. *Source*: From Ref. 41.

murine hair follicles (79). Interestingly, PPARα and PPARβ/δ expression is reactivated in the adult epidermis after various stimuli (tetradecanoylphorbol acetate topical application, hair plucking, or skin wound healing), resulting in keratinocyte proliferation and differentiation (79). Furthermore, expression of all the three isoforms has also been demonstrated in human hair follicles (84).

Further, mRNA expression of the three PPAR subtypes was demonstrated in cultured human sebocytes (39), as well as the protein expression of PPARγ. In accordance, mRNA and protein expression of PPARα, PPARβ/δ, and PPARγ was shown in isolated human sebaceous glands (Figs. 3 and 4, respectively) (41). Although no differences in mRNA levels could be observed, the level of protein PPARβ/δ was much more abundant compared to PPARα and PPARγ, which were only weakly expressed (41).

PEROXISOME PROLIFERATOR-ACTIVATED RECEPTORS ARE ACTIVATED BY A DIVERSE ARRAY OF COMPOUNDS

Nuclear transcription factors can achieve gene- or tissue-specific activity in several ways: (*i*) restriction of expression to a given tissue and/or at a given time, (*ii*) binding to specific DNA sequences and thus to specific genes, (*iii*) activation by tissue-specific ligands or activators, and (*iv*) modulation of the transactivation properties by physical or functional interactions with tissue specific cofactors. Thus, the predominant expression of PPARγ in adipose tissue and the high expression of PPARα in the liver correlate with their specific role in adipose

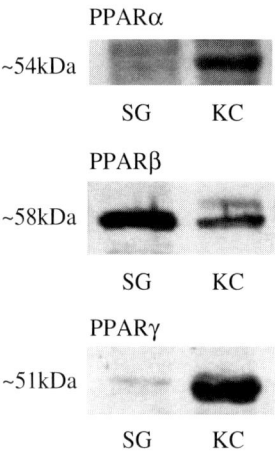

FIGURE 4   Peroxisome proliferator activated receptor (PPARα), PPARβ/δ, and PPARγ protein is detectable in freshly isolated human sebaceous glands. Sebaceous glands were isolated and processed for immunoblotting as previously described. Approximate protein sizes are indicated. This micrograph is representative of $n = 3$ subjects. *Abbreviations*: KC, primary human keratinocytes; PPAR, peroxisome proliferator activated receptor; SG, human sebaceous glands. *Source*: From Ref. 41.

differentiation and fatty acid catabolism, respectively. Further, fatty acids, leukotriene B_4, and hypolipidemic drugs (fibrates and $Wy_{14,643}$) preferentially activate PPARα, whereas the PPARγ subtype binds and is activated by prostaglandin derivatives and insulin-sensitizing thiazolidinediones such as pioglitazone, troglitazone, and BRL 49653 (42,52,65,85).

The identification of fatty acids as endogenous ligands for PPARs has provided a unique approach to study lipid homeostasis at the molecular level. Among the fatty acids, linoleic acid, linolenic acid, and arachidonic acid are potent activators of PPARα (86,87). Other natural ligands include leukotriene B_4 and 15-deoxy-$\Delta^{12,14}$-prostaglandin J_2, which are PPARα and PPARγ activators, respectively (88,89).

Most studies on PPAR ligand activation have involved transfection experiments. Obviously, in these experiments, the activation of the receptor may result from a cascade of events rather than a direct binding of the tested ligand. Furthermore, the potency of a given compound is dependent on the rate at which it is taken up and metabolized by the cell type used. Finally, due to structural similarity, exogenous applied ligands probably interfere with the metabolic processing of endogenous ligands, possibly fatty acids and/or eicosanoids. Thus, the measured PPAR response presumably results from the combined actions of direct receptor binding of the exogenous ligand and the indirect effects, owing to the perturbation of endogenous ligand levels (52).

PEROXISOME PROLIFERATOR-ACTIVATED RECEPTOR TARGET GENES

PPARs regulate gene expression by binding to specific PPRE in the promoter regions of target genes (64). PPREs have a core element called DR-1, in which PPAR–RXR heterodimers preferentially bind to. Since stimulation of peroxisomal fatty acidβ-oxidation is one of the key effects of peroxisome proliferators, genes encoding enzymes of this pathway represent prime candidate target genes of PPARs. The first gene described was acyl-CoA oxidase that is the rate-limiting and specificity-defining enzyme of peroxisomal fatty acidβ-oxidation (2). PPREs have since been found in regulatory sequences of a number of enzyme of this pathway, including enoyl-CoA hydratase/3-hydroxyacyl-CoA dehydrogenase, cytochrome P450 4A6 (CYP4A6) gene, fatty acid binding protein gene, acyl-CoA synthetase gene, mitochondrial 3-hydroxy-3-methylglutaryl-CoA synthase gene, and the malic enzyme gene (2,14,15,90–93). PPAR target genes identified to date belong largely to pathways of lipid transport and metabolism.

The target genes of PPARα, which have mostly been studied in the context of liver parenchymal cells where it is highly expressed, are a relatively homogenous group of genes that participate in aspects of lipid catabolism, such as fatty acid uptake through membranes, fatty acid binding in cells, fatty acid oxidation (in microsomes, peroxisomes, and mitochondria), and lipoprotein assembly and transport (94). Recently, novel PPARα regulated genes, including ubiquitin COOH-terminal hydrolase 37 and cyclin T1, have been described, which could be involved in the regulation of cell cycle and carcinogenesis (95).

Most of the PPARγ target genes in adipose tissue are directly implicated in lipogenic pathways, including lipoprotein lipase, adipocyte fatty acid-binding protein, acyl-CoA synthase, and fatty acid transport protein (94). Further, PPARγ ligands have been shown to inhibit the growth and induce apoptosis in cells from different cancer lineages, including liposarcoma, breast cancer, melanoma, and colon cancer, demonstrating antitumor effects (96–99).

PPARβ/δ has been shown to regulate the expression of acyl-CoA synthetase 2 in the brain (92) and has also been linked to colon cancer where it is a negative target of the adenomatous polyposis coli gene (100). Further, PPARβ/δ activation has been implicated in keratinocyte differentiation, regulating the expression of transglutaminase-1, involucrin, and CD36 (34), and wound healing (79).

PPARs also control the expression of genes implicated in the inflammatory response via negative interference with different inflammatory pathways such as nuclear factor kappa B, activator protein-1, CCAAT/enhancer-binding protein (C/EBP)β, signal transducer and activator of transcription-1, and nuclear factor of activated T-cell. As such, PPARs influence inflammatory cytokine production and cell recruitment to the inflammatory sites (46).

It is beyond the scope of this review to further discuss the role of PPARs in health and disease, in particular metabolic disorders such as hyperlipidaemia, atherosclerosis, diabetes, obesity, and coronary artery disease, and the reader is referred to a number of excellent reviews on these subjects (24,89,101,102).

PEROXISOME PROLIFERATOR-ACTIVATED RECEPTOR ACTIVITY IN THE EPIDERMIS AND PILOSEBACEOUS UNIT

Terminal differentiation of the cells of the human pilosebaceous unit is not dissimilar from that of the epidermal keratinocytes. Like epidermal keratinocytes, the matrix cells of the hair follicle and the sebocytes of the sebaceous gland terminally differentiate to die, forming the hair fibre or releasing their cell content as sebum, respectively. This program includes a biochemical differentiation, the expression of various structural proteins, and the processing and reorganization of lipids. A wealth of data has been collected to date, suggesting that PPARs have specific roles in these complex processes.

The epidermal expression of the three PPAR isoforms has prompted studies on the effects of PPAR ligands on keratinocyte differentiation. In human primary keratinocytes, PPARα activators, including putative endogenous ligands such as fatty acids, induce differentiation and inhibit proliferation, suggesting a regulatory role for PPARα in epidermal homeostasis (31). In addition, PPARα ligands are able to influence lipid metabolism in an in vitro human skin model (33). In contrast, in a more recent study, PPARα activators, like PPARγ activators, seemed to have little effect on human keratinocyte differentiation (30). However, a selective PPARβ/δ ligand induced the expression of keratinocyte differentiation markers (30). These apparent discrepancies remain to be elucidated. In the rat, PPARα ligands accelerate epidermal maturation in vitro (31,103,104) and in utero (32), whereas PPARβ/δ and PPARγ activators had no effects. In addition, PPARα ligands induce epidermal differentiation and restore epidermal homeostasis in hyperproliferative mouse epidermis (105).

PPAR mutant mouse models have contributed to our understanding of the role of PPARs in epidermal homeostasis. Using PPARα, PPARβ/δ, and PPARγ mutant mice, it was shown that PPARα and PPARβ/δ are important for the rapid epithelialization of a skin wound and that each of them plays a specific role in this process. PPARα was mainly involved in the early inflammation phase of the healing, whereas PPARβ/δ was implicated in the control of keratinocyte proliferation. In addition and very interestingly, PPARβ/δ mutant primary keratinocytes showed impaired adhesion and migration properties (77,79). However, PPARα, PPARβ/δ, and PPARγ mutations appear to have no obvious effects during normal foetal development of the epidermis (79,106,107).

Unfortunately, epidermal and sebaceous gland functions were not examined in the mouse mutant models. However, in rat preputial sebocytes, PPARγ and PPARα activation induced sebocyte lipogenesis in vitro but not in keratinocytes, whereas activators of PPARβ/δ induced lipid formation in both sebocytes and keratinocytes (36). PPARγ ligands promoted the differentiative effects of androgens on sebocytes and PPARγ1 was shown to be expressed more strongly in freshly dispersed sebocytes compared to cultured sebocytes, suggesting that androgen influences an early step in sebocyte differentiation, which is related to but distinct from that influenced by PPARγ1. Further, PPARβ/δ was abundantly expressed in sebocytes and keratinocytes (36). RXR agonists augmented the stimulation of sebocyte differentiation by PPAR agonists, as expected from PPAR–RXR heterodimerization; however, the evidence for PPAR–RXR cooperativity was limited (37). Moreover, in cultured human sebocytes, PPARβ/δ activation had a stimulatory effect on lipid production, whereas PPARγ and PPARα activation was ineffective (39). In addition, treatment with arachidonic acid resulted in increased lipid formation in cultured human sebocytes (38). Furthermore, treatment with arachidonic acid enhanced apoptosis in cultured human sebocytes, as determined by the presence of fragmented nuclei, indicating that apoptosis is part of the sebocyte differentiation process (38). Using a PPARβ/δ mutant mouse model, proinflammatory cytokines initiated the production of endogenous PPARβ/δ ligands, which were essential for PPARβ/δ activation and action, and activated PPARβ/δ regulated the expression of genes associated with apoptosis (108).

In contrast, in organ maintained human sebaceous glands, PPARγ and PPARα selective ligands inhibited total sebaceous lipogenesis (Table 1) and also reduced the production of the sebum-specific lipids, squalene and triacylglycerol (Table 2). Further, arachidonic, linoleic, linolenic, and oleic acid, which are less specific in their PPAR subtype activation, also inhibited sebaceous lipogenesis (41). Similar observations were made using the hamster flank organ where PPARα activation with clofibric acid produced a dose-dependent inhibition of lipogenesis (40). In addition, it has been demonstrated that the oral administration of eicosatetraynoic acid to human male volunteers significantly reduced sebum secretion (109). These findings indicate that PPAR effects are differentiation

TABLE 1 Peroxisome Proliferator Activated Receptor and FXR Ligands Differentially Inhibit Sebaceous Gland Lipogenesis

Ligand	8 mM [1,2-^{14}C]acetate uptake into total lipid (pmol//mg gland wet wt/hr), mean ± SD					
	0 μM	0.01 μM	0.1 μM	1 μM	10 μM	100 μM
Arachidonic acid	1318 ± 814	877 ± 546	562 ± 361[a]	870 ± 612	635 ± 421[a]	385 ± 175[b]
Bezafibrate	1253 ± 310	1132 ± 462	1194 ± 628	1142 ± 497	971 ± 520	
BRL49653	1454 ± 524	1175 ± 467	1224 ± 568	991 ± 735[c]	322 ± 131[a]	
Clofibrate	1470 ± 478	1400 ± 521	1332 ± 696	1043 ± 296	901 ± 292	
d-PGJ$_2$	1764 ± 952	1931 ± 1187	1196 ± 1174	1097 ± 838	716 ± 606[a]	
ETYA	1284 ± 498	1418 ± 524	986 ± 651	616 ± 497[d]	(48 ± 46[b])	
Juvenile hormone III	1353 ± 745	1414 ± 897	1190 ± 285	1015 ± 386	1404 ± 528	
Leukotriene B4	2001 ± 949	1564 ± 756	1224 ± 861	1217 ± 804		
Linoleic acid	1467 ± 1089	632 ± 580[d]	332 ± 186[b]	549 ± 258[d]	535 ± 361[d]	513 ± 233[d]
Linolenic acid	1900 ± 659	1073 ± 802[d]	1143 ± 626[a]	1035 ± 469[d]	678 ± 410[b]	809 ± 327[b]
LY171883	1376 ± 321	1782 ± 722	1085 ± 406	1223 ± 639	474 ± 199[a]	
Oleic acid	1761 ± 756	963 ± 802[c]	691 ± 329[d]	536 ± 145[b]	718 ± 417[d]	860 ± 360[a]
PGJ$_2$	1251 ± 519	1095 ± 420	1350 ± 365	1273 ± 574	752 ± 441	
Trans-farnesol	1042 ± 409	899 ± 379	1060 ± 627	994 ± 351	818 ± 327	
WY14643	1415 ± 682	1224 ± 622	1062 ± 369	923 ± 289[c]	480 ± 371[b]	

Notes: Sebaceous glands were isolated and maintained, incubated with 8 mM [1,2-^{14}C]acetate, and subsequently lipids were analyzed, as described in Materials and Methods. Experiments were carried out for $n = 5$ subjects. Data are expressed as mean ± SD. Statistical significance was determined using single factor ANOVA with blocking (subjects were blocked) followed by Dunnett's multiple comparison procedure.
[a]$P < 0.01$.
[b]$P < 0.001$.
[c]$P < 0.05$.
[d]$P < 0.005$; (), compound toxic at this concentration.
Abbreviation: ETYA, eicosatetraynoic acid.
Source: From Ref. 41.

TABLE 2 Peroxisome Proliferator Activated Receptor and FXR Ligands Differentially Inhibit Sebaceous Gland Lipid Classes

Ligand 10 μM	Squalene		Wax esters		TAG		Cholesterol		Phospholipid	
	Control	Ligand	Control	Ligand	Control	Ligand	Control	Ligand	Control	Ligand
Arachidonic acid	39.9±9.9	27.4±9.3[a]	8.7±2.9	6.3±2.7	28.2±6.7	19.2±4.7[b]	10.4±9.9	25.5±11.1[a]	7.3±2.8	10.4±2.8[a]
Bezafibrate	29.3±11.8	20.6±9.9	8.5±1.8	8.3±4.9	26.2±6.1	18.5±4.9	16.5±11.1	22.2±8.5	10.2±2.7	16.0±5.7[a]
BRL49653	37.5±3.9	18.9±7.4[a]	8.8±0.9	8.9±1.9	26.3±2.1	21.7±4.4	12.7±3.3	20.7±4.3	8.4±0.5	15.2±3.5[a]
Clofibrate	28.6±11.6	28.5±10.9	9.3±3.0	8.1±1.2	26.7±6.9	23.8±6.7	17.0±9.4	18.1±8.4	10.5±3.7	12.0±5.1
d-PGJ$_2$	30.1±5.8	20.3±12.1[a]	7.3±3.1	5.7±1.2	26.4±3.3	22.6±1.3	17.7±8.9	26.9±13.5[a]	10.1±3.4	14.3±6.0[a]
ETYA[a]	38.8±6.7	29.3±10.2[a]	8.8±1.0	7.2±1.7	31.3±5.1	21.9±1.8[c]	7.6±3.0	20.0±5.4[a]	7.9±1.8	12.0±4.0
Juvenile hormone III	34.8±3.8	31.6±4.7	11.0±5.1	11.9±1.5	29.6±1.4	30.5±3.1	9.7±2.6	7.7±2.4	9.9±0.9	11.2±2.3
Leukotriene B4[a]	36.0±7.1	33.6±10.2	9.9±2.0	8.1±1.8[a]	31.5±5.3	30.4±8.4	8.4±6.3	10.7±7.1	8.5±2.4	9.5±4.3
Linoleic acid	39.4±8.1	22.4±10.0[c]	7.9±1.5	6.3±2.4[a]	33.3±7.0	22.5±9.3[a]	8.4±5.8	24.1±9.2[d]	5.8±0.4	9.2±0.9[d]
Linolenic acid	36.5±5.8	31.8±4.3	7.4±1.5	5.5±0.5[a]	34.9±4.6	26.4±3.7[a]	6.0±4.2	14.6±2.9[a]	9.4±1.1	10.9±0.7
LY171883	29.6±7.7	7.6±7.3[b]	9.5±3.7	5.8±3.9	26.3±2.6	13.1±3.1[d]	14.9±6.3	37.6±9.1[b]	11.7±2.3	21.6±2.6[d]
Oleic acid	37.0±6.6	31.8±5.1[a]	9.9±0.6	6.8±1.2[b]	36.4±6.1	26.3±3.8[a]	4.0±1.7	15.7±4.5[b]	8.2±2.4	9.9±2.5[a]
PGJ$_2$	40.5±12.6	29.2±14.3	8.8±1.7	7.2±2.7	27.3±5.8	23.2±5.8[a]	10.1±2.5	20.7±13.0	7.5±2.5	9.6±2.5
Trans-farnesol	33.9±6.9	33.2±2.2	7.3±1.2	7.5±1.7	26.0±2.4	25.2±1.2	15.4±3.8	14.9±2.3	9.4±2.3	10.6±3.6
WY14643	37.0±4.5	14.3±8.9[b]	8.7±1.7	4.1±2.6	33.3±3.0	19.0±7.0[a]	7.3±2.0	27.6±8.1[a]	9.4±1.2	18.7±5.6[a]

Notes: Sebaceous glands were isolated and maintained, incubated with 8 mM [1,2-^{14}C]acetate and subsequently lipids were analyzed as described in Materials and Methods. Experiments were carried out for $n = 5$ subjects. Data are expressed as mean±SD. Statistical significance was determined using two-tailed paired student's t test.
[a] $P < 0.05$.
[b] $P < 0.005$.
[c] $P < 0.01$.
[d] $P < 0.001$.
[e] $1 \mu M$.
Abbreviations: ETYA, eicosatetraynoic acid; FXR, farnesoid X receptor; TAG, triacylglycerols.
Source: From Ref. 41.

sensitive, that is, one might postulate that structures that are missing in sebocyte monolayers but are present in whole organ cultures may be involved in PPAR agonist activity.

Further, there is an evidence that cutaneous inflammation can be reduced by PPAR agonists, such as linoleic acid, with clinical effects comparable to that of glucocorticoids (110). In addition, the PPARα activators, WY-14,643 and clofibrate, were shown to reverse ultraviolet-B-light-mediated expression of inflammatory cytokines, that is, interleukin (IL)-6 and IL-8 (43). This work suggests the possibility of PPARα activators as novel nonsteroidal anti-inflammatory drugs in the topical treatment of inflammatory skin diseases (43). Further, PPARα activation with clofibrate treatment resulted in the reduction of inflammatory cells and a decrease in tumor necrosis factorα and IL-1α in the epidermis of a mouse model of irritant and allergic contact dermatitis (44).

ACNE

Acne is a disease unique to humans. It affects up to 80 % of young adults, in whom it can induce stress, depression, and anxiety, as determined by psychometric scoring (47,111,112). Acne is a disease of the infundibulum or "pore" of the human sebaceous pilosebaceous unit and of the gland itself. This unit develops at puberty, appears only at the site of acne lesions (the chest, back, and face), and seems to have no other function than to sometimes produce acne lesions. The earlier forms of acne are characterized by microcomedones, which represent an intrainfundibular scaling-like phenomenon. As the disease progresses in severity, comedogenesis develops, as does inflammation. Duct rupture is a late event in the development of most inflammatory lesions (47–50).

Acne is generally accepted by clinicians to be a multifactorial disease and it is believed that acne is associated with seborrhea, the excess production of sebum by the sebaceous gland (49,113). Further, *Propionibacterium acnes* is a major bacterium implicated in the pathogenesis of acne (114). Acne is characterized by the presence of noninflammatory lesions, termed comedones (47,50). The earliest pathological change in acne is altered follicular epithelial differentiation, resulting in a follicular retention hyperkeratosis—the microcomedo (50). In addition to the noninflammatory lesions, inflammatory lesions can develop when such microcomedos are colonized by *P. acnes*. For inflammatory lesions such as papules, pustules, and nodulocystic lesions to occur, a variety of pathogenic factors are involved, including besides *P. acnes*, inflammatory mediators, and host immunity (115). In vitro experiments on organ maintained human infudibula have identified a number of cytokines that can model the morphological and inflammatory aspects of acne (116). These cytokines not only induce the infundibular changes in acne, namely (*i*) hypercornification (scaling) of the infundibulum, (*ii*) expression of intercellular adhesion molecule-1 and human leukocyte antigen-D related, and (*iii*) disruption of infundibular morphology, but will also inhibit the secretion of lipid from the sebaceous gland (117). Since acne seems to be provoked by *P. acnes* in sebum and since *P. acnes* depends on sebum for nutrition, the inhibition of sebum secretion would be expected to promote the remission of the disease by inhibiting *P. acnes* colonization (117).

A number of acne therapies are currently in use, including retinoids (e.g., isotretinoin, adapalene), antiandrogens (e.g., cyproterone acetate), contraceptives, antibacterials (e.g., clindamycin, erythromycin), benzoyl peroxide, and salicylic acid (118,119). In milder cases, topical therapy is sufficient, but in more severe

TABLE 3   Summary of Peroxisome Proliferator Activated Receptor Expression Profiles and Physiological Functions in Various Study Models

Study model	PPAR expression profiles	Physiological functions upon subtype activation
Rodent epidermis in vitro	PPARα = PPARα/δ = PPARγ in fetal epidermis, not present in the adult	PPARα: acceleration of epidermal maturation PPARα/δ and PPARγ: no effects
Human epidermis in vitro	PPAR$\alpha/\delta \gg$ PPARα = PPARγ	Not determined
Rodent keratinocytes in vitro	PPARα = PPARα/δ = PPARγ	PPARα: induction of differentiation PPARα/δ and PPARγ: no effects
Human keratinocytes in vitro	PPAR$\alpha/\delta \gg$ PPARα = PPARγ	PPARα: regulation of lipid metabolism, possible induction of differentiation and inhibition of proliferation PPARα/δ: induction of differentiation PPARγ: no effects
Murine hair follicles	PPARα = PPARα/δ = PPARγ	Not determined
Mutant mouse models	n/a	PPARα and PPARα/δ: promote rapid epithelialization of skin wound PPARα: involved in early inflammatory phase of healing PPARα/δ: contol of keratinocyte proliferation
Human hair follicles	PPARα = PPARα/δ = PPARγ	PPARα: enhanced hair follicle survival PPARα/δ and PPARγ: not determined
Rat sebocytes in vitro	PPAR$\alpha/\delta \gg$ PPARγ1 PPARα not determined	PPARα, PPARα/δ, and PPARγ: induction of sebocyte lipogenesis
Human sebocytes in vitro	PPARα = PPARα/δ = PPARγ	PPARα/δ: stimulation of lipid synthesis PPARα and PPARγ: no effects
Hamster sebaceous gland in vitro	Not determined	PPARα: inhibition of lipid synthesis PPARα/δ and PPARγ: not determined
Human sebaceous gland in vitro	PPAR$\alpha/\delta >$ PPARα = PPARγ	PPARα, PPARα/δ, and PPARγ: inhibition of lipid sythesis
Human clinical data in vivo	Not determined	PPARα: inhibition of sebum secretion PPARα/δ and PPARγ: not determined

Abbreviation: PPAR, peroxisome proliferator activated receptor.

cases where papulopustular or nodulocystic acne is present, there is a need of systemic treatment. However, there is a continued need for effective drugs for the therapy of acne, although judicious combined use of existing topical and systemic therapies offers great relief to many patients and a recent review of these therapies indicated that approximately 68% of treatment is effective (120). Nonetheless, PPARs may offer a solution for the development of novel effective drugs for acne therapy.

CONCLUSIONS

The study of PPAR expression profiles and the identification of target genes and ligands in the skin and its appendages as well as the utilization of PPAR mouse mutant models have unveiled distinct physiological functions of the PPARs (Table 3). In particular, activation of PPARs regulates differentiation and proliferation, lipid metabolism, inflammation, and apoptosis. However, the molecular mechanisms by which PPARs coordinate the regulation of these processes remain largely unknown, and thus PPARs represent a major research target for the understanding and treatment of many skin diseases including acne.

The research reviewed here focused on PPAR activity in human epidermis and its appendages. The data demonstrates that PPARs regulate many of the physiological processes that are involved in acne. However, it is also apparent that there is some discrepancies with regard to the physiological effects of PPAR ligands on sebaceous lipogenesis, which may be attributed to the different study models used, but this requires further elucidation. It would be of particular interest to evaluate the efficacy of PPAR ligands on acne and other skin disorders in the clinic.

Since the completion of this manuscript, more research has been done into examining the effects of PPAR ligands on sebaceous lipogenesis. The PPAR ligands GW7647, GW0742, GW2433, rosiglitazone, and GW4148 significantly increased lipogenesis in SEB-1 sebocytes (121), confirming earlier reports referenced in this chapter. Interestingly, patient data collected in the same paper showed increased sebum secretion in patients receiving fibrates for hyperlipidemia or thialzolidienediones for diabetes. However, this is in contrast to observation in healthy volunteers, and one might argue that these patients are treated for metabolic diseases of the liver and pancreas, which may also effect sebaceous gland metabolism, and therefore these data should be treated with caution. In addition, PPAR involvement in the prostaglandin pathway has been shown in a recent paper where PPARγ activation has been implicated in oxidative stress-mediated prostaglandin E(2) production in SX95 human sebaceous cells (122).

REFERENCES

1. Issemann I, Green S. Activation of a member of the steroid hormone receptor superfamily by peroxisome proliferators. Nature 1990; 347:645–650.
2. Dreyer C, Krey G, Keller H, et al. Control of the peroxisomal beta-oxidation pathway by a novel family of nuclear hormone receptors. Cell 1992; 68:879–887.
3. Göttlicher M, Widmark E, Li Q, et al. Fatty acids activate a chimera of the clofibric acid-activated receptor and the glucocorticoid receptor. Proc Natl Acad Sci U S A 1992; 89:4653–4657.
4. Schmidt A, Endo N, Rutledge SJ, et al. Identification of a new member of the steroid hormone receptor superfamily that is activated by a peroxisome proliferator and fatty acids. Mol Endocrinol 1992; 6:1634–1641.

5. Chen F, Law SW, O 'Malley BW. Identification of two mPPAR related receptors and evidence for the existence of five subfamily members. Biochem Biophys Res Commun 1993; 196:671–677.

6. Sher T, Yi HF, Mcbridge OW, et al. cDNA cloning, chromosomal mapping, and functional characterization of the human peroxisome proliferator activated receptor. Biochemistry 1993; 32:5598–5604.

7. Zhu Y, Alvars K, Huang Q, et al. Cloning of a new member of the peroxisome proliferator-activated receptor gene family from mouse liver. J Biol Chem 1993; 258:26817–26820.

8. Mukherjee R, Jow L, Croston GE, et al. Identification, characterization, and tissue distribution of human peroxisome proliferator-activated receptor (PPAR) isoforms PPARγ2 versus PPARγ1 and activation with retinoid X receptor agonist and antagonist. J Biol Chem 1997; 272:8071–8076.

9. Auboeuf D, Rieusset J, Fajas L, et al. Tissue distribution and quantification of the expression of mRNAs of peroxisome proliferator-activated receptors and liver X receptor-alpha in humans: no alteration in adipose tissue of obese and NIDDM patients. Diabetes 1997; 46:1319–1327.

10. Hess R, Stäubli W, Riess W. Nature of the hepatomegalic effect produced by ethyl-chlorophenoxy-isobutyrate in the rat. Nature 1965; 208:856–858.

11. Reddy JK, Rao MS, Azarnoff DL, et al. Mitogenic and carcinogenic effects of a hypolipidemic peroxisome proliferator, [4-chloro-6-(2,3-xylidino)-2-pyrimidinylthio]acetic acid (WY-14,643), in rat and mouse liver. Cancer Res 1979; 39:152–161.

12. Styles JA, Kelly M, Pritchard NR, et al. A species comparison of acute hyperplasia induced by the peroxisome proliferator methylclofenapate: involvement of the binucleated hepatocyte. Carcinogenesis 1988; 9:1647–1655.

13. Zhang X-K, Lehman J, Hoffmann B, et al. Homodimer formation of retinoid X receptor induced by 9-cis retinoic acid. Nature 1992; 358:587–591.

14. Bardot O, Aldridge TC, Latruffe N, et al. PPAR-RXR heterodimer activates a peroxisome proliferator response element upstream of the bifunctional enzyme gene. Biochem Biophys Res Commun 1993; 192:37–45.

15. Krey G, Keller H, Mahfoudi A, et al. Xenopus peroxisome proliferator activated receptors: genomic organization, response element recognition, heterodimer formation with retinoid X receptor and activation by fatty acids. J Steroid Biochem Mol Biol 1993; 47:65–73.

16. Dreyer C, Keller H, Mahfoudi A, et al. Positive regulation of the peroxisomal β-oxidation pathway by fatty acids through activation of peroxisome proliferator activated receptors (PPAR). Biol Cell 1993; 77:67–76.

17. Desvergene B, Wahli W. PPAR: a key nuclear factor in nutrient/gene interactions? Inducible Gene Expr 1995; 1:142–176.

18. Hihi AK, Michalik L, Wahli W. PPARs: transcriptional effectors of fatty acids and their derivatives. Cell Mol Life Sci 2002; 59:790–798.

19. Lock EA, Mitchell AM, Elcombe CR. Biochemical mechanisms of induction of hepatic peroxisome proliferation. Annu Rev Pharmacol Toxicol 1989; 29:145–163.

20. Reddy JK, Lalwani ND. Carcinogenesis by hepatic peroxisome proliferators: evaluation of the risk of hypolipidemic drugs and industrial plasticizers to humans. CRC Crit Rev Toxicol 1983; 12:1–58.

21. Conway JG, Tomaszewski KE, Olson MJ, et al. Relationship of oxidative damage to the hepatocarcinogenicity of the peroxisome proliferators di(2-ethylhexyl)phthalate and WY-14,643. Carcinogenesis 1989; 10:513–519.

22. Kasai H, Okada Y, Nishimura S, et al. Formation of 8-hydroxydeoxyguanosine in liver DNA of rats following long-term exposure to a peroxisome proliferator. Cancer Res 1989; 49:2603–2605.

23. Shoonjans K, Staels B, Auwerx J. The peroxisome proliferator activated receptors (PPARs) and their effects on lipid metabolism and adipocyte differentiation. Biochim Biophys Acta 1996; 1302:93–109.

24. Lee CH, Olson P, Evans RM. Minireview: lipid metabolism, metabolic diseases, and peroxisome proliferator activated receptors. Endocrinology 2003; 144:2201–2207.

25. Kliewer SA, Lehmann JM, Willson TM. Orphan nuclear receptors: shifting endrocrinology into reverse. Science 1999; 284:757–760.
26. Chawala A, Lazar MA. Peroxisome proliferator and retinoids signaling pathways co-regulate preadipocyte phenotype and survival. Proc Natl Acad Sci USA 1994; 91:1786-1790.
27. Tontonoz P, Hu E, Spiegelman BM. Stimulation of adipogenesis in fibroblasts by PPARγ2, a lipid-activated transcription factor. Cell 1994; 79:1147–1156.
28. Tontonoz P, Hu E, Spiegelman BM. Regulation of adipocyte gene expression and differentiation by peroxisome proliferators activated receptorγ. Curr Opin Genet Dev 1995; 5:571–576.
29. Adams M, Montague CT, Prins JB, et al. Activators of peroxisome proliferator-activated receptor gamma have depot-specific effects on human preadipocyte differentiation. J Clin Invest 1997; 100:3149–3153.
30. Sewter C, Blows F, Considine R, et al. Differential effects of adiposity on peroxisomal proliferator-activated receptor gamma1 and gamma2 messenger ribonucleic acid expression in human adipocytes. J Clin Endocrinol Metab 2002; 87:4203–4207.
31. Hanley K, Jiang Y, He SS, et al. Keratinocyte differentiation is stimulated by activators of the nuclear hormone receptor PPARα. J Invest Dermatol 1998; 110:368–375.
32. Hanley K, Komuves LG, Bass NM, et al. Fetal epidermal differentiation and barrier development *in vivo* is accelerated by nuclear hormone receptor activators. J Invest Dermatol 1999; 113:788–795.
33. Rivier M, Castiel I, Safonova I, et al. Peroxisome proliferator-activated receptor-α enhances lipid metabolism in a skin equivalent model. J Invest Dermatol 2000; 114:681–687.
34. Westergaard M, Henningsen J, Svendsen ML, et al. Modulation of keratinocyte gene expression and differentiation by PPAR selective ligands and tetradecylthioacetic acid. J Invest Dermatol 2001; 116:702–712.
35. Rosenfield RL, Deplewski D, Kentsis A, et al. Mechanisms of androgen induction of sebocyte differentiation. Dermatology 1998; 196:43–46.
36. Rosenfield RL, Kentsis A, Deplewski D, et al. Rat preputial sebocytes differentiation involves peroxisome proliferator-activated receptors. J Invest Dermatol 1999; 112:226–232.
37. Kim MJ, Deplewski D, Ciletti N, et al. Limited cooperation between peroxisome proliferator-activated receptors and retinoid X receptor agonists in sebocyte growth and development. Mol Genet Metab 2001; 74:362–369.
38. Wróbel A, Seltmann H, Fimmel S, et al. Differentiation and apoptosis in human immortalized sebocytes. J Invest Dermatol 2003; 120:175–181.
39. Chen W, Yang CC, Sheu HM, et al. Expression of peroxisome proliferator-activated receptor and CCAAT/enhancer binding protein transcription factors in cultured human sebocytes. J Invest Dermatol 2003; 121:441–447.
40. Venencie PY, Vantrou-Delaunay M, Bougaret S, et al. Modification of lipogenesis in the isolated hamster flank organ through clofibric acid. Skin Pharmacol 1995; 8:203–206.
41. Downie MMT, Sanders DA, Maier LM, et al. PPAR and FXR ligands differentially regulate sebaceous differentiation in human sebaceous gland organ cultures in vitro. Br J Dermatol 2004; 151:766–775.
42. Devchand PR, Keller H, Peters JM, et al. The PPARα-leukotriene B4 pathway to inflammation control. Nature 1996; 384:39–43.
43. Kippenberger S, Loitsch SM, Grundmann-Kollmann M, et al. Activators of peroxisome proliferator-activated receptors protect human skin from ultraviolet-B-light-induced inflammation. J Invest Dermatol 2001; 117:1430–1436.
44. Sheu MY, Fowler AJ, Kao J, et al. Topical peroxisome proliferator activated receptor-alpha activators reduce inflammation in irritant and allergic contact dermatitis models. J Invest Dermatol 2002; 118:94–101.
45. Houseknecht KL, Cole BM, Steele PJ. Peroxisome proliferator-activated receptor gamma (PPARgamma) and its ligands: a review. Domest Anim Endocrinol 2002; 22:1–23.

46. Blanquart C, Barbier O, Fruchart JC, et al. Peroxisome proliferator-activated receptors: regulation of transcriptional activities and roles in inflammation. J Steroid Biochem Mol Biol 2003; 85:267–273.
47. Kligman AM. An overview of acne. J Invest Dermatol 1974; 62:268–287.
48. Strauss JS, Kligman AM. Pathological patterns of the sebaceous gland. J Invest Dermatol 1958; 30:51–61.
49. Cunliffe WJ, Shuster S. Pathogenesis of acne. Lancet 1969; ii:685–687.
50. Knutson DD. Ultrastructural observations in acne vulgaris: the normal sebaceous follicle and acne lesions. J Invest Dermatol 1974; 62:288–307.
51. Enmark E, Gustafsson JA. Orphan nuclear receptors—the first eight years. Mol Endocrinol 1996; 10:1293–1307.
52. Lemberger T, Desvergne B, Wahli W. Peroxisome proliferator-activated receptors: a nuclear receptor signalling pathway in lipid physiology. Annu Rev Cell Dev Biol 1996; 12:335–363.
53. Beamer BA, Negri C, Yen CJ, et al. Chromosomal localization and partial genomic structure of the human peroxisome proliferator activated receptor-gamma (hPPAR gamma) gene. Biochem Biophys Res Commun 1997; 33:756–759.
54. Skogsberg J, Kannisto K, Roshani L, et al. Characterization of the human peroxisome proliferator activated receptor delta gene and its expression. Int J Mol Med 2000; 6:73–81.
55. Camp HS, Tafuri SR. Regulation of peroxisome proliferator-activated receptor γ activity by mitogen-activated protein kinase. J Biol Chem 1997; 272:10811–10816.
56. Shalev A, Siegrist-Kaiser CA, Yen PM, et al. The peroxisome proliferator-activated receptorα is a phosphoprotein: regulation by insulin. Endocrinology 1996; 137:4499–4502.
57. Blanquart C, Barbier O, Fruchart JC, et al. Peroxisome proliferator-activated receptor alpha (PPARalpha) turnover by the ubiquitin-proteasome system controls the ligand-induced expression level of its target genes. J Biol Chem 2002; 277:37254–37259.
58. Miyata KS, McCaw SE, Patel HV, et al. The orphan nuclear hormone receptor LXLα interacts with the peroxisome proliferator-activated receptor and inhibits peroxisome prolifarator signaling. J Biochem Chem 1996; 271:9189–9192.
59. Kliewer SA, Umesono K, Noonan DJ, et al. Convergence of 9-cis retinoic acid and peroxisome proliferator signaling pathways through heterodimer formation of their receptors. Nature 1992; 358:771–774.
60. Gearing KL, Gottlicher M, Teboul M, et al. Interaction of the peroxisome-proliferator-activated receptor and retinoid X receptor. Proc Natl Acad Sci USA 1993; 90: 1440–1444.
61. Issemann I, Prince RA, Tugwood JD, et al. The peroxisome proliferator activated receptor: retinoid X receptor heterodimer is activated by fatty acids and fibrate hypo-lipidemic drugs. J Mol Endocrinol 1993; 11:37–47.
62. Keller H, Dreyer C, Medin J, et al. Fatty acids and retinoids control lipid metabolism through activation of peroxisome proliferator-activated receptor-retinoid X receptor heterodimers. Proc Natl Acad Sci U S A 1993; 90:2160–2164.
63. Chawla A, Repa JJ, Evans RM, et al. Nuclear receptors and lipid physiology: opening the X-files. Science 2001; 294:1866–1870.
64. Green S. Promiscuous liaisons. Nature 1993; 361:590–591.
65. Juge-Aubry C, Pernin A, Favez T, et al. DNA binding properties of peroxisome proliferator-activated receptor subtypes on various natural peroxisome proliferator response elements. J Biol Chem 1997; 272:25252–25259.
66. Miyamoto T, Kaneko A, Kakizawa T, et al. Inhibition of peroxisome proliferator signaling pathways by thyroid hormone receptor. J Biol Chem 1997; 272:7752–7758.
67. Zhu Y, Qi C, Calandra C, et al. Cloning and identification of mouse steroid receptor coactivator-1 (mSRC-1), as a coactivator of peroxisome proliferator-activated receptor gamma. Gene Expr 1996; 6:185–195.
68. Zhu Y, Qi C, Jain S, et al. Isolation and characterization of PBP, a protein that interacts with peroxisome proliferator-activated receptor. J Biol Chem 1997; 272:25500–25506.
69. Zhu Y, Kan L, Qi C, et al. Isolation and characterization of peroxisome proliferator-activated receptor (PPAR) interacting protein (PRIP) as a coactivator for PPAR. J Biol Chem 2000; 275:13510–13516.

70. Gonzales FJ. The role of peroxisome proliferator activated receptorα in peroxisome proliferation, physiological homeostasis, and chemical cacinogenesis. Adv Exp Med Biol 1997; 422:109–125.

71. Su JL, Simmons CJ, Wisely B, et al. Monitoring of PPAR alpha protein expression in human tissue by the use of PPAR alpha-specific Mabs. Hybridoma 1998; 17:47–53.

72. Rosen ED, Spiegelman BM. PPARgamma: a nuclear regulator of metabolism, differentiation, and cell growth. J Biol Chem 2001; 276:37731–37734.

73. Peters JM, Lee SS, Li W, et al. Growth, adipose, brain, and skin alterations resulting from targeted disruption of the mouse peroxisome proliferator activated receptor beta (delta). Mol Cell Biol 2000; 20:5119–5128.

74. Lim H, Gupta RA, Ma WA, et al. Cyclo-oxygenase-2-derived prostacyclin mediates embryo implantation in the mouse via PPARdelta. Genes Dev 1999; 13:1561–1574.

75. Leibowitz MD, Fievet C, Hennuyer N, et al. Activation of PPAR-delta alters lipid metabolism in db/db mice. FEBS Lett 2000; 473:333–336.

76. Kuenzli S, Saurat JH. Peroxisome proliferator-activated receptor in cutaneous biology. Br J Dermatol 2003; 149:229–236.

77. Wahli W. Peroxisome proliferator-activated receptors (PPARs): from metabolic control to epidermal wound healing. Swiss Med Wkly 2002; 132:83–91.

78. Braissant O, Wahli W. Differential expression of peroxisome proliferator activated alpha, beta and gamma during rat embryonic development. Endrocrinology 1998; 139:2748–2754.

79. Michalik L, Desvergne B, Tan NS, et al. Impaired skin wound healing in peroxisome proliferator-activated receptor (PPAR) alpha and PPARbeta mutant mice. J Cell Biol 2001; 154:799–814.

80. Matsuura H, Adachi H, Smart RC, et al. Correlation between expression of peroxisome proliferator activated receptorβ and squamous differentiation in epidermal and tracheobronchial epithelial cells. Mol Cell Endocrinol 1999; 147:85–92.

81. Rivier M, Safonova I, Lebrun P, et al. Differential expression of peroxisome proliferator-activated receptor subtypes during the differentiation of human keratinocyte. J Invest Dermatol 1998; 111:1116–1121.

82. Michalik L, Desvergne B, Dreyer C, et al. PPAR expression and function during vertebrate development. Int J Dev Biol 2002; 46:105–114.

83. Braissant O, Foufelle F, Scotto C, et al. Differential expression of peroxisome proliferator-activated receptors (PPARs): tissue distribution of PPAR-alpha, -beta, and -gamma in the adult rat. Endocrinology 1996; 137:354–366.

84. Billoni N, Buan B, Gautier B, et al. Expression of peroxisome proliferator activated receptors (PPARs) in human hair follicles and PPAR alpha involvement in hair growth. Acta Derm Venereol 2000; 80:329–334.

85. Lehmann JM, Moore LB, Smith-Oliver TA, et al. An antidiabetic thiazolidinedione is a high affinity ligand for peroxisome proliferatior-activated receptorγ (PPARγ). J Biol Chem 1995; 270:12953–12956.

86. Forman BM, Chen J, Evans RM. Hypolipidemic drugs, polyunsaturated fatty acids, and eicosanoids are ligands for peroxisome proliferator-activated receptorsα and δ. Proc Natl Acad Sci USA 1997; 94:4312–4317.

87. Lin Q, Ruuska SE, Shaw NS, et al. Ligand selectivity of PPARα. Biochemistry 1999; 38:185–190.

88. Yu K, Bayona W, Kallen C, et al. Differential activation of PPAR by eicosanoids. J Biol Chem 1995; 270:23975–23983.

89. Forman BM, Tontonoz P, Chen J, et al. 15-Deoxy-delta 12, 14-prostaglandin J2 is a ligand for the adipocyte determination factor PPAR gamma. Cell 1995; 83:803–812.

90. Zhang B, Marcus SL, Sajjadi FG, et al. Identification of a peroxisome proliferator-responsive element upstream of the gene encoding rat peroxisomal enoyl-CoA hydratase/3-hydroxyacyl-CoA dehydrogenase. Proc Natl Acad Sci USA 1992; 89:7541–7545.

91. Meertens LM, Miyata KS, Cechetto JD, et al. A mitrochondral ketogenic enzyme regulates its gene expression by association with the nuclear hormone receptor PPARa. EMBO J 1998; 17:6972–6978.

92. Basu-Modak S, Braissant O, Escher P, et al. Peroxisome proliferator-activated receptorβ regulates acyl-CoA synthetase 2 in reaggreated rat brain cell cultures. J Biol Chem 1999; 274:35881–35888.

93. IJpenberg A, Jeannin E, Wahli W, et al. Polarity and specific sequence requirements of peroxisome proliferator-activated receptor (PPAR)/retinoid X receptor heterodimer binding to DNA. J Biol Chem 1997; 272:20108–20117.

94. Kersten S, Desvergne B, Wahli W. Roles of PPARs in health and disease. Nature 2000; 405:421–424.

95. Tien ES, Gray JP, Peters JM, et al. Comprehensive gene expression analysis of peroxisome proliferator-treated immortalized hepatocytes: identification of peroxisome proliferator-activated receptor alpha-dependent growth regulatory genes. Cancer Res 2003; 63:5767–5780.

96. Demetri GD, Fletcher CD, Mueller E, et al. Induction of solid tumor differentiation by the peroxisome proliferator-activated receptor-gamma ligand troglitazone in patients with liposarcoma. Proc Natl Acad Sci USA 1999; 96:3951–3956.

97. Lapillonne H, Konopleva M, Tsao T, et al. Activation of peroxisome proliferator-activated receptor gamma by a novel synthetic triterpenoid 2-cyano 3,12 dioxooleana-1,9-dien-28-oic acid induces growth arrest and apoptosis in breast cancer cells. Cancer Res 2003; 63:5926–5939.

98. Placha W, Gil D, Dembinska-Kiec A, et al. The effect of PPARgamma ligands on the proliferation and apoptosis of human melanoma cells. Melanoma Res 2003; 13:447–456.

99. Peek RM. The role of PPARgamma in colon cancer: is it as simple as APC? Gastroenterology 2003; 125:619–621.

100. He TC, Chan TA, Vogelstein B, et al. PPARdelta is an APC-regulated target of nonsteroidal anti-inflammatory drugs. Cell 1999; 99:335–345.

101. Plutzky J. The potential role of peroxisome proliferator-activated receptors on inflammation in type 2 diabetes mellitus and atherosclerosis. Am J Cardiol 2003; 92:34J–41J.

102. Gurnell M, Savage DB, Chatterjee VK, et al. The metabolic syndrome: peroxisome proliferator-activated receptor gamma and its therapeutic modulation J Clin Endocrinol Metab 2003; 88:2412–2421.

103. Hanley K, Jiang Y, Crumrine D, et al. Activators of the nuclear hormone receptors PPARalpha and FXR accelerate the development of the fetal epidermal permeability barrier. J Clin Invest 1997; 100:705–712.

104. Komuves LG, Hanley K, Jiang Y, et al. Ligands and activators of nuclear hormone receptors regulate epidermal differentiation during fetal rat skin development. J Invest Dermatol 1998; 111:429–433.

105. Komuves LG, Hanley K, Man MQ, et al. Keratinocyte differentiation in hyperproliferative epidermis: topical application of PPARalpha activators restores tissue homeostasis. J Invest Dermatol 2000; 115:361–367.

106. Barak Y, Nelson MC, Ong ES, et al. PPAR gamma is required for placental, cardiac, and adipose tissue development. Mol Cell 1999; 4:585–595.

107. Rosen ED, Sarraf P, Troy AE, et al. PPAR gamma is required for the differentiation of adipose tissue in vivo and in vitro. Mol Cell 1999; 4:611–617.

108. Tan NS, Michalik L, Noy N, et al. Critical roles of PPAR beta/delta in keratinocyte response to inflammation. Genes Dev 2001; 15:3263–3277.

109. Strauss JS, Pochi PE, Whitman EN. Supression of sebaceous gland activity with eicosa —5:8:11:14-tetraynoic acid. J Invest Dermatol 1967; 48:492–493.

110. Schurer NY. Implementation of fatty acid carriers to skin irritation and the epidermal barrier. Contact Dermatitis 2002; 47:199–205.

111. Jowett S, Ryan T. Skin disease and handicap: an analysis of the impact of skin conditions. Soc Sci Med 1985; 20:425–429.

112. Shuster S, Fisher GH, Harris E, et al. The effects of skin disease on self image. Br J Dermatol 1978; 99:18s–19s.

113. Pochi PE, Strauss JS. Sebum production, casual sebum levels, titratable acidity of sebum, and urinary fractional 17-ketosteroid excretion in males with acne. J Invest Dermatol 1964; 43:383–388.

114. Holland KT, Leeming JP. Follicular micro-organisms in acne. In: Marks R, Plewig G, eds. Acne and Related Disorders. London: Martin Dunitz Ltd, 1989:121–126.
115. Dolitsky C, Shalita AR. Pathogenesis of inflammatory acne. In: Marks R, Plewig G, eds. Acne and Related Disorders. London: Martin Dunitz Ltd, 1989:77–80.
116. Guy R, Green MR, Kealey T. Modeling acne *in vitro*. J Invest Dermatol 1996; 106:176–182.
117. Downie MMT, Sanders D, Kealey T. Modelling the remission of individual acne lesions *in vitro*. Br J Dermatol 2002; 147:869–878.
118. Gollnick H. Current concepts of the pathogenesis of acne: implications for drug treatment. Drugs 2003; 63:1579–1596.
119. Rosen MP, Breitkopf DM, Nagamani M. A randomized controlled trial of second-versus third-generation oral contraceptives in the treatment of acne vulgaris. Am J Obstet Gynecol 2003; 188:1158–1160.
120. Larsen TH, Jemec GB. Acne: comparing hormonal approaches to antibiotics and isotretinoin. Expert Opin Pharmacother 2003; 4:1097–1103.
121. Trivedi NR, Cong Z, Nelson AM, et al. Peroxisome proliferator-activated receptors increase human sebum production. J Invest Dermatol 2006; 126(9):2002–2009. Epub May 4, 2006.
122. Zhang Q, Seltmann H, Zouboulis CC, et al. Involvement of PPARgamma in oxidative stress-mediated prostaglandin E(2) production in SZ95 human sebaceous gland cells. J Invest Dermatol 2006; 126(1):42–48.

6   Antimicrobial Peptides and Acne

Michael P. Philpott

Centre for Cutaneous Research, Institute of Cell and Molecular Science, Barts and the London, Queen Mary's School of Medicine and Dentistry, University of London, London, U.K.

INTRODUCTION

It is well known that the epidermis forms an effective structural barrier and is also highly resistant to pathological infection by the many different types of microorganism that colonize its surface. If the epidermal barrier is breached by pathogens, the first line of defence is the hosts innate immune response followed by the adaptive immune response. The innate immune response consists of a number of pre-existing defence mechanisms including phagocytic and natural killer cells, mast cells as well as epithelial cells themselves (1). These cells respond to microbial pathogens in a number of ways including the release of antimicrobial peptides. More than 500 antimicrobial peptides have been described in plants, insects, amphibians, and mammals, with broad-spectrum activity against bacteria, fungi, and viruses, representing an integral part of innate immunity (2,3). Of these antimicrobial peptides, the defensins, adrenomedullin (AM), and cathelicidins are perhaps the most widely studied in skin, although to date only defensins and AM appear to have been investigated in acne.

DEFENSINS

Mammalian defensins are a family of cationic antimicrobial peptides, 28 to 42 amino acids long, containing three disulfide bonds. They have been divided into two subtypes, the α-defensins and the β-defensins (4). The α-defensins are found in neutrophil granules [human neutrophil proteins (HNP)1–3] or in the paneth cells [human defensin (HD)5–6] of the small intestine (5). The four β-defensins so far identified, human beta-defensin 1 to 4 (hBD1–4) are produced in various epithelia including keratinocytes of the epidermis (6,7). In keratinocytes, hBD1 is constitutive, whereas hBD2–4 are inducible and are produced by keratinocytes in response to pro-inflammatory stimuli such as interleukin 1 (IL-1), tumor necrosis factor (TNF), and lipopolysaccharide (LPS).

    The most widely studied defensins in skin are hBD1 and hBD2 (8,9). Strong constitutive expression of both hBD1 and hBD2 mRNA and protein can be detected in the distal outer root sheath (ORS) of the hair follicle, surrounding the hair canal and in the pilosebaceous duct (Fig. 1). It is of particular interest that hBD1 and hBD2 proteins appear to be strongly expressed in more suprabasal cells. These patterns of expression are consistent with the concept that these regions are highly exposed to microbial organisms, and it is most likely that hBD1 and hBD2 play a key role in protecting the pilosebaceous unit from microbial invasion. In contrast, hair follicle compartments that are rarely exposed to microbial invasion such as the proximal ORS and inner root sheath (IRS) as well as the hair follicle bulb, including the

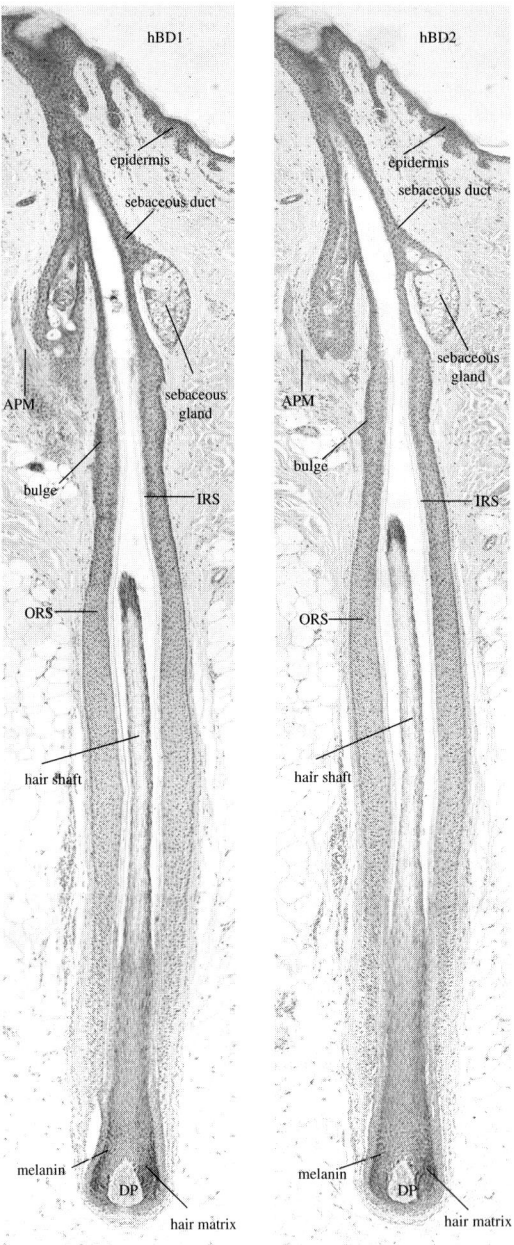

FIGURE 1   (*See color insert.*) Human beta-defensin 1 (hBD1) and hBD2 immunoreactivity in human hair follicles. hBD1 (**A**) and hBD2 (**B**) immunoreactivity is found in the suprabasal layers of the epidermis and the distal outer root sheath (ORS) of the hair follicle. Strong basal expression is seen in the bulge area, which contains a population of epidermal stem cells. Strong β-defensin expression is also found in the sebaceous gland and duct. Weaker expression is present in the suprabasal layers of the central and proximal ORS and in the proximal inner root sheath. hBD1 and hBD2 IR are not detected in the hair matrix or the dermal papilla. *Abbreviations*: APM, arrector pili muscle; DP, dermal papilla; IRS, inner root sheath; ORS, outer root sheath. *Source*: From Ref. 9.

dermal papilla (DP), showed only very weak hBD1 and hBD2 expression. More-over, as we shall discuss below it would also appear that as well as defensin expression in compartments with high exposure to microorganisms, defensins are also expressed in potential hair follicle stem cell compartments.

Perhaps, one of the most striking observations with regard to defensin expression in normal skin is that in contrast to the hair canal, pilosebaceous duct and interfollicular epithelium (8,9), where defensin expression is restricted to the cells of the suprabasal layers. In the central ORS and the buzlge region of the hair follicle, strong defensin expression is found in basal keratinocytes. This may be very important as it is accepted the central ORS and bulge of the hair follicle contain a population of epidermal stem cells (10–12). It is therefore tempting to speculate that the role of β-defensins in this region of the ORS may be to protect stem cells from microbial invasion. A similar role for defensins has recently been proposed in the gut, where marked defensins expression is detected in the paneth cells of the small intestine (2). Since paneth cells are located in the intestinal crypts, it has been suggested that paneth cell secretions might protect stem cells from pathogenic microbes. Whether defensins play an important role in protecting stem cells in the hair follicle remains to be investigated. However, it is also of note that the distal hair follicle containing the DP and hair follicle matrix are very weak expressers of defensins. The lower hair follicle is transient and during the hair growth cycle undergoes apoptotic driven regression (11,13,14). Moreover, if surgically removed, the lower follicle including the DP and matrix are able to regenerate (15,16). Therefore, lack of or weak defensin expression in these regions may reflect the transient nature of this part of the hair follicle, and the fact that if lost through mechanical injury and presumably infection they can regenerate. Whereas, the proximal hair follicle including the stem cell compartment cannot regenerate and must therefore be protected.

ADRENOMEDULLIN

AM is a 52-amino acid ringed structure peptide with C-terminal amidation that mediates vasodilatory and natriuretic properties through the second messenger cAMP, nitric oxide, and the renal prostaglandin system. In addition to these cardi-ovascular and renal effects, AM is involved in a remarkable range of other functions involving growth regulation, modulation of hormone secretion, neurotransmission, and antimicrobial defence (17). AM is synthesized as part of the larger precursor molecule preproAM, which contains an additional biologically active peptide termed preproAM N-terminal 20 peptide or PAMP (18). The effects of AM appear to be mediated by two different receptors: L1, a previously identified orphan receptor and calcitonin receptor like receptor (CRLR) which can bind either calcitonin gene related peptide or AM, depending on whether receptor activity modifying proteins are co-associated with CRLR (19,20).

In normal human skin, AM is expressed in suprabasal layers of the epidermis, in melanocytes, and in sweat and sebaceous glands (8,21). In the hair follicle, AM protein is expressed in the basal and suprabasal layers of the hair bulb and the proximal ORS. Whereas, in the distal ORS AM becomes increasingly supra-basal, especially in proximity to the bulge region. In contrast to defensins, AM immunoreactivity (IR) is absent from the basal cells of the bulge. The CRLR is expressed in a similar pattern to that of AM. In contrast, the L1 IR receptor is only expressed in suprabasal cells (21).

AM has antimicrobial effects against both Gram-positive and -negative bacteria isolated from the skin and oral cavity. Moreover, antimicrobial activity is most marked for *Propionibacterium acnes* and *Micrococcus luteus* with minimal inhibitory concentrations close to AM concentrations measured in sweat (22). AM also acts as an autocrine/paracrine growth factor in different tumor cell lines (23), Swiss 3T3 fibroblasts (24), vascular smooth muscle cells (25), as well as keratinocytes of skin (26), and oral mucosa (27). Based on these data, possible roles for AM in the innate unspecific immune system of the skin and a possible participation of AM in the regulation of skin proliferation, wound repair, hair growth, and tumor progression have been postulated.

ROLE OF ANTIMICROBIAL PEPTIDES IN ACNE

The epidermis forms an effective barrier, however, the hair canal, the distal ORS of the hair follicle, and the pilosebaceous duct constitute major ports of entry for microbial invasion in humans and harbor a rich residential microflora such as *P. acnes, Staphylococcus epidermidis, Demodex folliculorum*, and *Malassezia furfur*. The distal ORS and the pilosebaceous duct are also characterized by many features of innate and adaptive immunological activity such as classical and nonclassical MHC class 1 expression, ICAM-1 expression, and the presence of intraepithelial Langerhans cells and perifollicular macrophages (28–30). It is of considerable interest, therefore, that this area of the pilosebaceous unit is also a "hot spot" in the development of "acne vulgaris" lesions.

Acne, a disease of the pilosebaceous unit is characterized by hypercornification and hyperkeratosis of the ORS and sebaceous duct and perilesional infiltrate (PI). Lesions may be characterized as "non"inflammatory versus inflammatory and their increasing inflammatory infiltrate may be classified as: comedones, papules, and pustules. In acne (Fig. 2), there is marked upregulation of hBD1 and hBD2 as follows: hBD1, healthy follicular skin $\leq$ pustule $\leq$ comedo $<$ papule; hBD2, healthy follicular skin $\leq$ comedo $<$ papule $<$ pustule. The fact that intensity of upregulation of hBD2 is identical to the classification of inflammatory infiltrate correlates with other inflammatory disorders such as psoriasis and mastitis, which also exhibit marked upregulation of hBD2 (31–33).

From the published studies to date, it is clear that β-defensins are expressed in regions of the pilosebaceous unit that are exposed to microorganisms and moreover, in regions that may provide access routes for these organisms into the skin. Moreover, it is also apparent that some β-defensins are upregulated in acne (9). What, therefore, is the role of antimicrobial peptides in acne? Major factors in the pathogenesis of acne include hypercornification of the distal ORS and the pilosebaceous duct in concert with increased sebum production and abnormalities of the microbial flora (34).

There is increasing evidence that proinflammatory cytokines, such as IL-1β, TNF-α, and bacterial LPS, can upregulate β-defensins (4,6,32). *P. acnes* produces many likely candidates for inflammation such as lipases, neuramidases, phosphatases, and proteases (35). Therefore, the observed upregulation of β-defensins in acne vulgaris lesions is most likely a secondary response to the marked PI. It has been suggested that, variation in the microenvironment of the duct is likely to influence the production and activity of inflammatory mediators (36,37) and this may influence defensin production. Although hBD1 has been reported to be constitutively expressed and not upregulated under inflammatory conditions in oral

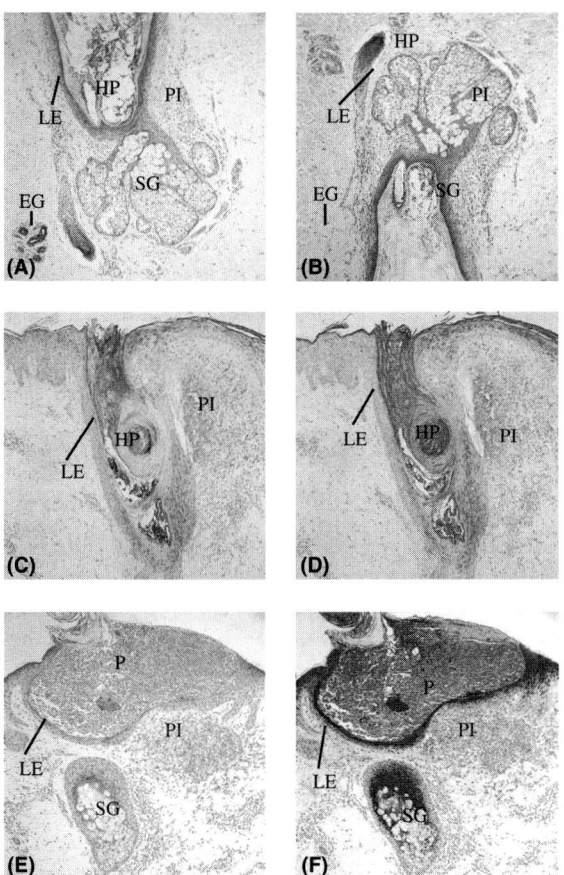

FIGURE 2 (*See color insert.*) Human beta-defensin 1 (hBD1) and hBD2 immunoreactivity in acne lesions. In comedones (**A** and **B**), hBD1 (**A**) is found in the hyperkeratotic plug (HP), the suprabasal layers of the lesional epithelium (LE), the pilosebaceous duct, and the sebaceous gland (SG). Strong hBD2 expression (**B**) is found in the suprabasal layers of the LE and the SG and duct. In papules (**C** and **D**), strong hBD1 expression is present in the HP, suprabasal layers of the epidermis, and LE, including the pilosebaceous duct and SG. Strong hBD2 expression (**D**) is present in the HP, the upper suprabasal layers of the epidermis, and LE including the pilosebaceous duct. In pustules (**E** and **F**), virtually no hBD1 (**E**) is found in the inflammatory area of the pustule. Moderate expression of hBD1 is present in the suprabasal layers of the epidermis, the LE and the pilosebaceous duct and SG. Intense hBD2 expression (**F**) is detected in the inflammatory area of the pustule, the suprabasal layers of the perilesional epidermis and LE, the pilosebaceous duct, and sebaceous gland. *Abbreviations*: EG, eccrine gland; HP, hyperkeratotic plug; LE, lesional epithelium; P, pustule proper; PI, perilesional infiltrate; SG, sebaceous gland. *Source*: From Ref. 9.

mucosa (38). Moderate upregulation of hBD1 has been reported in acne vulgaris lesions when compared to nonlesional skin of the same patient and also when compared to pilosebaceous follicles from healthy back skin controls (9). However, in contrast to the intense hBD2 upregulation found in and around pustules, including the area of maximal inflammation, relatively little upregulation of hBD1 IR is seen.

Because of the suggested antimicrobial function of AM in skin and in line with the proposed role of *P. acnes* in the pathogenesis of acne vulgaris, we have investigated AM immunoreactivity in inflammatory acne lesions compared to healthy pilosebaceous follicles. However, in contrast to β-defensins, AM does not appear to be upregulated in acne (21).

We have proposed (9,39) that acne vulgaris patients may suffer from a dysregulation of the production of innate and specific antimicrobial peptides. This is based on our own observations that substantial variations in the intensity of hBD1 and hBD2 IR occur between sex- and age-matched patients, between face and back skin as well as between different hair follicle types (terminal hair follicles and pilosebaceous follicles). Colonization of the pilosebaceous duct is a feature of established comedones and early inflammatory lesions (40,41). Why some colonized ducts become inflamed and others do not is uncertain. Variation in the microenvironment of the duct could be important. Likewise, it is possible that differences in levels or induction of defensins may explain why some colonized ducts become inflamed and others do not and may also explain why some individuals are prone to more severe acne than others. *P. acnes* is likely to be the major organism since selective antibiotic studies have shown that only those antibiotics which suppress *P. acnes* in vivo, are associated with clinical benefit. However, what is not clear is why some patients are good responders to antibiotic treatment and other not. An interesting line of study would be to investigate whether good responders to antibiotic antiacne treatment differ in their β-defensin levels and/or activity from bad responders.

From published studies, it is clear that there is marked variation in defensin expression, both between different body sites as well as between individuals. It has been reported that hBD-1 promotes keratinocyte differentiation in vitro (42). It is intriguing, therefore, to speculate whether defensins may play a role in the hypercornification of the sebaceous duct and whether perhaps individuals that are high producers of defensins may in fact be more prone to acne.

CONCLUSIONS

Defensins play a major role in innate immunity of epithelial tissues. It is clear that they are expressed in skin and are upregulated in inflammatory conditions. Their role in acne is still subject to much speculation and it is hoped that future studies will address whether individuals who suffer from severe acne or are poor responders to antibiotic treatment do produce lower levels of defensins.

ACKNOWLEDGMENTS

I would like to thank Dr. Sven Muller Roever and Catherine Chronnell for carrying out the research on defensins and acne in my laboratory; Professor Tony Quinn for many useful discussions; Dr. Bill Cunliffe and Dr. Diane Holland for supplying the acne biopsies; Dr. Thomas Ganz for donating the hBD1 and hBD2 antibodies, and Dr. Veronique Bataille for her valuable contributions to the study concept. I would also like to acknowledge the European Union (EU) for financial assistance.

REFERENCES

1. Oppenheim JJ, Biragyn A, Kwak LW, Yang D. Roles of antimicrobial peptides such as defensins in innate and adaptive immunity. Ann Rheum Dis 2003; 62(suppl II):17–21.
2. Boman HG. Innate immunity and the normal microflora. Immunol Rev 2000; 173:5–16.
3. Ganz T. Defensins and host defense. Science 1999; 286:420–421.

4. Diamond G, Bevins CL. Beta-defensins: endogenous antibiotics of the innate host defense response. Clin Immunol Immunopathol 1998; 88:221–225.
5. Ganz T, Lehrer RI. Antimicrobial peptides of vertebrates. Curr Opin Immunol 1998; 10:41–44.
6. Harder J, Bartels J, Christophers E, Schroder JM. A peptide antibiotic from human skin. Nature 1997; 387:861.
7. Valore EV, Park CH, Quayle AJ, Wiles KR, McCray PB, Ganz T. Human beta-defensin-1: an antimicrobial peptide of urogenital tissues. J Clin Invest 1998; 101:1633–1642.
8. Ali RS, Falconer A, Ikram M, Bissett CE, Cerio R, Quinn AG. Expression of the peptide antibiotics human beta defensin-1 and human beta defensin-2 in normal human skin. J Invest Dermatol 2001; 117:106–111.
9. Chronnell CMT, Ghali LR, Ali RS, et al. Human beta defensin-1 and -2 expression in human pilosebaceous units: upregulation in acne vulgaris lesions. J Invest Dermatol 2001; 117:1120–1125.
10. Cotsarelis G, Sun TT, Lavker RM. Label-retaining cells reside in the bulge area of pilosebaceous unit: implications for follicular stem cells, hair cycle, and skin carcinogenesis. Cell 1990; 61:1329–1337.
11. Cotsarelis G, Kaur P, Dhouailly D, Hengge U, Bickenbach J. Epithelial stem cells in the skin: definition, markers, localization and functions. Exp Dermatol 1999; 8:80–88.
12. Rochat A, Kobayashi K, Barrandon Y. Location of stem cells of human hair follicles by clonal analysis. Cell 1994; 76:1063–1073.
13. Stenn K, Parimoo S, Prouty S. Growth of the hair follicle: a cycling and regenerating biological system. In: Chuong CM, ed. Molecular Basis of Epithelial Appendage Morphogenesis. Austin, TX: Landes Bioscience Publ., 1998:111–124.
14. Lindner G, Botchkarev VA, Botchkarev NV, Ling G, van der Veen C, Paus R. Analysis of apoptosis during murine hair follicle regression (catagen). Am J Pathol 1997; 151(6):1601–1617.
15. Oliver RF. Whisker growth after removal of the dermal papilla and lengths of the follicle in the hooded rat. J Embryol Exp Morphol 1966; 15:331–347.
16. Paus R. Control of the hair cycle and hair diseases as cycling disorders. Curr Opin Dermatol 1996; 3:248–258.
17. Hinson JP, Kapas S, Smith DM. Adrenomedullin, a multifunctional regulatory peptide. Endocrine Rewiews 2000; 21:138–167.
18. Kitamura K, Sakata J, Kangawa K, et al. Cloning and characterization of cDNA encoding a precursor for human adrenomedullin [published erratum appears in Biochem Biophys Res Commun 1994; 202:643]. Biochem Biophys Res Commun 1993; 194:720–725.
19. McLatchie LM, Fraser NJ, Main MJ, et al. RAMPs regulate the transport and ligand specificity of the calcitonin-receptor-like receptor. Nature 1998; 393:333–339.
20. Kapas S, Catt KJ, Clark AJ. Cloning and expression of cDNA encoding a rat adrenomedullin receptor. J Biol Chem 1995; 270:25344–25347.
21. Muller FB, Muller-Rover S, Korge BP, Kapas S, Philpott MP. Adrenomedullin: expression and possible role in human skin and hair growth. Br J Dermatol 2003; 148:30–38.
22. Allaker RP, Zihni C, Kapas S. An investigation into the antimicrobial effects of adrenomedullin on members of the skin, oral, respiratory tract and gut microflora. FEMS Immunol Med Microbiol 1999; 23:289–293.
23. Miller MJ, Martinez A, Unsworth EJ, et al. Adrenomedullin expression in human tumor cell lines. Its potential role as an autocrine growth factor. J Biol Chem 1996; 271:23345–23351.
24. Withers DJ, Coppock HA, Seufferlein T, Smith DM, Bloom SR, Rozengurt E. Adrenomedullin stimulates DNA synthesis and cell proliferation via elevation of cAMP in Swiss 3T3 cells. FEBS Lett 1996; 378:83–87.
25. Iwasaki H, Eguchi S, Shichiri M, Marumo F, Hirata Y. Adrenomedullin as a novel growth-promoting factor for cultured vascular smooth muscle cells: role of tyrosine kinase-mediated mitogen-activated protein kinase activation. Endocrinology 1998; 139:3432–3441.
26. Martinez A, Elsasser TH, Muro-Cacho C, et al. Expression of adrenomedullin and its receptor in normal and malignant human skin: a potential pluripotent role in the integument. Endocrinology 1997; 138:5597–5604.

27. Kapas S, Brown DW, Farthing PM, Hagi-Pavli E. Adrenomedullin has mitogenic effects on human oral keratinocytes: involvement of cyclic AMP. FEBS Lett 1997; 418:287–290.

28. Paus R. Immunology of the hair follicle. In: Bos JD, ed. The Skin Immune System. Boca Raton: CRC Press, 1997.

29. Paus R, Müller-Röver S, Christoph T. Hair follicle immunology: a journey into *terra incognita*. J Invest Dermatol Symp Proc 1999; 4:226–234.

30. Christoph T, Müller-Röver S, Audring H, et al. The human hair follicle immune system: cellular composition and immune privilege. Br J Dermatol 2000; 142:1–13.

31. Schonwetter BS, Stolzenberg ED, Zasloff MA. Epithelial antibiotics induced at sites of inflammation. Science 1995; 267:1645–1648.

32. Stolzenberg ED, Anderson GM, Ackermann MR, Whitlock RH, Zasloff M. Epithelial antibiotic induced in states of disease. Proc Natl Acad Sci USA 1997; 94:8686–8690.

33. Schroder JM, Harder J. Human beta-defensin-2. Int J Biochem Cell Biol 1999; 31: 645–651.

34. Cunliffe WJ, Simpson NB. Disorders of the sebaceous gland [In: Rook, Wilkinson and Ebling: Diamond G, Russell JP, Bevins CL. Inducible expression of an antibiotic peptide gene in lipopolysaccharide-challenged tracheal epithelial cells]. Proc Natl Acad Sci USA 1996; 93:5156–5160.

35. Greenman J, Holland KT, Cunliffe WJ. Effects of pH on biomass, maximum specific growth rate and extracellular enzyme production by three species of cutaneous propionibacteria grown in continuous culture. J Gen Microbiol 1983; 129:1301–1307.

36. Holland KT, Cunliffe WJ, Roberts CD. The role of bacteria in acne vulgaris: a new approach. Clin Exp Dermatol 1978; 3:253–257.

37. Holland KT, Aldana O, Bojar RA, et al. Propionibacterium acnes and acne. Dermatology 1998; 196:67–68.

38. Mathews M, Jia HP, Guthmiller JM, et al. Production of beta-defensin antimicrobial peptides by the oral mucosa and salivary glands. Infect Immun 1999; 67:2740–2745.

39. Philpott MP. Defensins and acne. Mol Immunol 2003; 40:457–462.

40. Leeming JP, Holland KT, Cunliffe WJ. The pathological and ecological significance of microorganisms colonizing acne vulgaris comedones. J Med Microbiol 1985; 20:11–16.

41. Leeming JP, Holland KT, Cunliffe WJ. The microbial colonisation of inflamed acne vulgaris lesions. Br J Dermatol 1988; 118:203–208.

42. Frye M, Bargon J, Gropp R. Expression of human beta-defensin-1 promotes differentiation of keratinocytes. J Mol Med 2001; 79:275–282.

7   Hormonal Influences in Acne

Diane Thiboutot

Department of Dermatology, Pennsylvania State University College of Medicine, Hershey, Pennsylvania, U.S.A.

INTRODUCTION

The effects of hormones in acne are most notable in women. Androgens such as dihydrotestosterone (DHT) and testosterone, the adrenal precursor dehydroepiandrosterone sulfate (DHEAS), estrogen, and other hormones, including growth hormone or insulin-like growth factors (IGFs), may each be important. It is likely that the hormones affecting the sebaceous gland are both taken up from the serum in addition to being made locally within the gland.

Hormonal therapy is an option in women whose acne is not responding to conventional treatment or if signs of endocrine abnormalities are present. The greatest therapeutic benefit from hormonal therapy is achieved in combination with other effective anti-acne medications. This chapter focuses on the role of hormones in acne, the clinical presentation of adult female acne, the work-up of a suspected endocrine abnormality, and the available options for hormonal therapy.

ANDROGENS IN ACNE

Both clinical observation and experimental evidence confirm the importance of androgens in the pathophysiology of acne. The majority of circulating androgens are produced by the gonads and the adrenal gland. Androgens can also be produced locally within the sebaceous gland from the adrenal precursor hormone, DHEAS. The main androgens that interact with the androgen receptor are testosterone and DHT. Androgen receptors are found in the basal layer of the sebaceous gland and the outer root sheath keratinocytes of the hair follicle (1,2). DHT is approximately five to 10 times more potent than testosterone in its interaction with the androgen receptor.

An essential role for androgens in stimulating sebum production is supported by several lines of evidence. For example, the development of acne in the prepubertal period has been associated with elevated serum levels of DHEAS, a precursor for testosterone (3,4). Androgen-insensitive subjects who lack functional androgen receptors do not produce sebum and do not develop acne (5). Tumors of the ovary or the adrenal that produce androgens are often associated with the development of acne. Systemic administration of testosterone and dehydroepiandrosterone increases the size and secretion of sebaceous glands (6), and we know that severe acne is often associated with elevated serum androgens (7,8).

Androgen Metabolism Within the Skin

Acne may be mediated by serum androgens, locally produced androgens, or a combination of both. Insights have been gained regarding the local metabolism of androgens within sebaceous glands (9). Such insights may be of benefit in the design of new acne therapies. The skin and sebaceous gland are capable of producing and metabolizing androgens (9). DHEAS is the major adrenal androgen precursor. It circulates in the blood stream in relatively high levels compared with other hormones with the exception of cortisol. In fact, in for review, see Ref. postmenopausal women, all sex steroids made in the skin are from adrenal steroid precursors, especially DHEA. Secretion of this precursor steroid by the adrenals decreases progressively from age 30 to less than 50% of its maximal value at age 60 (10). The enzyme 3β-hydroxysteroid dehydrogenase (3β-HSD) acts on DHEA to convert it to androstenedione (Fig. 1). This conversion may take place in the adrenal gland and tissues such as the sebaceous gland, where activity of the 3β-HSD enzyme has been identified by several investigators (11–13). The reversible conversion of androstenedione into testosterone is then catalyzed in the human skin by 17β-HSD, a member of the short chain alcohol dehydrogenases that are related to retinol metabolizing enzymes (14–18). This is a reversible enzyme that can oxidize and reduce both androgens and estrogens. It is responsible for converting the weak androgen androstenedione into the more potent androgen testosterone. It can also interconvert weak and potent estrogens such as estrone and estradiol. The 17β-HSD enzyme may represent a regulatory point in androgen and estrogen metabolism within the skin.

DHT is produced from testosterone within peripheral tissues such as the skin by the action of the 5α-reductase enzyme. Two isozymes of 5α-reductase have been identified (19). The type 1 isozyme is active within the sebaceous gland (20,21). The type 2 isozyme is most active in the prostate gland, where it can be inhibited by drugs such as finasteride. Activity of 5α-reductase and 17β-HSD exhibits regional differences depending upon the source of the sebaceous glands (9). In skin that is prone to acne, such as facial skin, activity of the type 1 5α-reductase in sebaceous glands is greater than in sebaceous glands obtained from nonacne-prone skin (20). This implies that more DHT is being produced in sebaceous glands from facial skin compared with other areas of the body that are not prone to develop acne. The net effect of the activity of these two enzymes is the greater production of potent androgens such as testosterone and DHT within sebaceous glands of facial areas, which may in part account for the development of acne in these areas.

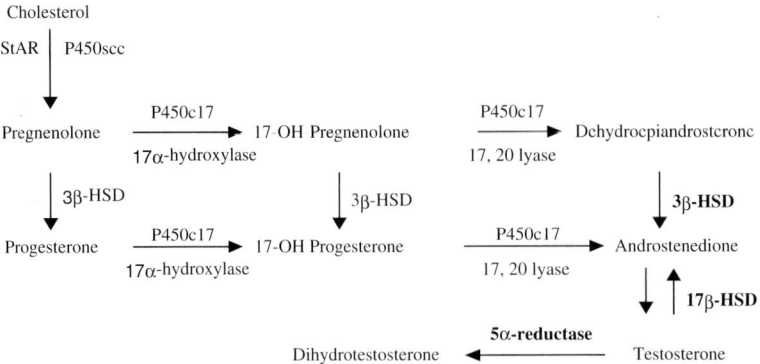

FIGURE 1 The steroidogenic pathway. *Abbreviations*: HSD, hydroxysteroid dehydrogenase; P450scc, P450 side chain cleavage enzyme; StAR, steroidogenic acute regulatory protein.

The Sebaceous Gland Is a Steroidogenic Tissue

The skin and sebaceous glands are capable of synthesizing cholesterol de novo from acetate (22–24). Although this cholesterol is utilized in cell membranes, in the formation of the epidermal barrier, and is secreted in sebum, its use as a substrate for steroid hormone synthesis had not been established until recently. In order for steroid synthesis to occur, cholesterol needs to be translocated from the outer to the inner mitochondrial membrane. This process is regulated by the steroidogenic acute regulatory protein (25). Additional enzymes and cofactors needed to convert cholesterol into a steroid include P450 cholesterol side chain cleavage, adrenodoxin reductase, cytochrome P450c17, and steroidogenic factor-1. Expression of each of these proteins was found in human facial skin, sebocytes, and in a recently developed simian virus (SV) 40-immortalized human sebocyte cell line (SEB-1) (26). These data demonstrate that the skin is in fact a steroidogenic tissue. The clinical significance of this finding in mediating androgenic skin disorders such as acne, hirsutism, or androgenetic alopecia remains to be established.

ESTROGENS IN ACNE

Very little is known about the role of estrogens in modulating sebum production. Any estrogen given systemically in sufficient amounts will decrease sebum production. The dose of estrogen required to suppress sebum production, however, is greater than the dose required to suppress ovulation (27). The major active estrogen is estradiol, which is produced from testosterone by the action of the enzyme aromatase. Aromatase is active in the ovary, adipose tissue, and other peripheral tissues. Estradiol can be converted to the less potent estrogen, estrone, by the action of the 17β-HSD enzyme. Both aromatase and 17β-HSD are present in the skin (17,28). Estrogens may act by several mechanisms; they may: (*i*) directly oppose the effects of androgens locally within the sebaceous gland, (*ii*) inhibit the production of androgens by gonadal tissue via a negative feedback loop on pituitary gonadotrophin release, and (*iii*) regulate genes that negatively influence sebaceous gland growth or lipid production.

GROWTH HORMONE AND INSULIN-LIKE GROWTH FACTORS IN ACNE

Growth hormone is secreted by the pituitary gland. It acts on the liver and peripheral tissues to stimulate the production of IGFs, formerly known as somatomedians. There are two forms of IGF, termed IGF-1 and IGF-2. IGF-1 is the more prevalent growth factor. It has been hypothesized that growth hormone may be involved in the development of acne (29). Acne is most prevalent in adolescents during a time when growth hormone is maximally secreted and serum levels of IGF-1 are highest. In addition, IGF-1 can be produced locally within the skin, where it can interact with receptors on the sebaceous gland to stimulate its growth. Furthermore, conditions of growth hormone excess such as acromegaly are associated with seborrhea and the development of acne. In some tissues, the actions of IGF-1 can be mediated by androgens. It is possible that androgens may influence IGF-1 action in the sebaceous gland as well.

CLINICAL PRESENTATION OF ADULT FEMALE ACNE

For reasons that are not understood, the distribution of facial acne in many adult females differs from that seen in adolescents and in males. Many adult women note that acne localizes to the lateral face, chin, and neck (Fig. 2). Oftentimes, acne in these women is not necessarily widespread or severe, but rather it may be low-grade, persistent, and consist of a few isolated deep-seated tender nodules.

Many women note flares of their acne just prior to their menstrual period with reports ranging from 27–60% to 70% of women (30–32). One study has been published that provides quantitative documentation of acne lesion counts over the menstrual period (33). In this study of women, who were followed over two menstrual cycles, 63% showed a 25% increase in inflammatory acne lesions prior to the menstrual period. Some women may feel that intermittent acne therapy prior to their menstrual period may be beneficial. There is no evidence for this approach. Since most acne therapy is designed to prevent the formation of lesions and since this process often takes several weeks, it seems unlikely that intermittent therapy would be beneficial. For this reason, it is important to have patients use their medications consistently and to avoid spot treatment.

WHEN TO SUSPECT AN ENDOCRINE DISORDER IN ACNE PATIENTS

Although hormones influence acne, most acne patients do not have an endocrine disorder. Hyperandrogenism should be considered in female patients whose acne is severe, sudden in its onset, or is associated with hirsutism, or irregular menstrual periods. Additional clinical signs of hyperandrogenism include Cushinoid features, increased libido, clitoromegaly, deepening of the voice, acanthosis nigricans, or androgenetic alopecia. Women with hyperandrogenism may also have insulin resistance. They are at risk for the development of diabetes and cardiovascular disease. It is therefore important for the long-term health of these patients to identify hyperandrogenism so that they can receive appropriate therapy from an endocrinologist or gynecologist.

SCREENING FOR AN ENDOCRINE DISORDER

A medical history and physical examination should be performed that is directed toward eliciting any symptoms or signs of hyperandrogenism. Screening laboratory tests for hyperandrogenism include a serum DHEAS, total testosterone, free testosterone, and luteinizing hormone/follicle-stimulating hormone (LH/FSH) ratio. These tests should be obtained apart from the time of ovulation in order to avoid the surge of hormones associated with ovulation. From a practical standpoint, it may be easiest to suggest that women have these tests performed either just prior to or during the menstrual period. It is important to note that if a patient is on oral contraceptives at the time of hormonal testing, an underlying hyperandrogenemia may be masked. This does not occur with antiandrogens such as cyproterone or spironolactone. Therefore, it is best that patients discontinue oral contraceptives four to six weeks prior to the endocrine evaluation.

Excess androgens may be produced by either the adrenal gland or the ovary. Serum levels of DHEAS can be used to screen for an adrenal source of excess androgen production. Patients with a serum DHEAS greater than 8000 ng/mL (units may differ depending upon the laboratory) may have an adrenal tumor and should be referred to an endocrinologist for further evaluation. Some adrenal tumors may also produce testosterone. Values of DHEAS in the range of 4000 ng/mL to 8000 ng/mL may be associated with congenital adrenal hyperplasia, which is most commonly due to a partial deficiency in the 21-hydroxylase or 11-hydroxylase enzyme in the adrenal gland.

Such an enzyme deficiency results in the shunting of steroids from the cortisol biosynthetic pathway into the androgen biosynthetic pathway.

An ovarian source of excess androgens can be suspected in cases where the serum total testosterone is elevated. Serum total testosterone in the range of 150 ng/dL to 200 ng/dL or an increased LH/FSH ratio (greater than 2 to 3) can be found in cases of polycystic ovary disease. This condition is a spectrum and is often, but not always, associated with irregular menstrual periods, reduced fertility, obesity, insulin resistance, or hirsutism. Greater elevations in serum testosterone may indicate an ovarian tumor and appropriate referral should be made. In some cases, there can be modest elevations in both DHEAS and testosterone. A serum level of 17-hydroxypregneneolone can be obtained to discern between an ovarian or adrenal source of androgens. If 17-hydroxypregneneolone is elevated, it indicates an adrenal source of excess androgens, most often secondary to late onset congenital adrenal hyperplasia. Of note is that there is a significant amount of variation in an individual's serum androgen levels. In cases where abnormal results are obtained, it is recommended to repeat the test before proceeding with therapy or a more extensive work-up.

Questions arise as to the importance of a pelvic ultrasound in the diagnosis of polycystic ovarian syndrome. This test can be nonspecific, in that women with normal androgens may have ovarian cysts and conversely, women with hyperandrogenism and other findings associated with polycystic ovarian syndrome may not have ovarian cysts at the time of pelvic ultrasound. For this reason, the diagnosis of polycystic ovarian syndrome is more heavily based upon the serum hormonal profile and associated clinical findings.

In the majority of women with acne, serum androgens are completely normal, yet these women will in fact respond if treated with hormonal therapy. Studies have shown that, as a group, women with acne may have higher levels of serum DHEAS, testosterone, and DHT than those without acne (7,34). However, although higher, these laboratory values may still be within the normal range. Serum levels of DHEAS, DHT, and IGF-1 are reported to correlate positively with acne lesion counts in women, whereas androstenedione and DHEAS correlate with lesion counts in men (35). Reduction of serum androgens or inhibition of their action, as obtained with oral contraceptives or antiandrogens, respectively, can lead to improvement in acne in women with normal serum androgen levels.

OPTIONS FOR THE HORMONAL THERAPY OF ACNE IN WOMEN

Once the decision has been made to initiate hormonal therapy, the various options to choose from include: (*i*) androgen receptor blockers, or antiandrogens (this class of drugs block the effect of androgens on the sebaceous gland); (*ii*) inhibitors of androgen production by the ovary or adrenal gland such as oral contraceptives or glucocorticosteroids, respectively; or (*iii*) in the future, it may be possible to inhibit the activity of androgen metabolizing enzymes in the skin or sebaceous gland itself.

Agents that Block the Androgen Receptor

Within the class of androgen receptor blockers, therapeutic options include spironolactone, cyproterone acetate, and flutamide. In the United States, spironolactone is the most commonly used drug, although flutamide is also available.

Spironolactone

Oral spironolactone decreases sebum excretion rate by 30% to 50%. Recommended doses are 50 to 100 mg taken with meals (36,37). However, many women with sporadic outbreaks of inflammatory lesions or isolated cysts respond well to 25 mg twice daily and some even respond to just 25 mg a day. These low doses in healthy young women are generally well-tolerated. However, if this drug is used in older women who may have other medical problems, or if higher doses are used for conditions such as hirsutism or androgenetic alopecia, serum electrolytes should be monitored. Side effects of spironolactone include breast tenderness and menstrual irregularities. Additionally, it is important that pregnancy be avoided during treatment with spironolactone due to the potential for abnormalities of the male fetal genitalia such as hypospadias.

Cyproterone Acetate

Cyproterone acetate is available in many parts of the world, but not in the United States. It possesses dual activity in that it serves as a progestogen in oral contraceptives in addition to its direct inhibition of the androgen receptor. It can be given in doses of 2 to 100 mg per day as a single agent, in which case there can be improvement in 75% to 90% of women with acne. Cyproterone acetate, however, is most commonly used in the form of an oral contraceptive combined with ethinyl estradiol in varying doses (38). Numerous clinical studies support the efficacy of these oral contraceptive preparations in women with acne.

Flutamide

Flutamide is a potent nonsteroidal antagonist of the androgen receptor. Although most commonly used to treat prostate cancer, flutamide has been reported to be efficacious in the treatment of acne, hirsutism, and androgenic alopecia (39). It can be given in doses of 250 mg twice daily in combination with an oral contraceptive. Fatal hepatitis has been reported with this drug. Liver function tests should be monitored and serious consideration should be given to the risk/benefit ratio of its use in acne (40). Additionally, because it is an antiandrogen, pregnancy issues are a concern.

Inhibitors of Adrenal Androgen Production

Another option in hormone therapy is to block the production of androgens either by the adrenal gland or ovary, which can be accomplished through the use of low-dose glucocorticoids or oral contraceptives, respectively.

Glucocorticoids

Low-dose glucocorticoids are most commonly used to treat patients with late onset congenital adrenal hyperplasia, which is an inherent defect in the 21-hydroxylase or the 11-hydroxylase enzyme. This defect causes a block in the cortisol biosynthetic pathway, which results in a buildup of steroid precursors that are shunted into the androgen biosynthetic pathway. Low-dose prednisone (2.5 to 5 mg a day, at bedtime) can be used. Low doses of dexamethasone can also be used, but the risk of adrenal suppression is higher. To ascertain if therapy with glucocorticoids is having the desired effect, serum DHEAS can be monitored for a decrease or normalization of the level of DHEAS. To check for adrenal suppression, an adrenocorticotrophin hormone (ACTH) simulation test can be performed. This consists of injecting

ACTH and assessing the plasma cortisol 30 minutes later. If plasma cortisol has risen by an appropriate amount, the adrenal gland is not suppressed.

Inhibition of Ovarian Androgen Production
Gonadotropin-Releasing Agonists
Androgen production in the ovary can also be blocked by gonadotropin-releasing hormone agonists such as buserelin, nafarelin, or leuprolide. These gonadotropin-releasing agonists block ovulation by interrupting the cyclic release of FSH and LH from the pituitary. These drugs are efficacious in acne and hirsutism, and are available as injectable drugs or nasal spray. However, in addition to suppressing the production of ovarian androgens, these drugs also suppress the ovarian production of estrogens, thereby eliminating the function of the ovary. Thus, the patient could develop menopausal symptoms and suffer from hypoestrogenism. Headaches can also develop, as well as the occurrence of bone loss, due to the reduction in estrogen.

Oral Contraceptives
Oral contraceptives generally contain an estrogen (most commonly ethinyl estradiol) and a progestin. In their early formulations, oral contraceptives contained over 100 μg of estrogen. In these and higher doses, estrogens themselves can suppress sebum production. Estrogens also act on the liver to increase the synthesis of sex hormone-binding globulin that binds testosterone and lowers the circulating levels of free testosterone. In addition, oral contraceptives inhibit the ovarian production of androgens by suppressing ovulation. This, in turn, decreases serum androgen levels and reduces sebum production. The concentrations of estrogen in oral contraceptives have decreased over the years from 150 to 35 μg, and in the most recent forms, to 20 μg, in order to reduce the side effects associated with estrogen (41). Oral contraceptives containing low doses of estrogen are listed in Table 1.

Progestins
The progestins contained in oral contraceptives include estranges and gonanes, which are derivatives of 19-nortestosterone, cyprotereone acetate, and a novel progestin, drosperinone. Members of the estrane and gonane class of progestins (Table 2) can cross-react with the androgen receptor, which can lead to increased androgenic effects and could aggravate acne, hirsutism, or androgenic alopecia. These progestins can also cause changes in lipid metabolism and can increase serum glucose, leading to glucose intolerance, as well as possibly interfering with the beneficial effect of estrogen on the sex hormone-binding globulin. However, the third generation progestins, including norgestimate, desogestrel, and gestodene, are more selective for the progesterone receptor rather than the androgen receptor. The biological relevance of these differences, however, is uncertain. For

TABLE 1   Oral Contraceptives Containing Low Doses of Estrogen

Ethinyl estradiol 20 μg/Levonorgestrel 0.1 mg (Alesse™)
Ethinyl estradiol 20, 10 μg/Desogestrel 0.15 mg (Mircette™)
Ethinyl estradiol 20, 30, 35 μg/norethindrone 1.0 mg (Estrostep®)
Ethinyl estradiol 20 μg/norethindrone acetate 1.0 mg (Lo-Estrin® 1/20)
Ethinyl estradiol 20 μg/drospirenone 3.0 mg (Yaz™)

TABLE 2   Progestins: 19-Nortestosterone Derivatives

Estranes	Gonanes
Norethindrone	Norgestrel
Norethindrone acetate	Levonorgestrel
Ethynodiol diacetate	Desogestrel
	Gestodene
	Norgestimate

years, it has been known that almost all oral contraceptives are beneficial in the treatment of acne (42). It is possible that some women are more sensitive to the androgenic effects of a progestin, but it is more likely that the effect of progestin may be offset by estrogen. All oral contraceptives, regardless of the type of progestin, will inhibit serum androgen levels. Moreover, although some progestins might be more androgenic than others, there is an increase in sex hormone-binding globulin with the use of any oral contraceptives and an improvement of the acne in women who are treated with them.

Drospirenone is a novel progestin that is derived from 17α-spironolactone. It possesses antiandrogenic and antimineralocorticoid activity, which can be of benefit in androgenic-related conditions such as acne and hirsutism and in the estrogen-related fluid retention associated with some oral contraceptives (43).

ORAL CONTRACEPTIVES STUDIED IN ACNE

Many oral contraceptives have been studied in the treatment of acne (Table 3). These include those containing ethinyl estradiol in combination with cyproterone acetate (Diane, Dianette), ethynodiol diacetate (Demulen), levonorgestrel (TriPhasil, Alesse), norgestimate (Ortho Tri-Cyclen®), desogesterel (Desogen), and drosperinone (Yasmin, Yaz). Numerous studies point to the efficacy of ethinyl estradiol/cyproterone acetate oral contraceptives (Diane and Dianette) in the treatment of acne. Reductions in inflammatory lesion count on the order of 50% to 75% have been reported (44,45). Two large studies involving a total of approximately 500 women with moderate acne were conducted with ethinyl estradiol 35 µg/norgestimate (Ortho Tri-Cyclen). Improvement in inflammatory lesions, total lesions, and global assessment was noted with this oral contraceptive after six months of treatment (46,47). There was a 50% to 60% improvement in inflammatory lesions. Decreases in serum free testosterone and an increase in sex hormone-binding globulin were noted in the active group. Two large, six-month, placebo-controlled trials (350 and 371 women, respectively) were conducted

TABLE 3   Oral Contraceptives Studied in Acne

Demulen (ethinyl estradiol 35 µg/ethynodiol diacetate)
Diane, Dianette (ethinyl estradiol 50, 35 µg/cyproterone acetate)
Estrostep (ethinyl estradiol 20, 25, 30 µg/norethindrone)
Alesse (ethinyl estradiol 20 µg/levonorgestrel)
Ortho Tri-Cyclen (ethinyl estradiol 35 µg/norgestimate)
Desogen (ethinyl estradiol 30 µg/desogestrel)
Yasmin (ethinyl estradiol 30 µg/drospirenone)
Yaz (ethinyl estradiol 20 µg/drospirenone)
Triphasil (ethinyl estradiol 30 µg, 40 µg/levonorgestrel)

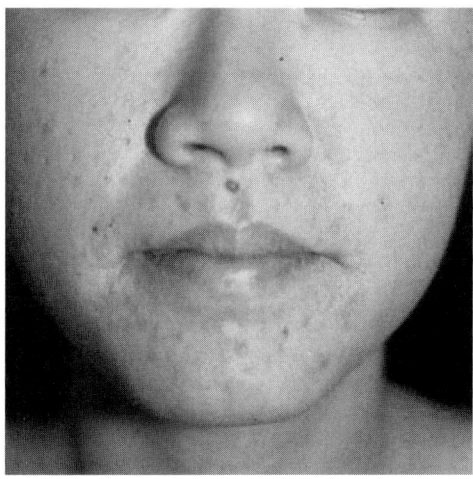

FIGURE 2   (*See color insert.*) Adult female with acne of the lower face.

using ethinyl estradiol 20 µg/levonorgestrel (Alesse) in the treatment of acne (48,49). In each study, the oral contraceptive demonstrated significantly greater reduction in acne lesion counts and improvement in global assessment scores compared with placebo. The reduction in inflammatory lesion count was on the order of 47%. A study of 128 women with mild-to-moderate acne compared the efficacy of ethinyl estradiol 30 µg/drospirenone (Yasmin) and ethinyl estradiol 35 µg/cyproterone acetate (Diane-35) in the treatment of acne for nine cycles (50). Both treatments produced comparable reductions in acne lesion counts, with an approximate 60% reduction in inflammatory lesion count. Both treatments also reduced sebum production and yielded comparable increases in sex hormone-binding globulin. Two large placebo-controlled studies involving a total of approximately 593 women with moderate acne, found improvement in inflammatory lesions, total lesions, global assessment, and quality of life in women who were treated for six months with a triphasic oral contraceptive that contains doses of 20 to 35 µg of ethinyl estradiol in combination with 1.0 mg norethindrone acetate (Estrostep) (51). In these studies, inflammatory lesion counts were reduced by approximately 47% (51).

Oral contraceptives that have been approved for the treatment of acne in the United States include ethinyl estradiol 35 µg/norgestimate (Ortho Tri-Cyclen) ethinyl estradiol 20 to 35 µg/norethindrone acetate (Estrostep), and ethinyl estradiol 20 µg/drospirenone (Yaz).

ORAL CONTRACEPTIVES AND ANTIBIOTICS

The concern regarding oral contraceptives and antibiotics is essentially theoretical, owing to the action of broad-spectrum antibiotics, which reduce the gut flora bacteria and thus may result in decreased absorption of estrogen. This could lead to a possible reduction in the efficacy of oral contraceptives, although pharmacokinetic studies suggest that serum levels of estrogen are unaffected by antibiotics such as tetracycline, doxycycline, and others (52,53). Nevertheless, there have been very few reports in the literature of pregnancies associated with the use of antibiotics in conjunction with oral contraceptives (54,55). Existing reports have focused on tetracycline, and the incidence was 1.2 to 1.4 pregnancies/100 woman years of use of the oral contraceptive. These data are no greater than the background failure rate of oral contraceptives (54,55).

NEWER FORMS OF CONTRACEPTIVES

Recently, newer forms of contraceptives have been developed, such as contraceptive patches, vaginal rings, and injectable combination hormones. Each of these is designed to suppress ovulation and in this regard will lower the ovarian production of androgens. As of yet, these formulations have not been studied in the treatment of acne. The contraceptive patch (Ortho Evra) contains 20 μg of ethinyl estradiol and 150 μg of the progestin, norelgestromin. The patch is worn for three weeks and removed for one week, during which time menstrual bleeding will occur. The advantages of this formulation are better patient compliance, dosing that is not affected by gastrointestinal disturbances, and more consistent serum levels of estrogen serum levels compared to oral dosing (56). The vaginal ring (NuvaRing) is a contraceptive vaginal ring that releases 15 μg of ethinyl estradiol and 120 μg of the progestin, etonogestrel. It is placed within the vagina for three weeks and removed for one week. In one study, the incidence of irregular bleeding was less compared with an oral combination contraceptive (57). An injectable combination of estradiol cypionate and medroxyprogesterone acetate (Lunelle) has been developed. This is given as a monthly contraceptive injection. Contraceptive efficacy was shown to be comparable to a triphasic oral contraceptive containing ethinyl estradiol and norethindrone (Ortho 7/7/7) (58).

APPROACH TO HORMONAL THERAPY IN FEMALE ACNE

Hormonal therapy is an excellent option for treatment of women whose acne is not responding to conventional therapy. If there are signs of hyperandrogenism, an endocrine evaluation is indicated, consisting of tests such as DHEAS, total- and free-testosterone, and an LH/FSH ratio. Although hyperandrogenism is an indication for hormonal therapy, women with normal serum androgen levels also respond well to treatment. The mainstays of hormonal therapy include oral contraceptives and spironolactone. Other agents to choose from include cyproterone acetate, flutamide, and glucocorticoids. Hormonal agents work best as part of a combination regimen including topical retinoids or topical or oral antibiotics depending upon the severity of the acne. In some women, the additional of hormonal therapy has improved acne to the point where subsequent treatment with isotretinoin was no longer necessary. As more is learned about the hormones involved in acne, their source of production and the mechanisms by which they influence sebaceous gland growth and sebum production, new opportunities will arise for the development of novel therapies aimed at the hormonal aspects of acne.

REFERENCES

1. Choudhry R, Hodgins M, Van der Kwast T, et al. Localization of androgen receptors in human skin by immunohistochemistry: implications for the hormonal regulation of hair growth, sebaceous glands and sweat glands. J Endocrinol 1991; 133:467–475.

2. Liang T, Hoyer S, Yu R. Immunocytochemical localization of androgen receptors in human skin using monoclonal antibodies against the androgen receptor. J Invest Dermatol 1993; 100:663–666.
3. Lucky AW, Biro FM, Huster GA, et al. Acne vulgaris in premenarchal girls. Arch Dermatol 1994; 130:308–314.
4. Stewart ME, Downing DT, Cook JS, et al. Sebaceous gland activity and serum dehydroepiandrosterone sulfate levels in boys and girls. Arch Dermatol 1992; 128:1345–1348.
5. Imperato-McGinley J, Gautier T, Cai LQ, et al. The androgen control of sebum production. Studies of subjects with dihydrotestosterone deficiency and complete androgen insensitivity. J Clin Endocrinol Metab 1993; 76(2):524–528.
6. Pochi PE, Strauss JS. Sebaceous gland response in man to the administration of testosterone, Δ4- androstenedione, and dehydroisoandrosterone. J Invest Dermatol 1969; 52:32–36.
7. Marynick SP, Chakmajian ZH, McCaffree DL, et al. Androgen excess in cystic acne. N Engl J Med 1983; 308:981–986.
8. Lucky A, McGuire J, Rosenfield R, et al. Plasma androgens in women with acne vulgaris. J Invest Dermatol 1983; 81:70.
9. Chen W, Thiboutot D, Zouboulis C. Cutaneous androgen metabolism: basic research and clinical perspectives. J Invest Dermatol 2002; 119:992–1007.
10. Labrie F, Luu-The V, Pelletier G, et al. Intracrinology and the skin. Horm Res 2000; 54:213–229.
11. Baillie A, Calman K, Milne J. Histochemical distribution of hydroxysteroid dehydrogenases in human skin. Br J Dermatol 1965; 7:610–616.
12. Sawaya ME, Honig JLS, Garland LD, et al. Δ5-3β-Hydroxysteroid dehydrogenase activity in sebaceous glands of scalp in male-pattern baldness. J Invest Dermatol 1988; 91:101–105.
13. Simpson NB, Cunliffe WJ, Hodgins MB. The relationship between the in vitro activity of 3β-hydroxysteroid dehydrogenase delta$^{4-5}$-isomerase in human sebaceous glands and their secretory activity in vivo. J Invest Dermatol 1983; 81(2):139–144.
14. Mason J. The 3β-hydroxysteroid dehydrogenase gene family of enzymes. TEM 1993; 4:199–202.
15. Chai Z, Brereton P, Suzuki T, et al. 17β-hydroxysteroid dehydrogenase type 11 localizes to human steroidogenic cells. Endocrinology 2003; 144:2084–2091.
16. Andersson S, Moghrabi N. Physiology and molecular genetics of 17ß-hydroxysteroid dehydrogenases. Steroids 1997; 62:143–147.
17. Hay JB, Hodgins MB, Donnelly JB. Human skin androgen metabolism and preliminary evidence for its control by two forms of 17 ß-hydroxysteroid oxidoreductase. J Endocrinol 1982; 93(3):403–413.
18. Thiboutot D, Martin P, Volikos L, et al. Oxidative activity of the type 2 isozyme of 17β-hydroxysteroid dehydrogenase (17β-HSD) predominates in human sebaceous glands. J Invest Dermatol 1998; 111:390–395.
19. Jenkins EP, Andersson S, Imperato-McGinley J, et al. Genetic and pharmacological evidence for more than one human steroid 5α- reductase. J Clin Invest 1992; 89:293–300.
20. Thiboutot D, Harris G, Iles V, et al. Activity of the type 1 5α-reductase exhibits regional differences in isolated sebaceous glands and whole skin. J Invest Dermatol 1995; 105(2):209–214.
21. Zouboulis C, Fritsch M, Seltmann H, et al. Allocated activity of androgen-metabolizing enzymes in human sebocytes and keratinocytes *in vitro*. J Invest Dermatol 2000; 114:796.
22. Cassidy D, Lee C, Laker M, et al. Lipogenesis in isolated human sebaceous glands. FEBS Lett 1986; 200:173–176.
23. Proksch E, Feingold KR, Elias PM. Epidermal HMG CoA reductase activity in essential fatty acid deficiency: barrier requirements rather than eicosanoid generation regulate cholesterol synthesis. J Invest Dermatol 1992; 99(2):216–220.
24. Smythe C, Greenall M, Kealey T. The activity of HMG-CoA reductase and acetyl- CoA carboxylase in human apocrine sweat glands, sebaceous glands and hair follicles is regulated by phosphorylation and by exogenous cholesterol. J Invest Dermatol 1998; 111:139–148.

25. Sugawara T, Lin D, Holt JA, et al. Structure of the human steroidogenic acute regulatory protein (StAR) gene: StAR stimulates mitochondrial cholesterol 27-hydroxylase activity. Biochemistry 1995; 34(39):12506–12512.
26. Thiboutot D, Jabara S, McAllister J, et al. Human skin is a steroidogenic tissue: steroidogenic enzymes and cofactors are expressed in epidermis, normal sebocytes, and an immortalized sebocyte cell line (SEB-1). J Invest Dermatol 2003; 120:905–914.
27. Strauss J, Kligman A. Effect of cyclic progestin-estrogen therapy on sebum and acne in women. JAMA 1964; 190:815.
28. Sawaya ME, Price VH. Different levels of 5α-reductase type I and II, aromatase, and androgen receptor in hair follicles of women and men with androgenetic alopecia. J Invest Dermatol 1997; 109:296–300.
29. Deplewski D, Rosenfield RL. Growth hormone and insulin-like growth factors have different effects on sebaceous cell growth and differentiation. Endocrinology 1999; 140(9):4089–4094.
30. Williams M, Cunliffe W. Explanation for pre-menstrual acne. Lancet 1972; 10:1055–1057.
31. Shaw JC. Low-dose adjunctive spironolactone in the treatment of acne in women: a retrospective analysis of 85 consecutively treated patients. J Am Acad Dermatol 2000; 43:498–503.
32. Stoll S, Shalita AR, Webster GF, Kaplan R, Danesh S, Penstein A. The effect of menstrual cycle on acne. J Am Acad Dermatol 2001; 45:957–960.
33. Lucky AW. Quantitative documentation of a premenstrual flare of facial acne in adult women. Arch Dermatol 2004; 140:423–424.
34. Thiboutot D, Gilliland K, Light J, et al. Androgen metabolism in sebaceous glands from subjects with and without acne [see comments]. Arch Dermatol 1999; 135(9):1041–1045.
35. Cappel M, Mauger D, Thiboutot D. Correlation between serum levels of insulin-like growth factor 1, dehydroepiandrosterone sulfate and dihydrotestosterone and acne lesion counts in adult women. Arch Dermatol 2005; 141:333–338.
36. Shaw J. Spironolactone in dermatologic therapy. J Am Acad Dermatol 1991; 24:236–243.
37. Lubbos HG, Hasinski S, Rose LI, et al. Adverse effects of spironolactone therapy in women with acne [letter]. Arch Dermatol 1998; 134(9):1162–1163.
38. Stewart ME, Greenwood R, Cunliffe WJ, et al. Effect of cyproterone acetate-ethinyl estradiol treatment on the proportions of linoleic and sebaleic acids in various skin surface lipid classes. Arch Dermatol Res 1986; 278(6):481–485.
39. Dodin S, Faure N, Cedrin I, et al. Clinical efficacy and safety of low-dose flutamide alone and combined with an oral contraceptive for the treatment of idiopathic hirsutism. Clin Endocrinol 1995; 43:575–582.
40. Wysowski D, Freiman J, Tourtelot J, et al. Fatal and nonfatal hepatotoxicity associated with flutamide. Ann Intern Med 1993; 118:860–864.
41. Thorneycroft IH, Stanczyk FZ, Bradshaw KD, et al. Effect of low-dose oral contraceptives on androgenic markers and acne. Contraception 1999; 60(5):255–262.
42. Leyden JJ. Therapy for acne vulgaris. N Engl J Med 1997; 336(16):1156–1162.
43. Thorneycroft I. Evolution of progestins. Focus on the novel progestin drospirenone. J Reprod Med 2002; 47(11 suppl):975–980.
44. van Vloten W, van Haselen C, van Zuuren E, et al. The effect of 2 combined oral contraceptives containing either drospirenone or cyproterone acetate on acne and seborrhea. Cutis 2002; 69(4 suppl):2–15.
45. Greenwood R, Brummitt L, Burke B, et al. Acne: double blind clinical and laboratory trial of tetracycline, oestrogen-cyproterone acetate, and combined treatment. Br Med J 1985; 291:1231–1235.
46. Lemay A, Dewailly SD, Grenier R, et al. Attenuation of mild hyperandrogenic activity in postpubertal acne by a triphasic oral contraceptive containing low doses of ethynyl estradiol and d,l-norgestrel. J Clin Endocrinol Metab 1990; 71(1):8–14.
47. Lucky A, Henderson T, Olson W, et al. Effectiveness of norgestimate and ethinyl estradiol in treating moderate acne vulgaris. J Am Acad Dermatol 1997; 37:746–754.

48. Redmond GP, Olson WH, Lippman JS, et al. Norgestimate and ethinyl estradiol in the treatment of acne vulgaris: a randomized, placebo-controlled trial. Obstet Gynecol 1997; 89:615–622.
49. Thiboutot D, Archer D, Lemay A, et al. A randomized, controlled trial of a low-dose contraceptive containing 20 mg of ethinylestradiol and 100 mg of levonorgestrel for acne treatment. Fertil Steril 2001; 76:461–468.
50. Leyden J, Shalita A, Hordinsky M, et al. Efficacy of a low-dose oral contraceptive containing 20 mg of ethinyl estradiol and 100 mg of levonorgestrel for the treatment of moderate acne: a randomized, placebo-controlled trial. J Am Acad Dermatol 2002; 47:399–409.
51. Maloney M, Arbit D, Flack M, et al. Use of a low-dose oral contraceptive containing norethindrone acetate and ethinyl estradiol in the treatment of moderate acne vulgaris. Clin J Women's Health 2001; 1:124–131.
52. Archer J, Archer D. Oral contraceptive efficacy and antibiotic interaction: a myth debunked. J Am Acad Dermatol 2002; 46:917–923.
53. Weaver K, Glasier A. Interaction between broad-spectrum antibiotics and the combined oral contraceptive pill. A literature review. Contraception 1999; 59:71–78.
54. Helms SE, Bredle DL, Zajic J, et al. Oral contraceptive failure rates and oral antibiotics. J Am Acad Dermatol 1997; 36(5 Pt 1):705–710.
55. London BM, Lookingbill DP. Frequency of pregnancy in acne patients taking oral antibiotics and oral contraceptives [letter]. Arch Dermatol 1994; 130(3):392–393.
56. Dittrich R, Parker L, Rosen J, et al. Transdermal contraception: Evaluation of three transdermal norelgestromin/ethinyl estradiol doses in a randomized, multicenter, dose-response study. Am J Obstet Gynecol 2002; 186:15–20.
57. Bjarnadottir R, Tuppurainen M, Killick S. Comparison of cycle control with a combined contraceptive vaginal ring and oral levonorgestrel/ethinyl estradiol. Am J Obstet Gynecol 2002; 186:389–395.
58. Kaunitz AM, Garceau R, Cromie M. Comparative safety, efficacy, and cycle control of Lunelle monthly contraceptive injection (medroxyprogesterone acetate and estradiol cypionate injectable suspension) and Ortho Novum 7/7/7 oral contraceptive (norethindrone/ethinyl estradiol triphasic). Lunelle Study Group. Contraception 1999; 60:179–187.

Antimicrobial Therapy in Acne

Guy F. Webster

Jefferson Medical College of Thomas Jefferson University, Philadelphia, Pennsylvania, U.S.A.

INTRODUCTION

Antibiotic therapy in acne is a time-honored practice whose mechanism is only recently thoroughly understood. Initially, it was assumed that the reduction in *Propionibacterium acnes* was the sole mechanism of antibiotic efficacy in acne, but it is now understood that certain antibiotic drugs are also potent anti-inflammatory agents via nonantibiotic mechanisms. In addition, the induction of resistance has made antibiotic therapy problematic in many patients.

BENZOYL PEROXIDE

Benzoyl peroxide (BP) is a topical disinfectant that was originally used as a peeling agent for acne. Its mechanism of action is through lowering *P. acnes* populations by oxidative killing, and the drug is extremely effective as a topical agent. When applied to the skin, BP breaks down into benzoic acid and hydrogen peroxide (1,2). It assumed that the peroxide accounts for the majority of bactericidal activity, but no studies have been performed to assess the activity of benzoic acid in acne.

The major side effect of BP is irritation, which usually is easily managed with moisturizers. However, BP has been reported as a contact sensitizer in as many as 4% of patients and can reach nearly 75% when applied to leg ulcers (3), but in clinical acne practice actual contact allergy is rarely noted. As a heavy prescriber of the drug, I see, at most, a case every few years.

Various concentrations of BP are available, but there is no convincing data to prove that high concentrations are more effective than lower ones. *P. acnes* reduction is as effective by 2.5% as 10% BP (4), and one small study shows therapeutic equivalence between 2.5%, 5%, and 10% BP gels and a lower rate of irritation with 2.5% than the higher concentrations (5). BP washes are useful in particular for trunk acne since they can cover a large area easily, but in the past have been of fairly low potency. Newer formulations have been designed to have greater substantivity and are capable of *P. acnes* reductions near that of traditional gels and creams. As a single agent, BP is superior to clindamycin (6). Combination products of BP plus erythromycin or clindamycin have been developed and are more effective clinically than either product alone (6,7).

MACROLIDES

Topical and oral erythromycin and topical clindamycin have been well-established acne treatments for decades, but have become much less effective in the past 15 years or so due to the acquisition of resistance by *P. acnes*. Resistant bacteria are now induced quickly by macrolide therapy because most patients have a portion of their normal skin flora that is genetically resistant, and that subgroup expands under the selective pressure of therapy (8–11). Resistant bacteria make for acne that resists therapy and erythromycin resistant strains are typically resistant to clindamycin and vice versa.

Resistance can be combated by the addition of BP to topical macrolide regimens. It has been clearly shown that such combination products are not only more effective than monotherapy with macrolides, but also do not permit the survival of resistant populations of *P. acnes* (6).

Other macrolides for example, azithromycin have been reported in small studies to be of value in acne (12), but no data is available on the effect of resistance on the utility of these drugs.

TETRACYCLINES

The tetracycline family of antibiotics are extremely useful in acne because they have multiple modes of action, functioning as antibiotics that reduce bacterial populations, and as anti-inflammatory drugs that attack acne from a second front.

Tetracyclines, especially doxycycline and minocycline are highly anti-inflammatory in many cell systems (Table 1). Neutrophil and monocyte chemotaxis is inhibited through calcium chelation, blunting the migration of cells to the follicle (13). Granuloma formation in vitro (14) and in vivo (15) is inhibited; with minocycline and doxycycline roughly 10-fold more active than tetracycline. In this model, macrolides and cephalosporines were inactive. Protein kinase C is inhibited (15), perhaps interfering with signal transduction. Generation of reactive oxygen species and the oxidative burst in neutrophils is decreased (16). Nitric oxide production is modulated (17). Matrix metalloprotease and collagenase activity is inhibited (18–20). In vivo, tetracyclines have been demonstrated to be highly active in treating purely inflammatory diseases including rheumatoid arthritis, bullous pemphigoid, and sarcoidosis (21). Nonantibiotic derivatives of doxycycline have been recently developed that are highly anti-inflammatory and even antineoplastic through inhibition of angiogenesis and may be of use in acne and other inflammatory diseases (22–24).

Concentrations of tetracyclines that are below the antibiotic threshold still have anti-inflammatory activity. Low doses of doxycycline and minocycine that do not affect bacterial growth decrease the production of neutrophil chemoattractants by *P. acnes* (25,26). Subminimal inhibitory doses also retain the ability to inhibit inflammation in vivo and improve diseases such as acne, rosacea, and periodontitis (27–29).

TABLE 1 Anti-inflammatory Activity of Antibiotic Classes

Inhibition of	Neutrophil chemotaxis	Granuloma formation	Protein kinase C	Nitric oxide	Sub-MIC chemotactic factor
Macrolides					++
Tetracyclines	+++	+++	+++	++	++
Ciprofloxacin		+	+		
Cephalosporines					

Abbreviation: MIC, minimal inhibition concentration.

TABLE 2 Significant Adverse Effects of Doxycycline and Minocycline

Doxycycline
Cutaneous: phototoxicity
Gastrointestinal: GI upset, nausea
Minocycline
Cutaneous: hyperpigmentation, especially in areas of chronic inflammation
Neurologic: light-headedness/vertigo
Allergic: urticaria, serum-sickness-like reactions, systemic hypersensitivity reactions

Abbreviation: GI, gastrointestinal.

Antibiotic resistance is less a problem with the tetracyclines than the macrolides, but resistance in *P. acnes* has been documented. In general, tetracycline resistant strains are cross-resistant to doxycycline but sensitive to minocycline (30).

Choice of oral antibiotic by dermatologists for treating acne has shifted over the past few decades. Currently, the once frequently prescribed tetracycline is used relatively infrequently, with the majority of patients treated with doxycycline or minocycline. Tetracycline has multiple disadvantages, including greatest effect of diet on absorption, lower anti-inflammatory and antibacterial activity, and lower effect on acne lesions (30–32). There are few studies that address the relative potency of these two drugs in treating acne, and the few that do are fairly small and do not involve the more severe patients and manage to show only equivalence (33). However, there is good reason to believe that minocycline is the stronger drug. In my experience, there have been many patients with significant acne who fail to respond to doxycycline yet have an excellent response when switched to minocycline. The reason for this may lie in the greater lipophilicity of minocycline and the greater activity in a lipid milieu. This is reflected in a 10-fold greater reduction of *P. acnes* by minocycline when compared with doxycycline (32).

The side effect profile (Table 2) of doxycycline and minocycline also differs, most notably in the incidence of photosensitivity with doxycycline and the occurrence of hypersensitivity reactions with minocycline. Photosensitivity is very common at higher doses of doxycycline. The minocycline hypersensitivity reactions are uncommon and include urticaria, serum sickness-like reactions, and what has been termed a lupus-like reaction that in reality is probably not an activation of systemic lupus erythematosus but a generalized drug-induced reaction that resembles lupus (34).

OTHER ANTIBIOTICS

Ciprofloxacin and trimethoprim-sulfamethoxazole are both sometimes useful in acne. No large, detailed studies exist to document efficacy, but there are sufficient anecdotes to believe that they are effective in acne (35,36). Whether these important drugs should receive wide usage in acne is a matter of some debate, but few would dispute that they should be reserved for patients who cannot be treated with conventional regimens.

TREATMENT REGIMENS

Because acne is a multifactorial disease, and because most acne treatments (isotretinoin excepted) are not completely effective, typical treatment regimens involve one or more medications. Multidrug treatment schemes are an undesirable fact of acne therapy. They make compliance difficult in a patient population that is

TABLE 3   Acne Treatment Regimens

Mild-to-moderate inflammatory acne
Benzoyl peroxide-clindamycin gel q.d. or b.i.d.
Topical clindamycin foam q.d. + benzoyl peroxide wash q.d.
Benzoyl peroxide-clindamycin gel q.d. + topical retinoid q.d.
Moderate-to-severe inflammatory acne
Doxycycline 75–100 mg b.i.d. + topical retinoid q.d.
Minocycline 75–100 mg b.i.d. + topical retinoid
Addition of a benzoyl peroxide wash is often useful for resistant areas on the trunk.
Women may benefit from addition of androgen blockers such as spironolactone
or cyproterone acetate.

fundamentally noncompliant, and add expense. Therefore, regimens should be as streamlined as possible. Table 3 presents useful antibiotic treatment plans for acne of varying severites.

THE PROBLEM OF ANTIBIOTIC OVERUSE AND A PHILOSOPHY FOR ACNE TREATMENT

Overuse of antibiotics has received increased attention from public health experts and the lay press for some time. The increase in resistant organisms is a real and a significant phenomenon that results in greater illness and expense in treatment of acne and other diseases as well. Moreover, chronic antibiotic use has been implicated in increasing the risk of breast cancer (37,38) and increasing the incidence of upper respiratory infections (39), all in single studies that have yet to be confirmed.

Whether or not this link to nonbacterial diseases proves to be real, there is sufficient reason to avoid long-term antibiotic therapy whenever possible. Acne, unfortunately, is neither a short-term disease nor one that is quickly controllable in many patients, and prolonged courses of antibiotics are often needed. Steps must be taken by the practitioner to minimize the need for chronic treatment by optimizing regimens so as to minimize antibiotic exposure. There are several methods that may be employed to achieve this end.

First, the use of combination therapy with topical retinoids should be begun early in treatment. It has been clearly shown by several studies that many patients treated with oral antibiotic and topical retinoid for 12 weeks may have long-term control of their acne with topical retinoids alone after 12 weeks (40,41). In my experience, almost 70% of patients with papular acne will have no need for oral antibiotic use after 12 weeks, if they have used topical retinoids aggressively for the first 12 weeks.

Second, patients who are severe enough to warrant isotretinoin therapy should get the drug sooner rather than later. A prolonged trial of antibiotics is not justifiable if the patient is a legitimate candidate for isotretinoin.

Third, when long-term antibiotic therapy is required, BP should be part of the regimen because of its ability to discourage the acquisition of resistance.

REFERENCES

1. Nacht S, Yeung D, Beasley JN, Anjo MD, Maibach HI. Benzoyl peroxide: percutaneous penetration and metabolic disposition. J Am Acad Dermatol 1981; 4:31–37.

2. Yeung D, Nacht S, Bucks D, Maibach HI. Benzoyl peroxide: percutaneous penetration and disposition II:Effect of concentration. J Am Acad Derm 1983; 9:920–924.
3. Bandmann HJ, Agathos M. Post-therapeutic benzoyl peroxidecontact allergyin ulcus cruris patients. Hautarzt 1985; 36:670–674.
4. Cotterill JA. Benzoyl peroxide. Acta Derm Venereol 1980; 60:57–63.
5. Mills OH, Kligman AM, Pochi P, Comite H. Comparing 2.5%, 5%, and 10% benzoyl peroxide in inflammatory acne vulgaris. Int J Dermatol 1986; 25:664–667.
6. Leyden J, Kaidbey K, Levy SF. The combination formulation of clindamycin 1% plus benzoyl peroxide 5% vs. three different formulations of topical clindamycin alone in the reduction of Propionibacterium acnes. Am J Clin Dermatol 2001; 4:263–266.
7. Ellis CN, Leyden J, Katz HI, et al. Therapeutic studies with a new combination benzoyl peroxide/clindamycin topical gel in acne vulgaris. Cutis 2001; 67:257–259.
8. Leyden JJ, McGinley KJ, Cavelieri S, Webster GF, Kligman AM. Propionibacterium acnes resistance to antibiotics in acne patients. J Am Acad Dermatol 1984; 8:41–45.
9. Ross JI, Snelling AM, Eady EA, et al. Phenotypic and genotypic characterization of antibiotic resistant Propionibacterium acnes isolated from acne patients attending dermatology clinicsin Europe, the USA, Japan and Australia. Br J Dermatol 2001; 144:339–346.
10. Mills O, Thornsberry C, Cardin CW, Smiles KA, Leyden JJ. Bacterial resistance and outcome following three months of topical acne therapy with 2% erythromycin gel vs. its vehicle. Acta Derm Venereol 2002; 82:260–265.
11. Vowels BR, Feingold DS, Sloughfy C, et al. Effects of topical erythromycin on the ecology of aerobic cutaneous bacterial flora. Antimicrob Agents Chemother 1996; 40:2598–2604.
12. Fernandez-Obregon AC. Azithromycin for the treatment of acne. Int J Dermatol 2000; 39:45–50.
13. Goodheart GL. Further evidence for the role of bivalent cations in human polymorphonuclear leukocyte locomotion. J Reticuloendothelial Soc 1979; 25:545–554.
14. Webster GF, Toso SM, Hegemann LR. Inhibition of in vitro granuloma formation by tetracyclines and ciprofloxacin: involvement of protein kinase C. Arch Derm 1994; 130:748–752.
15. Webster GF, Toso SM, Hegeman L. Inhibition of a model of granuloma formation by tetracyclines and ciprofloxacin: involvement of protein kinase C. Arch Dermatol 1994; 130:748–752.
16. Hand WL, Hand DL, King-Thompson NL. Antibiotic inhibition of the respiratory burst in human polymorphonuclear leukocytes. Antimicrob Agents Chemother 1990; 34:321–330.
17. Hoyt JC, Ballering J, Numanami H, Hayden JM, Robbins RA. Doxycycline modulates nitric oxide production in murine lung epithelial cells. J Immunol 2006; 176(1): 567–572.
18. Golub LM, Lee HM, Lehrer G, et al. Minocycline reduces gingival collagenolytic activity during diabetes. J Periodontal Res 1983; 18:516–526.
19. Maata M, Kari O, Tervahartiala T, et al. Tear fluid levels of MMP-8 are elevated in ocular rosacea: treatment effect of oral doxycycline. Graefes Arch Clin Exp Ophthalmol 2006; 244:957–962.
20. Sobrin L, Liu Z, Monroy DC, et al. Regulation of MMP-9 activity in human tear fluid and corneal epithelial culture supernatant. Invest Ophthalmol Vis Sci 2000; 41:1703–1709.
21. Sapadin AN, Fleishmajer R. Tetracyclines: non-antibiotic properties and their clinical implications. J Am Acad Dermatol 2006; 54:258–265.
22. Dezube BJ, Krown SE, Lee JY, Bauer KS, Aboulafia DM. Ramdomized pahse 2 trial of MMP inhibitor col-3 in AIDS-related Kaposi's sarcoma. J Clin Oncol 2006; 24:1389–1394.
23. Onoda T, Ono T, Dhar DK, Yamoanoi A, Nagasue N. Tatracyclines analogues doxycycline and col 3 induce caspase dependent and independent apoptosis in human colon cancer cells. Int J Cancer 2006; 118:1309–1315.
24. Acharya MR, Venitz J, Figg WD, Sparreboom A. Chemically modifiedtetracyclines as inhibitors f matrix metalloproteinases. Drug Resist Updat 2004; 7:195–208.
25. Webster GF, McGinlery KJ, Leyden JJ. Inhibition of lipase production in Propionibacterium acnes by sub minimal inhibitory concentrations of tetracycline and erythromycin. Br J Dermatol 1981; 105:453–457.

26. Webster GF, Leyden JJ, McGinley KJ, McArthur WP. Suppression of polymorphonuclear leukocyte chemotactic factor production by sub minimal inhibitory concentrations of tetracycline, minocycline, ampicillin and erythromycin. Antimicrob Agents Chemother 1982; 21:770–772.

27. Sanchez J, Somolinos AL, Almodovar PI, Webster G, Bradshaw M, Powala C. A randomized, double-blind, placebo-controlled trial of the combined effect of doxycycline hyclate 20-mg tablets and metronidazole 0.75% topical lotion in the treatment of rosacea. J Am Acad Dermatol 2005; 53(5):791–797.

28. Skidmore R, Kovach R, Walker C, et al. Effects of subantimicrobial-dose doxycycline in the treatment of moderate acne. Arch Dermatol 2003; 139(4):459–464.

29. Emingil G, Atilla G, Sorsa T, Luoto H, Kirilmaz L, Baylas H. The effect of adjunctive low-dose doxycycline therapy on clinical parameters and gingival crevicular fluid matrix metalloproteinase-8 levels in chronic periodontitis. J Periodontol 2004; 75(1):106–115.

30. Leyden JJ. Current issues in antimicrobial therapy for the treatment of acne. J Eur Acad Dermatol Venereol 2001; 15(suppl 3):51–55.

31. Hubbell CG, Hobbs ER, Rist T, White JW Jr. Efficacy of minocycline compared with tetracycline in treatment of acne vulgaris. Arch Dermatol 1982; 118(12):989–992.

32. Leyden JJ. The antimicrobial effects in vivo of minocycline, doxycycline and tetracycline in humans. J Dermatolog Treat 1996; 7:223–225.

33. Harrison PV. A comparison of doxycycline and minocycline in the treatment of acne vulgaris. Clin Exp Dermatol 1988; 13:242–244.

34. Elkayam O, Yaron M, Caspi D. Minocycline-induced autoimmune syndromes: an overview. Semin Arthritis Rheum 1999; 28(6):392–397.

35. Bottomly WW, Cunliffe WJ. Oral trimethoprim as a third line antibiotic in the management of acne vulgaris. Dermatology 1993; 187:193–196.

36. Sykes NL, Webster GF. Acne: a review of optimum treatment. Drugs 1994; 48:59–70.

37. Velicer CM, Heckbert SR, Rutter C, Lampe JW, Malone K. Association between antibiotic use prior to breast cancer diagnosis and breast tumor characteristics. Cancer Causes Control 2006; 17:307–313.

38. Velicer CM, Heckbert SR, Lampe JW, Potter JD, Robertson CA, Taplin SH. Antibiotic use in relation to the risk of breast cancer. JAMA 2004; 291:827–835.

39. Margolis DJ, Bowe WP, Hoffstad O, Berlin JA. Antibiotic treatment of acne may be associated with upper respiratory tract infections. Arch Dermatol 2005; 141(9):1132–1136.

40. Leyden J, Thiboutot DM, Shalita AR, et al. Comparison of tazarotene and minocycline maintenance therapies in acne vulgaris: a multicenter, double-blind, randomized, parallel-group study. Arch Dermatol 2006; 142(5):605–612.

41. Thiboutot DM, Shalita AR, Yamauchi PS, et al. Adapalene gel, 0.1%, as maintenance therapy for acne vulgaris: a randomized, controlled, investigator-blind follow-up of a recent combination study. Arch Dermatol 2006; 142(5):597–602.

9 Topical Retinoids

Daniela Kroshinsky and Alan R. Shalita
Department of Dermatology, SUNY Downstate Medical Center, Brooklyn, New York, U.S.A.

INTRODUCTION

Topical retinoids are singularly important agents in the treatment of acne vulgaris. Any molecule having a biological effect through the binding and activation of retinoid receptors is considered a retinoid (1). This class of medications includes vitamin A and all synthesized molecules that are derived from it (1). By influencing DNA transcription, retinoids can modify cellular growth and differentiation, immunomodulation, and tumor promotion. In turn, they improve acne vulgaris by inhibiting microcomedone formation, diminishing the number of mature comedones as well as inflammatory lesions, and normalizing follicular epithelium maturation and desquamation (2).

CLASSIFICATION

Three generations of retinoids exist. First-generation topical retinoids include vitamin A and its derivatives retinaldehyde, all-*trans*-retinoic acid (all-*trans*-RA) or tretinoin, and 13-*cis*-retinoic acid (13-*cis*-RA) or isotretinoin (3). The second generation retinoids comprise synthetic analogs where one aspect of the basic vitamin A structure has been changed, such as etretinate and acitretin, though no topical forms of these forms exist (3). Third-generation retinoids have significant modification of the original molecule, such as adapalene, tazarotene, arotinoid, arotinoid methyl sulfone, and arotinoid ethyl ester (3). Presently, there are seven topical retinoids: tretinoin, adapalene, tazarotene, topical isotretinoin, motretinide, retinaldehyde, and β-retinoyl glucuronide (3). Only all-*trans*-RA, adapalene, and tazarotene are available in the United States and are discussed in the text that follows.

ABSORPTION

Absorption of topical medications occurs transepidermally or transfollicularly, influenced by the size of the particles involved (4). Molecules 3 to 10 μm in diameter penetrate the follicular ducts, making this size the ideal target size for acne therapy (4). Particles larger than 10 μm become trapped on the skin surface, whereas particles less than 3 μm disperse over the stratum corneum and hair follicles and are, therefore, less efficacious (4).

MECHANISM OF ACTION

Topical retinoids act to clear and prevent the formation of the microcomedo, the precursor to acneiform lesions. The microcomedo is formed from the occlusion of the follicular ostium by the androgen-induced production of sebum and the accumulation of stratum corneum cells (5). In normal skin, the corneocytes of the hair follicle's infrainfundibular region are small and form a noncontinuous, incoherent layer of cells that easily desquamate individually into the follicular canal (1,2,6). They then travel to the surface of the skin through the secretion of lipid-rich sebum (6). In contrast, the follicular epithelium of the microcomedo demonstrates abnormal, hyperactive keratinization, resulting in hypergranulosis and hyperkeratosis (2,5). Corneocytes are more cohesive and less able to migrate to the skin surface and instead become lodged within the follicle, occluding the expulsion of sebum, distending the follicular ostia, and thus forming the comedo (1,6). The anaerobic environment created therein favors the proliferation of *Proprinibacterium acnes* (1,6), which subsequently creates an inflammatory response by secreting lipase, releasing chemotactic factors, and recruiting polymorphonuclear lymphocytes (PMNs) (1,2,6). Bacterial lipases break down sebum triglycerides into glycerol, a growth factor for the bacteria, and free fatty acids that are comedogenic and proinflammatory (1,6). The lipases and cytokines produced by the recruited PMNs each contribute to the breakdown of the follicular wall, eventually causing microcomedo rupture. The release of sebum, keratin, and free fatty acids induces an inflammatory foreign body reaction, resulting in the formation of inflammatory papules, pustules, and nodules (1,5,6). Therefore, by targeting the microcomedo, topical retinoids also help prevent the formation of inflammatory lesions that have the potential to heal with scarring. By preventing the formation of new microcomedones, topical retinoids produce acne remissions that can be successfully maintained for extended periods of time (2,7). These effects occur in what has be referred to as the "ideal state," in which retinoids could be used in sufficient concentrations and frequencies to obtain the desired effect. Unfortunately, for many patients, the irritant side effects of these drugs—erythema, xerosis, burning, desquamation—can impede 100% adherence and improvement (2). Unlike oral retinoids, the topical retinoids do not decrease production of sebum, but instead act by decreasing inflammation, normalizing keratinocyte differentiation, and increasing keratinocyte proliferation and migration (8,9).

Receptor Action

Topical retinoids regulate gene transcription through an interaction with nuclear retinoid receptors. Nuclear retinoid receptors are ligand-dependent transcription factors that regulate the transcription of target genes in two ways (10). One mechanism of action is via the direct binding to retinoid receptor cognate hormone response elements, direct repeats of six nucleotides, found in the promoter regions of retinoid-receptive genes (10,11). The second means of transcription modification is the antagonism of nuclear transcription factors that bind to alternate response elements (AREs), thereby preventing the expression of genes regulated by these AREs (10,11). For instance, when a retinoid binds to the retinoic acid receptor (RAR) subtype complexed with the jun/fos transcription factors, it disrupts the interaction between jun/fos and the ARE, activator protein-1 (AP-1), and prevents transcription of AP-1 regulated genes (11). It is thought that this results in the antiproliferative and anti-inflammatory effects seen with some of the retinoids (10–12).

Retinoid receptors, like thyroid hormone receptors, vitamin D receptors, and steroid receptors, are classified as nuclear receptors (12). There are two classes of nuclear retinoid receptors: RARs and retinoid X receptor (RXRs) (12). Each class of receptors consist of three subtypes: alpha, beta, and gamma, and in vivo, these receptors exist as dimers (12,13). RXRs can dimerize with RAR, thyroid hormone receptors, and vitamin D receptors. RARs, however, can only dimerize with RXR (12). RAR alpha subunits are found ubiquitously, RAR gamma subunits are found predominantly in the skin, and RAR beta subtypes are inducible by retinoids only in certain tissues, including the skin (6,10). RAR and RXR subtypes bind as heterodimers along with the retinoid ligand to the cognate hormone response elements. Each retinoid holds a different affinity for each receptor subtype. The clinical response to each retinoid differs on the basis of the affinity for specific receptors, the expression pattern of receptor subtypes, and the cognate response element (10,11). Gamma receptor is the most important receptor involved in epidermal differentiation, and tretinoin has a high affinity for these receptors.

Retinoid Types

The first developed topical retinoid was retinoic acid, or tretinoin. Tretinoin's flexible molecular structure allows it to bind all RAR and RXR subtypes, whereas tazarotene and adapalene are more rigid, and therefore demonstrate receptor specificity (13). Tretinoin also has the capacity to bind cytosolic retinoid-activating binding proteins (CRABPs) that exist in two forms, I and II, and act as buffers for retinoic acid by controlling free intracellular concentration (3,10,11). Retinoid potency correlates with affinity for the RARs but not for CRABPs (11).

Tretinoin is available as 0.025%, 0.05%, and 0.1% creams, 0.01% and 0.025% gels, and 0.05% solution, with 0.025% cream having the least and 0.05% solution having the most irritation potential (2,3,6). Newer microencapsulated tretinoin gel and polyolprepolymer 2 gel forms are less irritating than other formulations of tretinoin (2,6,14). The tretinoin microsphere, available in 0.4% and 0.1% gel forms, encapsulates the molecule within a porous acrylate copolyer microsphere (2,15). This packaging system allows selective, time-released delivery of tretinoin to the follicle, leading to a decreased available concentration and lower irritation without diminishing the efficacy (2,15). In fact, the maximum comedolytic activity of tretinoin is reached at a concentration 5 to 10 times lower when the drug is used in a microsphere form (15). In addition, potential percutaneous penetration to the blood vessels is diminished (2,15).

Similarly, novel vehicles can allow controlled release of topical retinoids. Polyolprepolymer-2 is a material designed to help retain drug molecules in and on the skin when applied topically and has been shown to distribute tretinoin over time with equivalent efficacy to vehicle-free analogous formulations (16). The incorporation of tretinoin into this vehicle prevents rapid and excess percutaneous absorption of tretinoin, decreasing irritation (16). In vitro absorption studies, guinea pig irritation models, human patch test studies, and acne clinical trials of tretinoin gel and cream containing polyolprepolymer-2 demonstrate that the absorption of tretinoin during the first six hours of delivery is significantly less than that of standard preparations of tretinoin, but becomes similar after this time (16). Additionally, the total penetration of polyolprepolymer-impregnated tretinoin is less than vehicle-free tretinoin (16). Human patch tests demonstrated that both tretinoin gel and cream formulated with polyolprepolymer-2 resulted in less irritation when compared to their tretinoin gel and cream forms (16). Human double-blind clinical trials comparing tretinoin 0.025% gel and cream containing polyolprepolymer-2 to their commercially available equivalents demonstrated diminished xerosis, erythema, and peeling in the tretinoin polyolpolymer gel and cream formulations

(16). This decrease in irritation was achieved without compromising treatment efficacy (16). Although the exact mechanism for these actions is unknown, one proposed mechanism is that the degree of irritation from tretinoin is related to the rate of initial penetration of drug and while the efficacy is more a consequence of mean molecular flux (16).

The second topical retinoid developed for the treatment of acne is adapalene, a stable naphthoic acid derivative with both significant anti-inflammatory and comedolytic properties (6,11,17). Adapalene has been shown to have a more favorable sideeffect profile than either tazarotene or tretinoin (6,17). It has a specific affinity for RAR beta and gamma subtypes in the terminal differentiation zone of the epidermis and does not bind to CRABP I and II due to steric hindrance (3,6,11,13,18,19). Adapalene treats acne by causing epidermal and follicular epithelium hyperplasia, increased desquamation, keratinocyte differentiation, and loosening of corneocyte connections (11,14,18).

Adapalene is available as 0.1% cream, gel, solution, and pledget forms and is in clinical trials as a newer 0.3% gel formulation (2,20). The 0.1% gel has been shown to be as effective as tretinoin 0.025% gel with decreased irritation (2,20). The 0.3% gel has been shown to be safe and well tolerated for long-term use with almost doubled success over adapalene 0.1% gel without a significant increase in clinically relevant side effects (20). The release of adapalene from solution formulations such as lotions and hydroalcoholic gels is greater than when dispersed in creams or aqueous gels (18,21).

The anti-inflammatory effects of adapalene result from inhibition of the oxidative metabolism of arachidonic acid by the 5 and 15 lipoxygenase pathways and through the inhibition of PMN chemotactic and chemokinetic responses (3,11). As such, adapalene has demonstrated superiority when compared to reference anti-inflammatory agents such as indomethacin and betamethasone valerate (22). Other contributing factors for the lower skin irritation induced by adapalene include its different RAR subtype-binding pattern and more neutral molecular structure, which makes it less likely to nonspecifically interact with cell membrane function (3). Its high melting point and low solubility result in low flux through the skin, leading to high concentrations in the stratum corneum and hair follicle, where it can best act to prevent and treat acne (11).

Tazarotene is a topical retinoid that has demonstrated superior efficacy when compared with other topical retinoids in the treatment of acne (23). Tazarotene is available in 0.05% and 0.1% cream and gel formulations (2). Tazarotene is selective for RAR beta and gamma subtypes (13). Although tazarotene does not directly bind to the RXRs, it does isomerize to 9-*cis*-RA, which weakly binds all RXRs leading to a degree of transactivation (21). The precise mechanism of action of tazarotene is unknown, however, it is postulated that through the activation of retinoid receptors, retinoid responsive genes are upregulated impacting the differentiation of keratinocytes. Similarly, by inhibiting proinflammatory transcription factors, tazarotene causes decreased cell proliferation and inflammation (21). Tazarotene penetrates the skin but accumulates in the upper dermis (24). The molecule remains concentrated here with very little absorption into blood vessels or lymphatics (24).

The topical retinoids induce specific changes in the structure and morphology of the skin. Normal epithelial cell differentiation is a vitamin A-dependent process (25). The presence of vitamin A alters the size of the keratin molecules synthesized by keratinocytes (25). When small keratin molecules are produced, a secretory-type epithelium is generated. A stratified squamous epithelium is induced when larger keratin molecules are synthesized (25). In the absence of vitamin A, cells differentiate toward keratinizing epithelium (25).

Keratinocytes within each layer of epidermis possess a distinct set of proteins unique to their stage of differentiation (26). As undifferentiated basal cells mature and migrate up through the epidermis, their pattern of protein expression changes (26). Once these cells arrive at the stratum corneum, the intracellular organelles have been catabolized and cytoplasmic and membrane proteins altered so as to produce a layer of dead corneocytes with thick keratin fibrils within a dense matrix (26). As a group, the retinoids alter this process by inducing dose-specific keratinocyte proliferation and reversing the abnormal keratinocyte desquamation found in acne (26). This helps form a thicker layer of suprabasal cells, but a thinned, loose stratum corneum (2,3,26). Topical retinoids increase the rate of keratinocyte turnover resulting in an increased rate of follicular proliferation and differentiation (24). This results in decreased follicular occlusion and faster microcomedone clearance (3,24). Specifically, topical retinoids cause basal and spinous epithelial cell proliferation and reduce the size and adhesion of corneocytes by decreasing filaggrin expression and suppressing the normal proteolysis of keratins 1 and 14 (1). In addition, retinoids thin the stratum corneum by causing desmosomal shedding, decreasing tonofilaments, and increasing keratinocyte autolysis (1,8,27).

Epidermal cell commitment to proliferation and differentiation can be altered by the topical retinoids. Normal keratinocyte differentiation involves the expression of keratins K1 and K10 (26). An alternative pathway of differentiation compatible with hyperproliferation occurs upon suprabasal expression of K6, K16, and K17 (26). Cells expressing K6 and K16 enlarge as they migrate to the surface and do not produce keratohyalin granules or lose their nuclei before desquamating (26).

The dose-dependent epidermal acanthosis results from increased number of cell layers, not from hypertrophy of individual cells (9). There is no change in structure or size of sebaceous glands after treatment with topical retinoids (9). All of the above factors demonstrate that comedolysis is retinoid-specific, not simply secondary to desquamation (3).

Retinoids also have secondary effects that facilitate acne clearance. By weakening and loosening the cornified layer and decreasing the number of corneocytes, skin permeability is increased (2). This facilitates the absorption of other topical agents, such as antimicrobials or benzoyl peroxide (2). Increased cell turnover within the follicular epithelium also allows more oral antibiotic to enter the follicular canal where *P. acnes* is concentrated (2). This increases antimicrobial activity, lowering the potential for antibiotic resistance from inadequate concentrations (2). By increasing the rate of acne clearance, the overall duration of antibiotic treatment and chance for antibiotic resistance can be reduced (2,6). In addition, this modification of skin morphology creates a more aerobic environment and decreases the ability of *P. acnes* to proliferate (2).

USE AND SIDE EFFECTS

Proper selection and usage of the topical retinoids is crucial to maximize efficacy and patient adherence and satisfaction. Treatment should begin with the lowest concentration of medication, usually in a cream-based form if available (21). Application should occur at night to dry skin, 20 to 30 minutes after the face has been washed with a mild, nonsoap cleanser (21). A pea-sized amount should be dispensed and equally divided over two index fingers, which then dab the medication evenly onto opposite sides of the face and spread the medication into a thin layer until no visible product remains (21). Hands should be washed afterwards to avoid retinoid dermatitis (21). Application should first occur every other night for one to two weeks depending on the skin type so as to minimize the initial irritation that may otherwise discourage adherence to the treatment regimen (1,21). Oily skin is better able to tolerate the potential irritating effects of the retinoids and, as such, a shorter introductory period may be utilized (21). Non-comedogenic moisturizers can be used to minimize xerosis, erythema, and stinging (2). Patients should be instructed that as long as four to six weeks of use may be required before the onset of efficacy and that an initial flare in acne may occur following two to four weeks of use due to an accelerated evolution of pre-existing microcomedones (3). Periodic encouragement and reassurance may be necessary. Four to six weeks of nightly application should occur, after which the concentration may be increased if the desired results are not obtained (21). An additional benefit to topical retinoid use is the potential to improve and prevent the postinflammatory hyperpigmentation often seen in darker skin types as acne lesions heal.

MINIMIZING SIDE EFFECTS

Side effects of topical retinoid use include initial local irritation, including erythema, burning, stinging, peeling, and xerosis (1). These symptoms usually peak after two weeks of use, and subsequently diminish and then resolve once the skin adapts to the use of the product (1,3,18). Factors influencing the extent and duration of irritation include concentration of the medication used, vehicle of delivery, frequency and amount of application, skin type, and environmental factors such as use of abrasive cleansers or other topical alcoholic agents, ambient xerosis, and exposure to the sun (1,6,14,18,28). Higher concentratations or use of a gel or solution vehicle predisposes to the most irritation. Topical retinoids produce more irritation when used by patients with eczema, rosacea, or other conditions of skin sensitivity, including exposure to extreme weather (2,14). In these patients and during the winter, lower concentrations and the milder forms and vehicles should be utilized (2,28). Individual patient variation does, however, occur and some patients may actually tolerate gels better than creams, perhaps because they are more difficult to apply. Adapalene and tretinoin are photoirritants, not photosensitizers, meaning that there is an increased susceptibility to irritation upon sun exposure, and therefore minimizing sun exposure through sun avoidance and the use of sunscreen or physical blockers is imperative (14,28).

For patients who are unable to tolerate even the gradual introduction of the mildest topical retinoids, short contact therapy can be utilized. Short contact therapy is a safe and effective method that involves applying the topical agent for a brief period and then washing it off (13). Patients should initially leave the retinoid on the skin for two minutes each day, increasing by one minute at least every three days as tolerated and without causing adverse effects (13). If irritation occurs, time of exposure should be decreased by 30 seconds for at least three days and then incremental increases can be resumed (13). Studies have demonstrated somewhat diminished efficacy than overnight tazarotene, but overall good results without irritation in patients who otherwise would be unable to benefit from topical retinoid therapy (13).

VEHICLES

The type of vehicle used to deliver the retinoid influences the degree of skin penetration, the clinical effect, and the side effect profile, including the degree of photoirritance (1,6). Future formulations suspending topical retinoids in a foam vehicle could potentially create a nongreasy, no-residue, less-drying formulation to more effectively deliver the medication over hair-bearing sites such as the back and chest (29).

EFFICACY

Acne vulgaris is an almost ubiquitous condition. When antimicrobials are used alone, there is a risk of creating widespread, multidrug resistance of *P. acnes* as well as other skin flora such as *Staphylococcus aureus* (2,5,30). This potential resistance can be limited by combining agents that act on different steps in the mechanism of acne pathogenesis. When topical retinoids are used in combination with oral or topical antimicrobials, excessive ductal cornification, *P. acnes* proliferation, and inflammation can be simultaneously targeted for increased efficacy, faster onset of effects, decreased total antibiotic use and risk of resistance, and shorter overall duration of treatment (2). The combination tretinoin with topical or oral antibiotics has been shown to be superior to either alone in decreasing lesion count, increasing rate of improvement, and decreasing levels of *P. acnes* and free fatty acids (8,14). Similarly, the combination of adapalene with topical doxycycline or clindamycin shows increased efficacy in improving total, inflammatory, and noninflammatory lesions including a faster onset of action without an augmentation in side effects (17). In addition, combination use of adapalene offers an anti-inflammatory benefit, which minimizes the increased risk of irritation that occurs upon increasing the number of topical treatments (17).

Similar results were found upon combining retinoic acid and antibiotics, with a reduction in the initial retinoid-induced flare of lesions through the antibiotic use (3). When combined with a benzoyl peroxide oxidizing wash—which demonstrates an effective bacteriostatic concentration after only 20 seconds of use—tretinoin 0.1% micro gel decreased *P. acnes* counts without increasing irritation (6,31).

With long-term use, however, overall improvement is similar with combination therapy as compared with topical retinoid use alone (14,23,32). Increased reductions in open and closed comedones, papules, and pustules were demonstrated when tazarotene or tretinoin creams were combined with clindamycin/benzoyl peroxide as compared to either retinoid alone (14,32).

Finally, it has been shown that combining topical retinoid therapy with oral antibiotics for inflammatory acne is more cost-effective than using an oral retinoid alone when accounting for pretreatment and treatment laboratory tests, pregnancy tests, and diagnostic fetal tests after a potential unintended pregnancy (33).

A new combination clindamycin 1%/tretinoin 0.025% gel, Velac, has demonstrated greater and faster treatment success in initial clinical trials when compared to clindaymycin or tretinoin gel alone and provides a convenient means of application, which may improve patient adherence (12). The side effect profile of Velac was similar to that of tretinoin gel alone, with only slightly higher irritancy than clindamycin gel alone (12).

And as previously discussed, the use of topical retinoid in combination with oral antibiotics can decrease time of use of antibiotics, decreasing risk of resistance, adverse response, or drug interaction.

SYSTEMIC ABSORPTION AND TERATOGENICITY

The teratogenic effects of oral retinoid therapy are well-documented. Tretinoin penetrates the skin and accumulates in the upper dermis with very little absorption into blood vessels or lymphatics (24). Several studies have evaluated the systemic effects of topical retinoid therapy. Tretinoin 0.1% to 0.2% applied for extended periods demonstrates minimal to no increase in tretinoin levels above endogenous and these level changes have not been associated with teratogenicity (1,21). Worobec et al. (34) studied the percutaneous absorption of 0.05% tretinoin by using radioactive labeling and measuring the levels of retinoid found in the urine, stool, and plasma, after repeated applications. An absorption level of 1.38% to 2.13% was found, correlating to an insignificant increase in the endogenous level of tretinoin and a very low risk of systemic toxicity (34). When 0.1% tretinoin cream, 0.1% Tazarotene gel, and 0.1% adapalene gel were applied over 26 days, the respective mean maximal plasma levels of were 4.7, 0.14, 0.04 ng/mL, which are all well below the mean endogenous level of 6.6 ng/mL of all-*trans*-, 13-*cis*- + 13-*cis*-4-oxo-RA (21). Other studies have also found that overnight tazarotene use produces levels of tazarotene and tazarotenic acid levels lower than endogenous, with the highest rate of absorption shown to occur after tazarotene was applied under occlusion for 10 hours resulting in <6% absorption of total applied dose (13). In fact, diurnal and nutritional factors alter endogenous plasma levels of retinoids more than widespread topical use of all-*trans*-RA (35). Buchan et al. (35) evaluated the daily use of radiolabeled 0.025% all-trans-RA over the face, shoulder, and upper chest and demonstrated a percutaneous absorption in the range of 0.1% to 7.2%, considered to be an insignificant increase in endogenous levels. Daily ingestion of the 50,000 IU of vitamin A, however, tripled the endogenous level of all-*trans*-RA, doubled the level of 4-oxo-13-*cis*-RA, and increased 13-*cis*-RA six times (35). The recommended daily allowance of vitamin A for male adults is 900 mg/day and fornonpregnant, nonlactating women 700 mg/day of vitamin A, with the recommended dosage actually increasing to 770 mg/day in preganancy and to 1300 mg/day in lactation (36). On the basis of this information, it is very unlikely that topical retinoid use could cause systemic toxicity.

Although there is a lack of studies on humans, topical retinoids have not demonstrated teratogenic effects in animals (24,37,38). Nevertheless, tretinoin should be used cautiously in pregnancy and lactation while tazarotene is contraindicated.

CONCLUSIONS

Topical retinoid therapy is a safe, effective, economical means of treating all but the most severe cases of acne vulgaris. The retinoids serve as the cornerstone of treatment and should be the initial therapeutic step, either alone or in combination with topical or oral antibiotic therapy and benzoyl peroxides. Once a patient has achieved adequate results, the topical retinoid should be continued alone as maintenance therapy to maintain lesion remission (2,20,33).

REFERENCES

1. Biro DE, Shalita AR. Clinical aspects of topical retinoids. Skin Pharmacol 1993; 6(suppl 1): 53–60.
2. Gollnick H, Cunliffe W, Berson D, et al. Management of acne: a report from a global alliance to improve outcomes in acne. J Am Acad Dermatol 2003; 49:S1–S373.

3. Verschoore M, Bouclier M, Czernielewski J, et al. Topical retinoids: their uses in dermatology. Dermatol Clin 1993; 11:107–115.
4. Allec J, Chatelus A, Wagner N. Skin distribution and pharmaceutical aspects of adapalene gel. J Am Acad Dermatol 1997; 36:S119–S125.
5. Wolff H, Plewig G, Braun-Falco O. Ultrastructure of human sebaceous follicles and comedones following treatment with vitamin A acid. Acta Dermatovenerol (Stockholm) 1975; 74:99–110.
6. Brown SK, Shalita AR. Acne vulgaris. Lancet 1998; 351:1871–1876.
7. Leyden JJ. A review of the use of combination therapies in the treatment of acne vulgaris. J Amer Acad Dermatol 2003; 49(3 suppl):S200–S210.
8. Leyden JJ. Retinoids and Acne. J Am Acad Dermatol 1988; 19:164–168.
9. Asthon RE, Connor MJ, Lowe NJ. Histologic changes in the skin of the rhino mouse induced by retinoids. J Invest Dermatol 1984; 82:632–636.
10. Shalita A. Clinical Management of Topical Retinoids for Acne. A presentation at the Annual Valley of the Sun Meeting, Pheonix, AZ 2005.
11. Shroot B, Michel S. Pharmacology and chemistry of adapalene. J Am Acad Dermatol 1997; 36(6):S96–S103.
12. Velac Phase III study efficacy results (combined analysis): primary outcome measures, Data on File Connetics Laboratories.
13. Bershad S, Kranjac Singer G, Parente JE, et al. Successful treatment of acne vulgaris using a new method: results of a randomized vehicle-controlled trial of short-contact therapy with 0.1% tazarotene gel. Arch Dermatol 2002; 138:481–489.
14. Weiss JS, Shavin JS. Adapalene for the treatment of acne vulgaris. J Am Acad Dermatol 1998; 39(2):50–54.
15. Dinarvand R, Rahmani E, Farbod E. Gelatin microspheres for the controlled release of all-trans-retinoic acid topical formulation and drug delivery evaluation. Iranian J Pharm Res 2003; 2:47–50.
16. Quigley JW, Bucks DA. Reduced skin irritation with tretinoin containing polyolprepolymer-2, a new topical tretinoin delivery system: a summary of preclinical and clinical investigations. J Am Acad Dermatol 1998; 38(4):S5–S10.
17. Thiboutot D, Shalita A. Combination therapy with adapalene gel 0.1% and doxycycline for severe acne vulgaris: a multicenter, investigator-blind, randomized, controlled-study. Skinmed 2005; 4(3):138–146.
18. Brogden R, Goa K. Adapalene: a review of its pharmacological properties and clinical potential in the management of mild to moderate acne. Drugs 1997; 53(3):511–519.
19. Cunliffe WJ, Poncet M, Loesche C, et al. A comparison of the efficacy and tolerability of adapalene 0.1% gel versus tretinoin 0.025% gel in patients with acne vulgaris: a meta-analysis of five randomized trials. Br J Dermatol 1998; 139(suppl 52):48–56.
20. Thiboutot, D. Clinical Experience With Adapalene 0.3% Gel, Presented at Satellite Symposium at the American Academy of Dermatology Meeting 2006, San Francisco, CA.
21. Topical Retinoids in the Treatment of Acne Vulgaris. A presentation.
22. Hensby C, Cavey D, Bouclier M, et al. The in vivo and in vitro anti-inflammatory activity of CD271: A new retinoids-like modulator of cell differentiation. Agents and Actions 1990; 29:56–58.
23. Shalita AR. Tazarotene cream in facial acne vulgaris the best in acne trial: balancing efficacy, speed, and tolerability. Cutis 2004; 74(suppl 4):4–8.
24. Stuttgen G. Historical perspectives of tretinoin. J Am Acad Dermatol 1986; 15(4):735–740.
25. Fuchs E, Green H. Regulation of terminal differentiation of cultured human keratinocytes by vitamin A. Cell 1981; 25:617–625.
26. Eichener MK, Capetola RJ, Gendimenico GJ, Mezick JA. Cytoskeletal effects of topical retinoids. J Invest Dermatol 1992; 98:154–161.
27. Bolognia JL, Jorizzo JL, Rapini RP. Dermatology. 1st ed. New York: Mosby, 2003.
28. Skov MJ, Quigley JW, Bucks DW. Topical delivery system for tretinoin: research and clinical implications. J Pharm Sci 1997; 86(10):1138–1143.
29. Shalita A. A novel clindamycin foam formulation for the treatment of acne vulgaris: focus of phase three clinical trials, presented at the 2004 American Academy of Dermatology Summer Meeting, New York, NY.

30. Iyer S, Jones D. Community-acquired methicillin-resistant Staphylococcus aureus skin infection: a retrospective analysis of clinical presentation and treatment of a local outbreak. J Am Acad Dermatol 2004; 50(6):854–858.

31. Shalita AR, Elyse SR, Anderson DN, et al. Compared efficacy and safety of tretinoin 0.1% microsphere gel alone and in combination with benzoyl peroxide 6% cleanser for the treatment of acne vulgaris. Ther Clin 2003; 72:167–172.

32. Shalita A, Tanghetti E, Abramouits W, Solomon B. Tazarotene versus tazarotene plus clindamycin/benzoyl peroxide in the treatment of acne vulgaris. Abstract for a poster presentation at the 63rd annual meeting of the American Academy of Dermatology, New Orleans, L.A. February 2005.

33. Harper J. The use of topical retinoids for inflammatory acne: a review of the pharmacoeconomic considerations. Manag Care Interface 2005; 18(3):51–55.

34. Worobec SM, Wong FA, Tolman EL, et al. Percutaneous absorption of 3H-tretinoin in normal volunteers. J Invest Dermatol 1991; 257:574.

35. Buchan P, Eckhoff C, Caron D, et al. Repeated topical administration of all-trans-retinoic acid and plasma levels of retinoic acids in humans. J Am Acad Dermatol 1994; 30:428–434.

36. RDA Dietary Reference Intakes: Vitamins website http://www.iom.edu/Object.File/Master/7/296/0.pdf

37. Latriano L, Tzimas G, Wong F, et al. The percutaneous absorption of topically applied tretinoin and its effect on endogenous concentrations of tretinoin and its metabolites after single doses or long-term use. J Am Acad Dermatol 1997; 36:S37–S46.

38. Johnson EM. A risk assessment of topical tretinoin as a potential human developmental toxin based on animal and comparative human data. J Am Acad Dermatol 1997; 36:S86–S90.

10 Phototherapy and Laser Therapy of Acne

Guy F. Webster

Jefferson Medical College of Thomas Jefferson University, Philadelphia, Pennsylvania, U.S.A.

INTRODUCTION

Light-based treatments for acne are not new. A tan has long been known to help teens with pimples, and it would not be surprising to find reports of acne phototherapy dating from the 1930s. In my youth, a local dermatologist was treating many of us with what must have been a cold quartz lamp along with various creams and oral antibiotics. He told me that he knew that the light was helpful, but could not say more than that about its mechanism. Since that time, there have been great advances in the understanding of acne and in laser and light technology, but the level of understanding of how light might help acne has not progressed much.

In the past 10 years or so, there have been many reports of different light-based acne regimens (1), but all are small (or very small) studies and most can best be categorized as organized anecdote. The typical report describes a handful of patients who have treatment with light plus antibiotics plus other interventions (such as peels). Controls, blinding, and randomization are lacking, and the phototherapy regimen differs from patient to patient. It is tempting to dismiss the reports as worthless, but that would be missing what could be an important new direction in acne treatment.

POTENTIAL TARGETS FOR LIGHT IN ACNE
Propionibacterium acnes

Propionibacterium acnes is an obvious target for acne phototherapy since it is central to the inflammatory process. The organism makes porphyrins, which are present in the follicle, in proportion to its population (2). These photoactive compounds can be excited by light to generate reactive oxygen, which is toxic to *P. acnes* (3). An inherent limitation is that to reduce *P. acnes* effectively, the therapy would have to be given very frequently since the organism proliferates rapidly and would quickly repopulate after being reduced by a phototoxic reaction. How frequently might be necessary? There are no data available to directly answer the question, but one can predict in vitro from the organism's generation time that populations would double every roughly 30 minutes, and a *P. acnes* suppressive therapy would have to be given at least every two or three days.

A study by Pollock et al. (4) sheds some light on the potential mechanism of porphyrin phototherapy in acne. They studied the effect of topically applied aminolevulinic acid (ALA) on acne, which is a precursor to porphyrins that are converted by skin enzymes and is more potent than the effects of endogenous porphyrin. The porphyrin was excited by a 635-nm diode laser. Ten patients had four areas of their back treated with ALA alone, ALA + light, light alone, or no treatment. After three treatments over three weeks, the acne improvement was noted only in the ALA +

light sites. Although there was a clear clinical benefit, sebum secretion and *P. acnes* populations were measured to be unchanged.

Similarly, blue-light treatment of acne patients reduces *P. acnes* levels after several treatments, but acne begins to improve before bacterial reduction can be noted (5). So, theoretically, and in acne trials, porphyrin-based photodynamic therapy is unlikely to exert its effects through reducing *P. acnes*.

Inhibition of Sebum Production

Sebum is, in a sense, the central problem in acne. Without it, *P. acnes* cannot proliferate and acne would not exist. The most effective drug for the disease isotretinoin exerts the majority of its effects on sebum secretion. A light-based treatment that targets sebum production would have the potential to cure acne. Could one do without sebaceous glands? Most likely. The function of sebum is unknown; it may serve to inhibit invading bacteria such as dermatophytes and streptococci, but children do well with no sebum and adults have little-to-no sebaceous activity on the extremities with no ill effects.

The challenge in a therapeutic photon attack on the sebaceous gland is its distance from the skin surface. Between the gland and the surface is up to 3 mm of tissue that can absorb light and be damaged. The key would seem to be to develop a chromophore that homes to the sebaceous gland and then can be activated by an otherwise innocuous wavelength of light.

Anderson et al. (6) have reported a series of 22 patients with acne of the back, who were sensitized aggressively with ALA and then irradiated with a potent dose of broadband (550–700 nm) light. Pain, erythema, and evidence of epidermal damage were common. Patients experienced a flare of acne that was suppressed by following treatments. Although the adverse effects were significant, there was histologic evidence of damage to sebaceous glands and patients had suppressed sebum production for at least 20 weeks after treatment. Although the adverse effects of this regimen are probably too severe for a practicable therapy, the report serves as a wonderful proof-of-principle study, documenting that the sebaceous gland can be destroyed by a limited number of light treatments. Similarly, Lloyd and Mirkov (7) demonstrated that indocyanine green accumulates in the sebaceous gland and can be activated by 810-nm light to damage the sebaceous gland, yet relatively spare the epidermis. All that remains is to develop a chromophore that is sebaceous gland specific, cosmetically practical, and excitable by a wavelength that can be delivered several millimeters into the skin.

Modulation of Keratinization

Formation of the comedo results from defective keratinization in the epidermal lining of the follicle and is the target of topical retinoids in acne. Could light alter the epidermis sufficiently to stop comedo formation and thus halt acne? So far, there is no evidence that this might be possible, but no theoretical reason why it might not.

Modulation of Immune Responsiveness

Toll-like receptors (TLRs) have been shown to be involved in the development of acne lesions (8). Might light-based techniques be able to improve acne through modulation of epidermal innate immunity? There is some evidence that this may be possible. It is well-described that sun and phototherapy decrease the reactivity of epidermal Langerhans cells (9), which could be involved in acne inflammation at some level. Omi et al. (10) have shown that a nonablative 585-nm laser increases IL-2 and IL-4. The relevance to acne of this observation is not certain.

Schnitkind et al. (5) studied the anti-inflammatory properties of narrow band blue light on cultured keratinocytes. They found that cytokine-induced production of IL-1a and ICAM-1 was inhibited, which gives credence to the concept that current phototherapy techniques exert an anti-inflammatory effect in acne.

NOTABLE OBSERVATIONS AND STUDIES

In contrast to a loosely controlled study showing that a single low-dose, nonpurpuric treatment with the pulsed-dye laser resulted in acne improvement up to 12 weeks after therapy (11), Orringer et al. (12) performed a blinded split-face study of similar low-dose pulsed-dye laser therapy for acne and found no effect on the number of lesions or on the clinical grade of the acne.

Alexiades-Armenakas (13) reported a series of acne patients, among whom 13 patients with what was described as severe or cystic acne were treated with long-pulsed 585-nm pulsed-dye laser and ALA. All patients received either topical retinoids or azaleic acid and either a sulfur- or benzoyl peroxide-based cleanser. All patients in this group achieved a complete clearance after a mean of 2.9 treatments and a mean follow-up of 6.9 months. Adverse effects were minimal and limited to erythema and "slight" pain. Several clinical photographs were shown documenting clearance of significant inflammatory acne [but acne that falls short (in these pictures) of what many would usually classify as "cystic"]. In spite of quibbling about the definition of cystic acne, and in spite of the use of other medications such as topical retinoids and benzoyl peroxide, it is clear that in this report, the use of ALA photodynamic therapy (PDT) resulted in an improvement in significant acne.

Weigell and Wulf (14) evaluated the efficacy of methyl aminolevulenate PDT on moderate-to-severe acne in a randomized, controlled trial. Twenty-one patients were treated and 15 served as controls. Two treatments separated by two weeks were administered and acne graded at 4, 8, and 12 weeks. Improvement was noted at 4 weeks and reached statistical significance at 8 and 12 weeks after therapy. Most patients developed "severe" pain during the first treatment, fewer complained during the second treatment. Exfoliation and crusting were common.

Although rigorous studies are limited in number, it is clear that there is great potential for a photodynamic approach to acne.

FUTURE DIRECTIONS FOR INVESTIGATION

Clinical trials where phototherapy is the only agent used. Even though most acne treatments are not used as a monotherapy in the clinic, in the development phase, it is important to test laser or PDT as monotherapy in order to ascertain whether it actually has any effect on acne and to be able to define the best regimen.

Investigation of the ability of phototherapy to modulate inflammatory systems. Selective modulation of TLRs in the skin, e.g., the TLR2 that is involved in acne, may be the explanation for the effects of phototherapy on acne. If so, perhaps less traumatic regimens can be designed.

Development of sebaceous gland—specific phototherapy. This could be a magic bullet for acne and is theoretically possible. Perhaps, the biggest obstacle would be the cost of development of a one-time treatment, which would have to be very expensive to offset development costs.

REFERENCES

1. Ross EV. Optical treatments for acne. Dermatol Ther 2005; 18:253–266.
2. McGinley KJ, Webster GF, Leyden JJ. Facial follicular porphyrin fluorescence: correlation with age and density of Propionibacterium acnes. Br J Dermatol 1980; 102(4):437–441.
3. Ashkenazi H, Malik Z, Harth Y, Nitzan Y. Eradication of Propionibacterium acnes by its endogenic porphyrins after illumination with high intensity blue light. FEMS Immunol Med Microbiol 2003; 35:17–24.
4. Pollock B, Turner D, Stringer MR, et al. Topical aminolaevulinic acid photodynamic therapy for the treatment of acne vulgaris: a study of clinical efficacy and mechanism of action. Br J Dermatol 2004; 151:616–622.
5. Schnitkind E, Yaping E, Geen S, Shalita AR, Lee W-L. Anti-inflammatory properties of narrow band blue light. J Drugs Dermatol 2006; 5:605–610.
6. Hongcharu W, Taylor CR, Chang Y, et al. Topical ALA-photodynamic therapy for the treatment of acne vulgaris. J Invest Dermatol 2000; 115:183–192.
7. Lloyd JR, Mirkov M. Selective photothermolysis of sebaceous glands for acne treatment. Laser Surg Med 2002; 31:115–120.
8. McInturff JE, Kim J. The role of toll-like receptors in the pathophysiology of acne. Semin Cutan Med Surg 2005; 24(2):73–78.
9. Belsito DV, Baer RL, Gigli I, Thorbecke GJ. Effect of combined topical glucocorticoids and ultraviolet B irradiation on epidermal Langerhans cells. J Invest Dermatol 1984; 83(5):347–351.
10. Omi T, Kawana S, Sato S, et al. Cutaneous immunological activation elicited by a low fluence pulsed dye laser. Br J Dermatol 2005; 153(suppl 2):57–62.
11. Seaton ED, Charakida A, Mouser PE, et al. Pulsed dye laser treatment for inflammatory acne vulgaris: randomized controlled trial. Lancet 2003; 362:1347–1352.
12. Orringer JS, Kang S, Hamilton T, et al. Treatment of acne vulgaris with a pulsed dye laser: a randomized controlled approach. JAMA 2004; 291:2834–2839.
13. Alexiades-Armenakas M. Long pulsed dye laser mediated photodynamic therapy combined with topical therapy for mild to severe comedonal, inflammatory or cystic acne. J Drugs Dermatol 2006; 5:1–11.
14. Weigell SR, Wulf HC. Photodynamic therapy of acne vulgaris using methyl aminolevulinate: a blinded, randomized, controlled trial. Br J Dermatol 2006; 154:969–976.

11 Benzoyl Peroxide and Salicylic Acid Therapy

Gabi Gross

Department of Research and Development, Reckitt Benckiser PLC, Hull, U.K.

INTRODUCTION

Nearly, everyone is affected by acne sometime in their lifetime. This is most prevalent among teenagers when, shortly after the onset of puberty, spots and blackheads start to appear. However, acne may continue or start in adulthood and, indeed, it is reported that an increasing number of people within this age group are affected by the condition (1).

When discussing acne, it is important to distinguish the varying degrees of severity of the disease because the selection of a therapeutic regime is dependent on this severity grading (Table 1). Pathophysiology and classification systems of acne have been described in detail in other chapters; however, before starting to discuss its therapy with benzoyl peroxide (BPO) and salicylic acid (SA), it is worth providing a brief overview of this in order to understand acne active selection.

Acne, or acne vulgaris, is a common disease of the pilosebaceous unit. The disease is localized to the skin regions such as face, back, and chest, where numerous pilosebaceous units are located. The pathogenesis of acne has not yet been fully established. Several factors contribute to the development of acne: increased sebum production (mainly influenced by hormones), ductal cornification, bacterial colonization of the pilosebaceous duct, and inflammation (2–5). *Propionibacterium acnes*, an anaerobic bacteria, is a member of the skin and pilosebaceous follicle microflora. It is thought to play a significant role in acne because it can proliferate within the obstructed duct, modifying the components of sebum and producing enzymes, including lipases, that increase fatty acids and, consequently, cause inflammation. Inflammatory events, however, occur as a consequence of the bacterial colonization and the subsequent reactions. Recent research revealed that inflammatory events could arise before or after hyperproliferative changes. There is evidence for vascular endothelial cell activation and involvement of inflammatory responses in the very earliest stages of acne lesion development (6). Whether a poor diet of excess chips or chocolate play a role in acne is rather questionable. Although this impact has been observed in individual cases, no scientific evidence has been provided up to now (2–5). Another factor that is often suspected to exacerbate acne is psychological stress. In the past, reports of the influence of emotional stress were mainly anecdotal. However, recently, a study revealed that changes in acne severity correlate highly with increasing stress, suggesting that emotional stress from external sources may have a significant influence on acne, which might be useful for understanding the pathophysiology of acne and its therapy (7).

Because of increased sebum production and ductal cornification, the so-called comedo clinically develops first. Depending on whether the comedo is open or closed determines whether they are called blackheads or whiteheads, respectively. If the comedo becomes inflamed, pustules, papules, or even nodules will develop, which are described as pimples or spots by most consumers.

TABLE 1 Grade of Acne and Its Therapy

Acne severity	Definition	Therapy
Mild-to-moderate acne	Predominantly noninflammatory lesions (comedones), few inflammatory lesions (papules, pustules), no scars	Cosmetic products and/or drug products; Potential actives: antibacterials, mainly BPO — Salicylic acid — Sulfur — Resorcinol
Moderate-to-severe acne	Predominantly inflammatory lesions (papules, pustules, few nodules), scars	Drug products that mostly require prescription by physician; Potential actives: BPO — Antibiotics, also in combination with BPO (topical and systemic: clindamycin, erythromycin, tetracycline) — Antiandrogens — Retinoids (tretinoin, adapalene, tazarotene) — Azelaic acid
Severe acne	Inflammatory lesions (papules, pustules), extensive nodules and cysts, scars	Drug products that require prescription by physician; Potential actives: Isotretinoin — Antiandrogens — Antibiotics (topical and systemic)

Abbreviation: BPO, benzoyl peroxide.
Source: Adapted from Ref. 7.

WHAT IS THE GOAL OF ACNE THERAPY?

The most important thing is to minimize or remedy the negative psychological effects caused by the disease and to prevent scar formation. This is achieved by removing existing lesions and preventing the formation of new ones (the existence of spots among acne sufferers might be due to psychological discomfort). But how can one get rid of spots? Based on the pathophysiology of acne, there are only few ways that a successful acne therapy can follow:

1. controlling increased sebum production/reducing excess sebum,
2. affecting the ductal cornification/hyperkeratinization,
3. acting on the bacteria that are deemed to be involved in acne pathophysiology,
4. reducing inflammation.

There are numerous substances available that provide one or more of the mentioned actions and are therefore effective in acne therapies. The choice of active, however, depends upon the severity of acne.

Table 1 shows that cosmetic acne products are only dedicated for mild-to-moderate acne. In general, they are predominantly used for dealing with mild acne lesions first or as accompanying skin care regime. More severe acne requires medical consultation and advice, and, in most of the cases, "stronger" actives that are available on prescription only.

TABLE 2 Selected Acne Products

Trade name	Primary ingredients
Benzoyl peroxide products	
Clean and Clear® Persa-Gel 10[a]	Benzoyl peroxide 10%
Clearasil® Maximum Strength Lotion[b]	Benzoyl peroxide 10%
Neutrogena® Clear Pore Mask[c]	Benzoyl peroxide 3.5%
PanOxyl® Acne Gel 10[d]	Benzoyl peroxide 10%
PanOxyl® W Emulsion[d]	Benzoyl peroxide 10%
Salicylic acid products	
Clean and Clear® Blackhead Clearing Astringent[a]	Salicylic acid 1%
Clean and Clear Blackhead Clearing Scrub[a]	Salicylic acid 2%
Clearasil® Acne Fighting Cleansing Wipes[b]	Salicylic acid 2%
Clearasil® 3-in-1 Acne Defense Cleanser[b]	Salicylic acid 2%
Neutrogena® Clear Pore Treatment[c]	Salicylic acid 2%

[a]Johnson and Johnson Corporation, New Jersey, U.S.A.
[b]Reckitt Benckiser, Inc., New Jersey, U.S.A.
[c]Neutrogena Corporation, California, U.S.A.
[d]Stiefel Laboratories, Inc., Florida, U.S.A.

This chapter focuses on two actives that are indicated for mild-to-moderate acne: BPO and SA. BPO and SA have been used for a long time in the treatment of various skin diseases. Over the last years, many acne ranges have been launched by many companies, consisting of cosmetics as well as over-the-counter (OTC) drugs that have included one of these actives, making use of their good reputation. Nowadays, many formats, including cleansing, treatment and care products, are available in the mass market, drugstores, or pharmacies (Table 2).

BENZOYL PEROXIDE
History
BPO, which is derived from a by-product of coal tar, was first used as a nonirritating oxidizing antiseptic by Loevenhart (8) in 1905. Subsequently, there was little dermatological interest in this compound and its main use was as a bleaching agent for flour. Lyon and Reynolds (9), in 1929, claimed that BPO promoted wound healing. In 1934, Peck and Chargin (10) described the use of topical BPO in sycosis vulgaris; and Leake (11), in 1942, claimed that BPO, when applied locally to wounds, acted as a long-lasting oxidizing antiseptic without any local irritant effects. In addition, healing was promoted and there was also a local anesthetic action relieving pain and local irritation.

Modern interest in BPO was stimulated by Pace in 1965, when BPO, combined with sulfur in a cream formulation, was first used in the treatment of acne vulgaris (12). Following this development, the pharmaceutical industry found a way of preparing stable lotions of BPO. Combination therapy was also developed using sulfur and chlorhydroxyquinoline. BPO was registered for the treatment of acne in the United States in 1960 and in Germany in 1974. Due to formulation stability issues, it did not become popular until the late 1970s, when much-improved products became available. More recent developments have included BPO in gels, creams, and wash bases.

Chemistry
A synonym for BPO is dibenzoyl peroxide. The empirical formula of BPO is $C_{14}H_{10}O_4$ (Fig. 1) The hydrous form of BPO is a white or granular powder with a

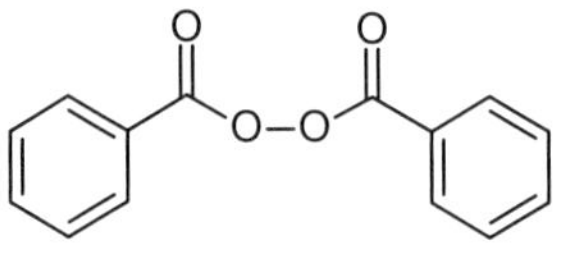

FIGURE 1   Chemical structure of benzoyl peroxide.

characteristic phenolic odor. It is practically insoluble to sparingly soluble in water, slightly to sparingly soluble in alcohol, and soluble in acetone, chloroform, and ether. It is a powerful oxidizing agent and is widely used in the industry as a catalyst and as a bleaching agent, for edible oils and flour (13,14). As BPO is heat-labile, stability is a major concern when developing new formulations. This issue, however, is discussed elsewhere.

Pharmacokinetic and Pharmacodynamic
What Happens with Benzoyl Peroxide After Application on the Skin?
BPO is well-absorbed into the stratum corneum and tends to concentrate in the pilosebaceous units (15). If an active can easily penetrate into the stratum corneum, the likelihood of systemic action increases. Therefore, it is important to know the absorption rate and metabolism of the drug in order to assess the safety. Using a bovine udder system, it was demonstrated that BPO, applied in an acetone vehicle, was absorbed by 22% after a topical application (16) and was converted within the skin layers mainly to benzoic acid (Fig. 2) (17,18).

The metabolite is then absorbed into the systemic circulation and rapidly excreted in urine, thereby circumventing hepatic conjugation. In vivo investigations with rhesus monkeys revealed that at in no time did the urine samples contain hippuric acid. Had any significant amount of the benzoic acid formed by the intracutaneous metabolism of BPO been circulated to the liver, it would have been conjugated with glycine and excreted as hippuric acid. This indicated that topical BPO should engender no systemic toxic effects due to drug accumulation since there would be no appreciable opportunity for either the drug, or its metabolites, to accumulate in body tissues or organs (18). In order to determine the penetration rate in human beings, in vivo investigations on patients with ulcus cruris were carried out. After application of a 20% BPO formulation, less than 5 µmol/L benzoic acid were detected in the serum and after three days no metabolite could be found (19). Transferring these results to acne therapy, a lower penetration rate could even be expected since the skin barrier in acne patients is normally not broken as in ulcus cruris patients and the applied concentration is much lower than the one used for antiseptic purpose.

Safety
As discussed in the earlier section, it is unlikely that BPO causes systemic adverse reactions or intoxications due to its rapid renal clearance. The main adverse reaction in acne therapy is the occurrence of skin irritation such as dryness, erythema, and scaling, which is dependent on the BPO concentration and vehicle base (20). A high BPO level and an alcoholic base, for example an alcoholic gel, has a higher associated irritation than low levels of BPO in an emulsion base. For instance. in order to avoid skin irritation, one should start with the lowest concentration and, having

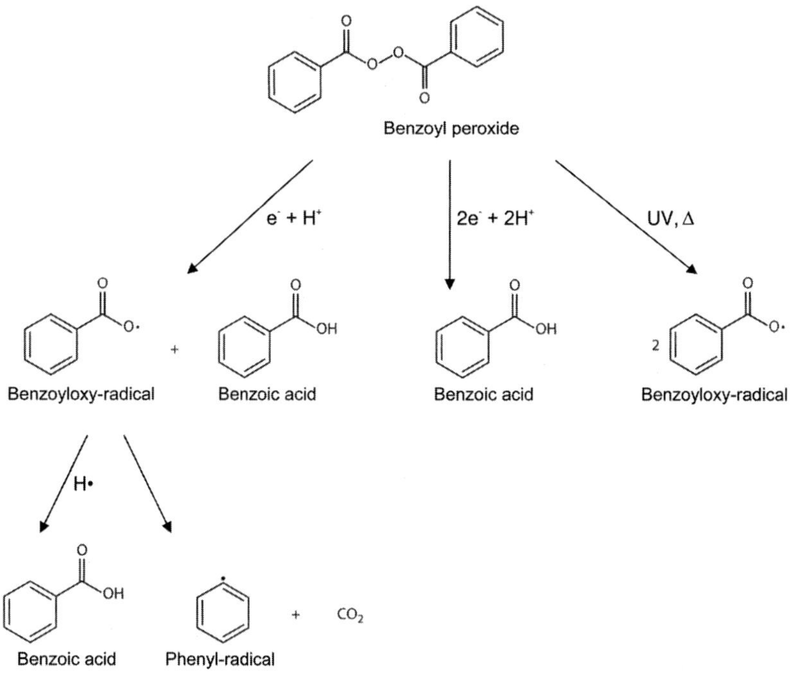

FIGURE 2 Metabolism of benzoyl peroxide in keratinocytes of SENCAR-mice. *Source*: Adapted from Ref. 18.

accustomed the skin to BPO, continue with increased strength formulations. In general, a lower strength or less frequent application of the preparation may reduce irritation. A further possible way of reducing irritation is through usage of BPO washes, where the contact time with the skin is limited to seconds. Consequently, the irritation potential may also be lessened.

Another noteworthy side effect that needs to be considered is contact sensitization that has been observed occasionally among acne patients during treatment with topical preparations of BPO (21). Under the guinea pig maximization test, which is designed for testing the contact allergenic potential of chemicals, 76% contact sensitization was observed. A high sensitization potential is observed during treatment of ulcus cruris; however, under the treatment of acne, the sensitization rate is disproportionally less. Numerous investigators have assessed the likelihood of sensitization after use of BPO in acne treatment and have found an incidence of less than 1/500 (22), which is not significant. (14,23).

It is also important to mention the data on toxicity of the active. Investigations regarding acute, subacute, and chronic toxicity demonstrated that toxicity could be regarded as harmless (24). Although BPO does not show toxicity, it is still considered to be a carcinogen. Over the last 30 years, many studies were conducted to evaluate the safety of BPO (in general, the results of epidemiology studies and animal carcinogenicity tests serve as important markers for cancer risk assessment). Epidemiology studies have provided evidence that its use to treat acne is not associated with any increased risk of skin cancer (25–27).

Furthermore, it was investigated in several studies whether BPO has complete carcinogenic potential, differentiated among complete carcinogenic activity, initiator activity, promotor activity, or progressor activity. Studies were conducted in mice, rats, and hamsters where BPO was administered by the oral, subcutaneous, and dermal route for up to 120 weeks duration. These studies revealed extensive data supporting the conclusion that BPO does not have complete carcinogenic activity (28). Two further studies revealed that BPO is not a tumor initiator (29). Contrary to this, tumor promotion was demonstrated in chemical-induced tumors in animal studies. This tumor promotion seems to be limited to chemical-induced tumors. There is no evidence that BPO promotes or enhances UV radiation-induced carcinogenesis (28,30). The human relevance of tumor promotor or progressor activities has not been established up to now. In contrast, the human relevance of initiating activity is more certain, because initiators are genotoxic carcinogens that are likely to pose a hazard to humans. BPO has, at most, a weak genotoxic potential in some in vitro systems, but this does not appear to be manifested in vivo based on a lack of initiating or complete carcinogenic activity.

Overall, based on the current data, the safety of BPO use in nonprescription acne medications can be supported (28,31). This is also confirmed by the American Academy of Dermatology and the German BGA-Monograph (32), where BPO is evaluated as safe and effective in acne therapy. However, it should be kept in mind that in order to obtain more data, further investigations are still going on. Because of its carcinogenic potential, the Food and Drug Administration (FDA) assigned BPO to the category III to OTC products, which means that more information is required to make a final determination on safety and efficacy of BPO for OTC use. Such drugs are on the market awaiting either the development of new data or for that drug's monograph to make its way through to the final rule (BPO is included in tentative monograph at the moment). Therefore, the safety of BPO needs to be carefully followed up until final results are available.

Efficacy and Use of Benzoyl Peroxide

BPO is still the gold standard for mild-to-moderate acne. It is the leading OTC antiacne agent (in the United States) and it is available in several formulation types including gels, creams, lotions, soap bars, and liquid cleansers, at a concentration ranging from 2.5% to 10% in strength.

Why Is Benzoyl Peroxide So Successful in Acne Therapy?

Antibacterial formulations that suppress *P. acnes* are a mainstay in the treatment of acne. As BPO's activity is primarily antibacterial against *P. acnes*, its use in acne therapy is corollary. The mechanism of action is presumably due to its strong oxidizing action, as explained further in Figure 2. The release of free radical oxygen causes oxidation of bacterial proteins and the development of oxygen creates a milieu in the follicle, where anaerobic bacteria like *P. acnes* cannot survive. The antibacterial efficacy is reported in a large body of literature (13,33–36) and is proven in numerous studies. BPO has a broad-spectrum activity and rapid bactericidal effects. It is active against gram-positive and gram-negative bacteria, yeasts, and various fungi (34). In vitro investigations using the agar diffusion method demonstrated strong antibacterial efficacy against gram-positive bacteria

(Table 3). The minimal inhibitory concentration (MIC) of BPO was found to be about 100 μg/mL (35,36).

In addition to this in vitro data, antibacterial action within the sebaceous follicle was also shown in vivo using the cyanoacrylate technique. After a seven-week treatment with a 5% BPO-gel, reduction of propionibacteria was demonstrated (37). Further studies have revealed a very fast antibacterial action that, however, does not increase with the continued use of BPO. After application of 5% BPO in an aqueous gel (daily use on the face), mean numbers of propionibacteria recovered from the skin surface and follicular casts were significantly reduced after two days of treatment. In the following days, the population was maintained, but no further decrease was observed (38). The same rapid effects could be observed in another study where the effect of BPO against *P. acnes* after only three days was proven, but no further decrease was observed at day 7 (39).

One major advantage of BPO over common antibiotics, used in acne therapy, is its full activity against antibiotic-resistant propionibacteria as well as sensitive strains (36). This might be due to its mechanism of antibacterial action, which is probably mediated by its powerful oxidizing property. This nonspecific mode of antibacterial action means that BPO does not induce resistance like antibiotics during long-term therapeutic use (38). Therefore, in order to preserve the efficacy of antibiotics in the therapy of acne, one obvious way could be to treat patients either concomitantly or sequentially with a broad-spectrum antibacterial agent such as BPO.

As acne is not only caused by bacterial colonization, efficacy of BPO against other factors is also of interest and has been investigated. One question is whether BPO has any impact on sebum production or secretion. It was found that BPO has a lack of direct effect on sebum production per se and does not reduce skin surface lipids, but it is effective in reducing the free fatty acids, known as comedogenic agents, and triggers of inflammation, in sebum. It inhibits hydrolysis of fatty esters and dramatically lowers the free fatty acid content in

TABLE 3 Inhibitory Efficacy of 5% Benzoyl Peroxide and Placebo Against Different Bacteria/Germs; Punched Hole 15 mm

Bacteria/germs	5% BPO inhibition zone in mm	Placebo[a] (without BPO and natrium lauryl sulfate) inhibition zone in mm
Staphylococcus aureus	18	—
Micrococcus epidermidis	18	—
Streptococcus faecalis	19	—
Sarcinen	18	—
Propionibacterium acnes HIK 07	32	—
P. acnes HIK 23 A	30	—
Escherichia coli	—	—
Proteus	—	—
Pseudomonas aeruginosa	—	—
Candida albicans	22	—

[a]The placebo preparation without BPO, but with natrium lauryl sulfate acts against the gram-positive bacteria *P. acnes* due to the content of 1.823% natrium lauryl sulfate.
Abbreviation: BPO, benzoyl peroxide.
Source: Adapted from Ref. 37.

sebum, concomitantly leading to an increase of triglycerides (Table 4) (37,40,41). This was also found in a further study (42). The same study revealed contrary results in the way that a sebo-suppressive effect was demonstrated by investigations on cell kinetics. A prolongation of the S-phase of sebaceous follicle cells and a diminution of the sebum glands were observed, which would be regarded as a direct sebo-suppressive effect and, therefore, the skin surface lipids would need to be reduced in consequence. As this, however, was not observed, the practical relevance of these data remains uncertain. Therefore, due to these contrary results, the impact of BPO on sebo-suppression in acne therapy is still under discussion.

Having discussed the questions of antibacterial and sebo-suppressive activity of BPO, it is still open whether BPO can also act against another factor of acne—the comedolytic activity. Before going on, it is necessary to define the terms comedolytic, keratolytic, or corneodesmolytic. Although these terms are often used for the same action, they are, strictly speaking, not identical. Comedolytic means lysis of a comedo caused by loosening of sticked corneocytes, whereas keratolytic is defined as lyses of superficial corneocytes, nails, or hair due to lyses of keratin. Corneodesmolytic is a newer terminology, which expresses nearly the same action, as it results in desquamation due to degradation of corneodesmosomes, which are proteinaceous complexes that effectively rivet corneocytes together. As a keratolytic action, however, can be defined as reducing cohesion between corneocytes in a broader sense, the terms comedolytic, corneodesmolytic, and keratolytic will be used for the same action from here on.

The keratolytic efficacy of BPO has widely been investigated in the past. On the one hand, this drug was considered to be moderately comedolytic in the rabbit ear model, whereas it looked rather inactive in the human assay. Using the rabbit ear model, which is used for comedonegicity assessment, BPO was shown to moderately reduce the development of comedones (24). Recent studies, using a new technique for quantifying the number and size of microcomedones, also demonstrated comedolytic activity of BPO (43). However, using the follicular biopsy technique, the anticomedogenic effect is only comparatively slight in contrast to tretinoin or SA (4,22). One explanation for this mismatch may reside in

TABLE 4 Thin-Layer Chromatographic and Densitometric Analysis of Skin Surface Lipids (Volunteers $n = 5$) Before and After Application of 5% Benzoyl Peroxide and Placebo (Half-Faced Comparison). Ratio of Triglycerides to Free Fatty Acids

Time	Verum (TG/FFS)	Placebo (TG/FFS)	Significance
Baseline	1.25	1.25	—
Day 4	1.87	2.15	ns
After 1 wk	2.01	1.46	ns
After 2 wk	3.11	2.39	ns
After 3 wk	5.57	1.76	$P \leq 0.1$
After 4 wk	9.02	2.14	$P \leq 0.05$
After 5 wk	12.08	2.27	$P \leq 0.02$
After 6 wk	14.59	2.61	$P \leq 0.1$
1 wk after treatment	7.60	1.86	ns

Abbreviations: FFS, free fatty acids; ns, not significant; TG, triglycerides.
Source: Adapted from Ref. 37.

the nature of comedones. In the follicular biopsy technique, native microcomedones were studied, which may well be different from the tar- or azetulen-induced comedones used in the rabbit studies (43). Overall, a weak comedolytic activity of BPO can be stated.

Another supplementary benefit of BPO in acne therapy is its anti-inflammatory action. BPO, however, does not have significant direct in vivo anti-inflammatory potency. It had been suggested that protein kinase C might serve as an additional pharmacological target of BPO. Therefore, the effects of BPO were investigated on the release of reactive oxygen species, regulated by protein kinase C and calmodulin, from human neutrophils, a potential important step in acne inflammation. Micromolar concentrations of BPO were found to inhibit the release of reactive oxygen species from human neutrophils but associated with a marked drug-induced cytotoxicity. When, in cell-free assays, the effects of BPO on protein kinase C and calmodulin as regulators of the release of reactive oxygen species were investigated, there was only a marginal inhibition of protein kinase C and no detectable inhibition of calmodulin. Thus, the inflammatory activity of BPO is unlikely to be mediated by protein kinase C or calmodulin (44,45). A potential explanation for the anti-inflammatory effects of BPO could be the mediation by the antibacterial or oxidizing action of BPO. Following the decrease in the population of *P. acnes* in the follicles and the reduction of free oxygen radicals, one source of inflammation is cut and therefore inflammatory reactions are suppressed (4,22).

The anti-inflammatory benefit of BPO, regardless of being direct or indirect, is reflected in several studies (37,46,47). BPO products are indicated for mild-to-moderate acne with occurrence of predominantly inflamed lesions.

One study tested gel formulations with different concentrations of BPO (3, 5, or 10%) depending on the skin condition. After four weeks of treatment, the different BPO formulations were proven to be effective in the treatment of moderate acne. BPO was shown to decrease the number of papules and pustules and, to a smaller degree, the number of comedones (48).

Interestingly, not only efficacy in mild-to-moderate acne but also a quick onset of action can be observed after BPO application, which accompanies the quick antibacterial action. A double-blind study showed that a 5% BPO lotion used topically for only five days significantly reduced the number of inflamed lesions (49). Since acne usually responds slowly to treatment, these results are very surprising. Another study also demonstrated the effect of short-duration treatment with a BPO aqueous gel. Compared to baseline, a statistically significant reduction of inflamed-lesions was determined after nine days and a reduction of noninflamed lesions after four days of treatment. Over the whole study period (28 days), improvement in the reduction of inflamed lesions could be observed (50).

Is There a Difference in Efficacy Between Various Benzoyl Peroxide Levels?
As mentioned earlier, BPO products are not only available in a variety of formulations such as gel, cleanser, or emulsion but also in a variety of concentrations. But is a higher level of active really more efficacious than a lower one? In general, one would expect superior efficacy from a product with the higher concentration. Surprisingly, a 2.5% gel formulation of BPO was proven to be equivalent in

reducing the number of inflammatory lesions to 5% or 10% BPO gel preparations. With respect to the side effects, however, a difference could be observed. Desquamation, erythema, and symptoms of burning with the 2.5% gel were less frequent than with the 10% preparation but equivalent to the 5% gel. The 2.5% formulation also significantly reduced *P. acnes* and the percentage of free fatty acids in the surface lipids after two weeks of topical application (51). So why are not the lowest strengths in favor? The answer is probably consumer psychology. Folklore has established the belief that products with higher levels of active are generally better and more efficacious than those with a lower concentration (52). Which preparation should be used then? In practical use, people with delicate or irritable skin should start with preparations of lower strength and, when this preparation is tolerated, can continue with higher strength formulations.

SALICYLIC ACID
History
SA can be regarded as an old-timer in acne therapy. Its benefits in treating skin disorders and other diseases have been known for generations. SA is a natural ingredient in numerous plants like the willow tree, sweet birch bark, wintergreen leaves, or chamomile flowers. The Romans knew of the efficacy of willow bark in treating ailments such as pain and fever, and the salicylic word in salicylic acid is derived from the Latin for willow, salix. For the first time, in 1838 the chemist Raffaele Piria succeeded in synthesizing Salicin from willow bark components. In 1860, Kolbe synthesized pure SA and proposed its use as a preservative and drug. Due to better tolerability of stomach, (SA is highly irritating to gastric mucosa if ingested orally, and therefore is used only as a topical agent), SA was enhanced and the derivate acetyl salicylic acid was born 30 years later (53). This well-established active, better known under the trade name of Aspirin® (Bayer Healthcare AG, Leverkusen, Germany), has been used systemically for pain relief and fever for over 100 years. For topical use, however, the pure acid is used for several skin disorders like acne, dandruff, psoriasis, or ichthyosis.

Chemistry
The systematic name for SA is a 2-hydroxybenzoic acid with the empirical formula $C_7H_6O_3$ (Fig. 3). It belongs to the group of hydroxyacids, which are carboxylic acids, classified into the α- and β-types according to their molecular structure (α-acids are the so-called fruit acids, whereas SA represents the only β-type).

SA is a white, odorless, crystalline powder, or occurs as white or colorless acicular crystals. It is slightly soluble in water and freely soluble in alcohol and ether (54).

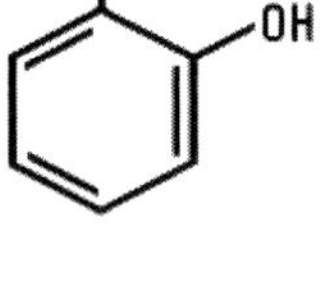

FIGURE 3   Chemical structure of salicylic acid.

Pharmacokinetic and Pharmacodynamic
What Does Happen to Salicylic Acid After Application of a Salicylic Acid-Containing Product to the Skin?

Numerous studies have demonstrated that following deposition onto the skin, SA will readily penetrate the stratum corneum and enter the systemic circulation (55). However, the nature of the vehicle influences both the rate and extent of absorption. For instance, a hydroalcoholic vehicle allows for a higher percutaneous absorption than a cream (56), and the addition of PEG 400 to aqueous solutions decreases the in vivo absorption. Ethanol has been shown to enhance penetration into guinea pig epidermis (57). It is the vehicle that influences the absorption rate. It also depends on the structure of the skin and skin hydration condition. A broken or weak skin barrier will allow higher penetration than a healthy one. For instance, SA absorption is significantly higher in psoriatic skin than in healthy skin. After application of 10% SA in vaseline, 40% SA of the applied amount was recovered in the urine of psoriatic people, whereas only 20% were recovered in people with healthy skin (58) (Table 5).

Besides the skin condition, the penetration or release rate also depends on the pH of the formulation. Using a membrane model, it could be demonstrated that penetration of SA increases with lower pH values (59).

In terms of penetration, it is also noteworthy that SA has the ability to build up a depot in the skin, specifically in the stratum corneum. It has been demonstrated that SA can be detected 13 days after the last application (60). Investigations on swine skin indicate that SA mainly penetrates through the transfollicular route (61), leading to the sebaceous follicle, the target site for delivery of SA, and other anti-acne drugs. This can be verified using the follicular biopsy technique where SA was shown to be delivered to the follicle (62). Having spoken about the penetration and the penetration way of SA, the next question arises about the distribution and metabolism. In contrast to BPO, SA is not metabolized within the skin, but absorbed unchanged. It is distributed in the extracellular spaces (150 mL/kg body weight) with maximum SA plasma levels occuring six to 12 hours after application. Patients with a contracted extracellular space due to dehydration or diuretics for example, have higher SA levels than those with a normal extracellular space. The extracellular space is smaller on a weight basis in infants and children, which suggests a basis for the relative increase in SA levels and intoxication in this group for a given dose. In this context, it is important to know that SA plasma levels absorbed percutaneously are additive with salicylates absorbed orally or rectally (57). In contrast to BPO metabolism, the metabolism of SA takes part in

TABLE 5 Total Body Application of 10% SA in Vaseline® on Psoriatic Skin and Healthy Skin

SA detection	Psoriatic skin	Healthy skin
Detection rate, mean value (%)	40	19
SA blood level, mean value (mg/L)	56	18
Detection after therapy start (hr)		
Plasma	2.0	9.5
Urine	4.5	13.5
Detection after therapy finish (hr)		
Plasma	16.1	5.8
Urine	30.3	19.0

Abbreviation: SA, salicylic acid.
Source: Adapted from Ref. 58.

the liver by conjugation with glycine to salicyluric acid, with glucuronic acid to etherglucuronide, and by hydroxylation to gentisinic acid and benzoic acid. The half-life of SA is about two or three hours if a normal dosage is used. However, if overdosed, or due to limited liver metabolism capacity, half-life could be prolonged to 15 to 30 hours, which should be considered when using SA containing products while suffering with liver diseases. About 65% to 85% of a topically administered SA dose is recoverable from the urine. Almost 95% of a single dose of SA is excreted within 24 hours of its entrance into the extracellular space.

Safety

SA is likely to cause some degree of local skin peeling and discomfort, such as burning or skin reddening, as it is a mild irritant (54,63). Beside this topical adverse event, one major adverse reaction is the potential intoxication caused by increased penetration of SA. Intoxication has been shown in patients with a damaged skin barrier who received a treatment on the whole body over several days (such as psoriatic or ichthyotic patients). This can be explained due to high penetration of SA through a damaged skin barrier. Clinically, the patients have thirst, tinnitus, headache, lethargy, confusion, nausea, vomiting, diaphoresis, depression, and disorientation (54,57). According to the opinion of the Scientific Committee on Cosmetic Products and Non-Food Products (SCCNFP), however, this event is rare and depends on various factors, such as the age of patient, the intensity of the skin damage, the concentration of SA in the formulation, or the surface of the application. Ointments containing 3% to 6% SA have caused nausea, dyspnoea, hearing loss, confusion, and hallucinations in three patients with extensive psoriasis. They had two soap and water baths daily combined with UV therapy and six ointment applications. Under these conditions, the symptoms developed in four days and were associated with significant SA plasma levels (46–64 mg/100 mL). Fortunately, the symptoms disappeared rapidly after discontinuation of the ointment applications (63). The application of SA to extensive areas, particularly in children, may involve a risk of toxicity from absorption. As discussed earlier, children are particularly susceptible (63). Having a greater proportion of body surface and weight, they are exposed to a higher risk of systemic effects during large surface treatment. However, the number of reported cases of intoxication of children is quite lower than one would expect. This could be due to the fact that the horny layer barrier of children over one year is nearly identical to the one of adults and therefore their skin has nearly the same absorption rates, or because SA formulations were only rarely used on infants and children.

As salicylate plasma levels can be indicative of SA intoxication, plasma levels should be measured first in case of any intoxication suspicion. Symptoms occur at a plasma level of 35 mg/100 mL or higher (63,64).

Overall, the correlation between body salicylate and clinical severity of the intoxication is poor. Severe manifestations are linked with diseased skin and multiple applications on large body areas of formulations containing high concentrations of SA (63). Therefore, to prevent a toxic reaction, three factors should be kept in mind: the quantity of SA used should not be excessive (repeated, large areas of the body), the available extracellular fluid volume should not be limited (smaller children, because their extracellular fluid volume is much smaller in comparison to the potential surface area available for treatment), and the ability to metabolize and excrete the absorbed medication should not be impaired (64).

In terms of safety, the question of sensitization potential is as important as the adverse topic reaction. In the past, there have been numerous discussions on the sensitization potential of SA. Studies and literature research reveal that only in rare cases a sensitization potential was detected (65). According to the SCCNFP, SA is also not classified as a sensitizer. The results of human repeated insult patch tests conducted with formulation up to 2% SA confirm that topical application does not cause skin sensitization. On the other hand, other scientists doubt the available data. Although there are many examples of positive patch tests, no example was found that fulfilled the operational definition of clinically relevant allergic contact dermatitis. Allergic contact dermatitis to SA in man probably remains unproven in their opinion (66). However, based on data and current thinking, SA can be regarded as not being a sensitizer, or at most a weak sensitizer.

Overall, the safety of SA can be taken as granted when considering the given precautions and contraindications. SCCNFP considers that SA is safe for "other uses" than as a preservative, at a concentration up to 2% for the leave-on and rinse-off cosmetic products, and at a concentration up to 3% for rinse-off hair products (63).

Efficacy and Use of Salicylic Acid

Keratolytics like SA are commonly used as first-line therapy in mild cases of acne because of their widespread availability OTC. SA is widely used as a topical therapeutic agent for a variety of skin diseases, including acne, psoriasis, dandruff, and ichthyosis. Concentrations of SA ranging from 0.5% to 10% have been recommended for acne, but the maximum strength allowed in nonprescription acne products in the United States is up to 2% by the FDA Final Acne Monograph. At higher concentrations up to 40%, SA is also used for wart and corn removal.

Why Does Salicylic Acid Have Such a Good Reputation in Acne?

As the microcomedone is believed to be the precursor to all acne lesions, it is logical to treat it with a comedolytic agent that will counteract the plugging of the follicles. SA is an effective drug for this due to its keratolytic activity. Although SA has long been used as a keratolytic agent, the mechanism of action remains unsolved. The action may occur due to the reduced cohesion between corneocytes, resulting in the shedding of epidermal cells, rather than "lysing" of keratin. This was investigated in numerous studies. In 1943, it was first claimed that SA acts by producing epidermal irritation, but there has been no substantiation of this finding (67). Further studies suggested that the keratolytic effect of SA consists of a reduction of intercellular stickiness, thereby reducing corneocyte adhesion. The so-called cementing substances are the site of action and not the stratum corneum itself (68–70). No damage of the living epidermis is caused by SA and it has been shown to cause no epidermal change beneath the stratum corneum (68). Furthermore, there is no evidence that it works by lysing keratin. Keratin is a tough fibrous protein that remains in the intracellular region and it is regarded as unlikely that agents that promote desquamation do so by attacking this material (71). SA has no effect on the mitotic activity of the normal epidermis (69) and therefore does not influence the disordered cornification itself.

While the mechanism of action of SA's main property remains uncertain, an additional action is well-established. Besides the keratolytic action of SA within the pilosebaceous unit, the value of the antibacterial action is often neglected. Since antibacterial colonization in the pore is deemed to be a main cause for spot formation, the use of antibacterials in acne treatment or prevention plays a major role, as discussed earlier.

The antibacterial action of SA against *P. acnes* has been demonstrated in both in vitro and in vivo studies. MIC was determined at 0.25% (w/w) using the plate method. In vivo measurement also reveals the efficacy of SA within the pore, expected as penetration occurs through the transfollicular root to the follicle (72–75). Having penetrated into the pore, SA can start to work and inhibit bacteria growth.

SA also offers anti-inflammatory benefits in acne therapy, which have been reported in the literature (73,74,76). Anti-inflammatory activity was investigated using the UV model (76). Upon topical application to the skin of guinea pigs with UV dermatitis, SA exerted a distinct anti-inflammatory effect, which was most pronounced at concentrations between 0.5% and 5%. Its integrated activity over the range of concentrations tested, that is, from 0.05% to 5% and over a period from 4 to 26 hours after irradiation, equals that of the contact antiphlogistic agent bufexamac, which is a well-established active in clinical use (76).

The anti-inflammatory effect of SA might be adjuvant in acting not only against non-inflammatory but also against inflammatory lesions. Many clinical studies have proven the anti-acne efficacy of SA-containing products (77,78).

For instance, one study demonstrated that twice daily application of 2% SA alcohol-detergent lotion impregnated into pads was significantly better than the placebo in the treatment of mild-to-moderate acne. Significant benefit from the active therapy was evident at four, eight, and 12 weeks when total lesion counts were assessed. Regarding noninflamed lesions superiority over placebo could be demonstrated after eight and 12 weeks and for inflamed lesions after 12 weeks. These results strengthen the suggestion that SA has a primary effect on comedogenesis. The observation that inflamed lesions were reduced at a later date could be explained by the fact that inflamed lesions arise from noninflamed lesions. Therefore, the efficacy against comedones will prevent the development of inflamed lesions, though this a lagged efficacy (77).

Another double-blind, controlled study evaluated the efficacy of 0.5% SA in an alcohol-detergent solution and placebo (pads soaked in buffered water). SA was shown to be more effective in reducing open and inflamed lesions than placebo (78).

Furthermore, efficacy has been proven in a comparative study with BPO, which will be discussed separately.

Is There Another Use for Salicylic Acid Other than in Anti-acne Cosmetics?

SA can also be used as a peeling agent in high concentrations. However, at these high levels of SA, irritation or other adverse events are very likely and therefore such peelings must be done under the supervision and strict control of a physician.

SA peels are available in 20% and 30% concentrations. In general, superficial chemical peels are an invaluable accoutrement for dermatologists when treating fine wrinkles, photoageing, keratoses, acne, and dyspigmentation. It could be shown that SA peels facilitated the clearing of pustules, papules, and comedones. Moderate-to-significant clearing of acne vulgaris was also demonstrated (79). A further study using 20% to 30% SA in a hydroethanolic vehicle demonstrated that SA is useful as a single or multiple peeling agent for acne as well as for photodamage and hyperpigmentation. SA as a peeling agent was useful for both comedonal and papular acne. Areas of intense inflammation showed decreased erythema, and pustules were rapidly dried at one or two days postpeel. Many closed and open comedones were extruded by several days postpeel (80). When applied under strict control and indication, the SA peels can be regarded as safe and efficacious, and offer adjunctive benefit when treating acne vulgaris.

Comparison of Benzoyl Peroxide and Salicylic Acid

BPO and SA are both indicated for use in mild-to-moderate acne, but their main action of mechanism is different. While BPO has a strong antibacterial action, SA acts through a keratolytic action. Does this different action have any impact on the efficacy of the products? Is BPO more effective against inflamed lesions while SA predominantly acts against noninflamed lesions? Comparative studies demonstrated similar efficacy of both products or even slight superior efficacy of SA.

In a four-week crossover study, the efficacy of a 2% SA acne cleanser was compared with that of 10% BPO wash in the treatment of 30 patients with mild-to-moderate acne. The results demonstrated that only patients treated with the SA cleanser had a significant reduction in the number of comedones. However, when patients crossed over to BPO, acne worsened over the following two weeks and the number of comedones slightly increased. In contrast, the number of comedones decreased in patients who first used BPO and then crossed over to SA. These results suggest that SA is more effective than BPO for the treatment of comedonal acne (81).

In another, 12-week double-blind study with 180 subjects, 2% SA, the vehicle solution, and a 5% BPO cream were compared. Surprisingly, SA was not only found to produce a substantially greater reduction from baseline in the number of comedones but also a reduction in inflammatory lesions when compared with 5% BPO (Fig. 4) (82).

The observed superiority of SA might be due to its mode of action. Since the primary lesion of acne is the microcomedo, a treatment that is effective in preventing its formation will be effective in preventing inflammatory lesions into which the microcomedo can progress. As the action of SA is mainly keratolytic, it interferes in an earlier stage than BPO, and in consequence it seems to be superior in acting against later steps, the inflamed lesions. When evaluating the results of these

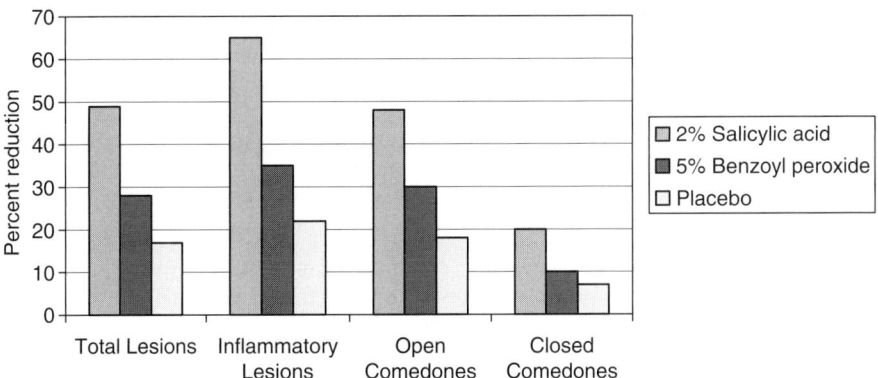

FIGURE 4 Percentage reductions in total number of lesions, inflammatory lesions, open comedones, and closed comedones in patients treated with salicylic acid, placebo, or benzoyl peroxide. *Source*: Adapted from Ref. 82.

TABLE 6 Comparison of Benzoyl Peroxide and Salicylic Acid

	Benzoyl peroxide	Salicylic acid
Antimicrobial	$++$	$(+)$
Keratolytic	$(+)$	$+$
Sebo-supressive	—	—
Concentration	2.5–10%	0.5–2%
Adverse effects	Skin irritation, bleaches hair and clothing	Skin irritation

Note: $++$, strong activity; $+$, moderate activity; $(+)$, weak activity; —, no activity.

studies, it is also important to consider the different bases of the formulations. In order to obtain comparable data, identical formulation bases would have needed to be used to avoid any impact or efficacy of the base itself. Taken as a whole, BPO and SA are expected to have a similar efficacy in the treatment of mild-to-moderate acne with slight superiority of SA against comedones (Table 6).

CONCLUSIONS

The mainstay of acne treatment, particularly for mild-to-moderate acne, is topical medication. Most cases of comedonal or papular acne can be controlled without systemic therapy. Several actives exist for acne therapy, some of them can be used in cosmetic products and some are only available by prescription.

Although there are numerous newer antiacne actives available with different mechanisms of action, the old-timers BPO and SA are still the gold standard in mild-to-moderate acne treatment, particularly for cosmetics or OTC drugs. They can be used as mono-therapy or combined with other acne products, in order to achieve better efficacy or better tolerability.

A comprehensive range of data shows that both actives have been well-established in dermatology. They are effective and safe for use in mild-to-moderate acne.

ACKNOWLEDGMENTS

The author would like to thank Nadine Selle, Carmen Matthies, Ed Owen, and Friedrich Wolf for their help in preparing this manuscript.

REFERENCES

1. Goulden V, Stables I, Cunliffe WJ. Prevalence of facial acne in adults. J Am Acad Dermatol 1999; 41:577–580.
2. Cunliffe WJ. Akne-Klinik, Differentialdiagnose, Pathogenese, Therapie. Stuttgart: Hippokrates Verlag GmbI I, 1993:250–251.
3. Plewig G, Kligman AM. Acne und Rosacea. 3rd ed. Springer, 2000:28–29.
4. Zouboulis CC. Moderne aknetherapie. Akt Dermatol 2003; 29:49–57.
5. Gollnick H, Cunliffe WJ. Management of Acne: a report from a global alliance to improve outcomes in acne. J Am Acad Dermatol 2003; 49:1–38.
6. Jeremy AHT, Holland DB, Roberts SG, et al. Inflammatory events are involved in acne lesion initiation. J Invest Dermatol 2003; 121(1):20–27.
7. Chiu A, Chon SY, Kimball AB. The response of skin disease to stress. Arch Dermatol 2003; 139:897–900.
8. Loevenhart CS. Benzoylperoxid, ein neues therapeutisches agens. Cited by Ther Mh. 1905; 12:426.

9. Lyon RA, Reynolds TE. Promotion of healing by benzoyl peroxide and other agents. Proc Soc Exp Biol Med 1929; 27(2):122–124.
10. Peck SM, Chargin L. Sycosis vulgaris: a new method of treatment. Arch Dermatol Sysp 1934; 29:456.
11. Leake CD. Advantages of benzoyl peroxide over zinc peroxide or sulfonamides in treating wounds or burns. JAMA 1942; 119:101.
12. Pace WE. A benzoyl peroxide-sulfur cream for acne vulgaris. Can Med Assoc J 1965; 93:252–254.
13. Sweetman SC. Martindale: The Complete Drug Reference: Benzoyl Peroxide. London-Chicago: Pharmaceutical Press, 2002:1111.
14. Cotterill JA. Benzoyl peroxide. Acta Derm Venereol 1980; 89:57–62.
15. Orth DS, Widjaja J, Wortzman MS. Benzoyl peroxide concentration in follicular casts. Cosmetics & Toiletries Magazin 1997; 112:87.
16. Kietzmann M, Löscher W, Arens D, et al. The isolated perfused bovine udder as an in vitro model of percutaneous drug absorption—skin viability and percutaneous absorption of dexamethasone, benzoyl peroxide and efonemate. J Pharmacol Toxicol Methods 1993; 30:75–84.
17. Binder RL, Aardema MJ, Thompson ED. Benzoyl peroxide: review of experimental carcinogenesis and human safety data. Prog Clin Biol Res 1995; 391:245–294.
18. Yeung D, Nacht S, Buchs D, et al. Benzoyl peroxide: percutaneous penetration and metabolic circulation. II Effect of concentration. J Am Acad Dermatol 1983; 6:920–924.
19. Holzmann H, Morsches R, Benes P. The absorption of benzoyl peroxide from leg ulcers. Arzneimittelforschung 1979; 29:1180–1183.
20. Brown SK, Shalita AR. Acne vulgaris. Lancet 1998; 351:1871–1876.
21. Poole RL, Griffith JF, MacMillan FSK. Experimental contact sensation with benzoyl peroxide. Arch Dermatol 1970; 102:635–639.
22. Gollnick H, Schramm M. Topical drug treatment in acne. Dermatology 1998; 196:119–125.
23. Bandmann HJ, Agathos M. Die posttherapeutische benzoylperoxid-kontaktallergie bei Ulcus cruris-patienten. Hautarzt 1985; 35:670–674.
24. Gloor M. Benzoylperoxid in der dermatologischen Lokaltherapie. Zentralbl Hautkr 1990; 157:1010–1015.
25. Hogan DJ, To T, Wilson ER, et al. A study of acne treatments as risk factors for skin cancer of the head and neck. Br J Dermatol, 1991; 125:343–348.
26. Hogan DJ, To T, Wilson ER. Drug and non-drug risk factors associated with facial skin cancer. A report to the Non-prescription Drug Manufacturers Association, Non-prescription Drug Manufacturers Association of Canada on the Saskatchewan Study, 1990.
27. To T, Hogan DJ, Wilson ER, et al. Benzoyl peroxide and facial skin cancer. Am J Epidermiol 1991; 134:772.
28. Binder RL, Aardema MJ, Thompson ED. Benzoyl peroxide: review of experimental carcinogenesis and human safety data. Prog Clin Biol Res 1995; 319:245–294.
29. Gloor M, Thoma K, Fluhr J. Benzoylperoxid (BPO) and Azelainsäure (AZ). In: Dermatologische Externatherapie. Berlin, Germany: Springer-Verlag, 1995:205.
30. King JK, Egner PA, Kensler TW. Generation of DNA base modification following treatment of cultured murine keratinocytes with benzoyl peroxide. Carcinogenesis 1996; 17(2):317–320.
31. Zbinden G. Scientific opinion on the carcinogenic risk due to topical administration of benzoyl peroxide for the treatment of acne vulgaris. Pharmacol Toxicol 1988; 63:307–309.
32. Benzoylperoxid. In: Aufbereitungsmonographien Kommission B7, BGA. PZ 1990; 27:1841–1842.
33. Beasley JN. Chemistry and metabolism of benzoyl peroxide and other antiacne drugs. Clin Res 1982; 30(3):698.
34. Kligman AM, Leyden JJ, Stewart R. New uses for benzoyl peroxide: a broad-spectrum antimicrobial agent. Int J Dermatol 1977; 16:413–417.
35. Patane AM, Pistillo M. Sull'azione antimicrobica del benzoilperossido. Ann Sclavo 1982; 24(5):513–522.
36. Farmery MR, Jones CE, Eady EA, et al. In vitro activity of azaleic acid, benzoyl peroxide and zinc acetata against antibiotic resistant propionibacteria from acne patients. J Dermatol Treat 1994; 5:63–65.

37. Puschmann M. Klinisch-experimentelle untersuchungen zum wirkungsnachweis von benzoylperoxid. Hautarzt 1982; 33:257–265.

38. Bojar RA, Holland KT, Cunliffe WJ. The in-vitro antimicrobial effects of azelaic acid upon Propionibacterium acnes strain P37. J Antimicrob Chemother 1991; 28(6):843–853.

39. Pagnoni A, Kligman AM, Kollias N, et al. Digital flourescence photography can assess the suppressive effect of benzoyl peroxide on Propionibacterium acnes. J Am Acad Dermatol 1999; 41(4):710–716.

40. Fulton JE, Farzad-Bakshandeh A, Bradley S. Studies on the mechanism of action of topical benzoyl peroxide and vitamin A acid in acne vulgaris. J Cutan Pathol 1974; 1:191–200.

41. Gloor M, Hummel A, Friedrich HC. Experimentelle untersuchungen zur Benzoylperoxidtherapie der acne vulgaris. Z Hautkr 1975; 50(15):657–663.

42. Wirth H, Spürgel D, Gloor M. Untersuchungen zur Wirkung von Benzoylperoxid auf die Talgdrüsensekretion. Dermatol Monatsschr 1983; 169:289–293.

43. Pierard GE, Peirard-Franchimont C, Goffin V. Digital image analysis of microcomedones. Dermatology 1995; 190:99–103.

44. Gollnick H, Krautheim A. Topical treatment in acne: current status and future aspects. Dermatology 2003; 206:29–36.

45. Hegemann L, Toso SM, Kitay K, et al. Anti-inflammatory actions of benzoyl peroxide: effects on the generation of reactive oxygen species by leucocytes and the activity of protein kinase C and calmodulin. Br J Dermatol 1994; 130(5):569–575.

46. Norris JFB, Hughes BR, Basey AJ, Cunliffe WJ. A comparison of the effectiveness of topical tetracycline, benzoyl-peroxide gel and oral oxytetracycline in the treatment of acne. Clin Exp Dermatol 1991; 16:31–33.

47. Lookingbill DP, Chalker DK, Lindholm JS, et al. Treatment of acne with a combination clindamycin/benzoyl peroxide gel compared with clindamycin gel, Benzoyl peroxide gel and vehicle gel: combined results of two double blind investigations. J Am Acad Dermatol 1997; 37:590–595.

48. Lassus A. Local treatment of acne. A clinical study and evaluation of the effect of different concentrations of benzoyl peroxide gel. Curr Med Res Opin 1981; 7:370–373.

49. Schutte H, Cunliffe WJ, Forster RA. The short-term effects of benzoyl peroxide lotion on the resolution of inflamed acne lesions. Br J Dermatol 1981; 106:91–94.

50. Bojar RA, Cunliffe WJ, Holland KT. The short-term treatment of acne vulgaris with benzoyl peroxide: effects on the surface and follicular cutaneous microflora. Br J Dermatol 1995; 132:204–208.

51. Mills OH, Kligman AM, Pochi P, et al. Comparing 2.5%, 5%, and 10% benzoyl peroxide on inflammatory acne vulgaris. Int J Dermatol 1986; 25(10):664–667.

52. Kligman AM. Acne vulgaris: tricks and treatments. Part II: the benzoyl peroxide saga. CUTIS 1995; 56(5):260–261.

53. Schmid-Wendtner MH. Salicylsäure. In: Korting HC, Sterry W, eds. Therapeutische Verfahren in der Dermatologie. Berlin: Blackwell Wissenschafts-Verlag Wien, 2001.

54. Sweetman SC. Martindale: The Complete Drug Reference: Salicylic Acid. London-Chicago: Pharmaceutical Press, 2002:1122–1123.

55. Taylor JR, Halprin KM. Percutaneous absorption of salicylic acid. Arch Dermatol 1975; 111:740–743.

56. Davis AP, Kraus AL, Thompson GA, et al. Percutaneous absorption of salicylic acid after repeated (14-day) in vivo administration on normal, acnegenic or aged human skin. J Pharm Sci 1997; 86(8):896–899.

57. Goldsmith LA. Salicylic acid. Int J Dermatol 1979; 18:32–36.

58. Arnold W, Trinnes F, Schroeder I. Zur hautresorption von salicylsäure bei psoriatikern und hautgesunden. Beitr Gerichtl Med 1979; 37:325–328.

59. Samuelov Y, Donbrow M, Friedman M. Effect of pH on salicylic acid permeation through ethyl cellulose PEG 4000 films. J Pharm Pharmacol 1979; 31:120–121.

60. Washitake M, Yajima T, Amno T, et al. Studies on percutaneous absorption of drugs. II Time course of cutaneous reservoir of drugs. Chem Pharm Bull 1972; 20:2429–2435.

61. Takahashi H, Ishii T, Tanabe K, et al. The percutaneous absorption of salicylic acid. J Dermatol 1976; 3:135–138.

62. Mills OH, Berger RS, Cardin C, et al. Analysis of salicylic acid levels in the sebaceous follicle. J Invest Dermatol 1995; 104(4):661–661.
63. Opinion of the scientific committee on cosmetic products and non-food products intended for consumers concerning Salicylic acid adopted by the SCCNFP during the 20th plenary meeting of 4 June 2002. SCCNFP/0522/01, final.
64. Lin AN, Nakatsui T. Salicylic acid revisited. Int J Dermatol 1998; 37:335–342.
65. Goh CL, Ng SK. Contact allergy to salicylic acid. Contact Dermatitis1986; 14:114.
66. Gallacher G, Hostynek JJ, Maibach HI. Salicylic acid: human allergic. Contact Dermatitis 1998; 46(3):129–130.
67. StrakoschEA. Studies on ointments. II. Ointments containing salicylic acid. Arch Dermatol Syphilol 1943; 47:16.
68. Huber C, Christophers E. "Keratolytic" effect of salicylic acid. Arch Dermatol Res 1977; 257(3):293–297.
69. Roberts DL, Marshall R, Marks R. Detection of the action of salicylic acid on the normal stratum corneum. Br J Dermatol 1980; 103:191–196.
70. Mills OH,Kligman AM. Assay of comedolytic activity in acne patients. Acta Derm Venereol 1983; 63:68–71.
71. Davies M, Marks R. Studies on the effect of salicylic acid on normal skin. Br J Dermatol 1976; 95:187–192.
72. Gloor M, Steinbacher M, Franke M. Über die antimikrobielle Wirkung der Salicylsäure auf die Propionibakterien im Talgdrüseninfundibulum bei der Lokalbehandlung der Acne vulgaris. Z Hautkr 1979; 54(19):856–860.
73. Gloor M, Wirth H, Schnyder UW. Pharmakologie der Salicylsäure bei topischer Applikation—eine Übersicht über die Literatur der letzten 20 Jahre. In: Hornmann OP, Schnyder UW, Schönfeld J, eds. Neue Entwicklungen in der Dermatologie. Berlin, Germany: Springer-Verlag, 1984:74–81.
74. Plewig G, Kligman AM. Exfoliants. In: Acne-Morphogenesis And Treatment. Berlin-Heidelberg-New York: Springer, 1975:277–279.
75. Hartmann AA, Hackel H, Elsner P, et al. Antibakterielle Wirkung der Salicylsäure—eine zu wenig beachtete Wirkung. Zbl Haut-GeschlKrankh 1990; 157:983.
76. Weirich EG, Longauer JK, Kirkwood AH. Dermatopharmacology of salicylic acid. Dermatologica 1979; 152:87–99.
77. Eady EA, Burke BM, Pulling K, et al. The benefit of 2% salicylic acid lotion in acne—a placebo-controlled study. J Dermatol Treat 1996; 7:93–96.
78. Shalita AR. Treatment of mild and moderate acne vulgaris with salicylic acid in an alcohol-detergent vehicle. CUTIS 1981; 28:556–561.
79. Grimes PE. The safety and efficacy of salicylic acid chemical peels in darker racial-ethnic groups. Dermatol Surg 1999; 25:18–22.
80. Kligman D, Kligman AM. Salicylic acid as a peeling agent for the treatment of acne. Cosmetic Dermatol 1997; 10:44–47.
81. Shalita AR. Comparison of a salicylic acid cleanser and a benzoyl peroxide wash in the treatment of acne vulgaris. Clin Ther 1989; 11(2):264–267.
82. Zander E, Weismann S. Treatment of acne vulgaris with salicylic acid pads. Clin Ther 1992; 14(2):247–253.

12 Treating Acne with Octadecenedioic Acid: Mechanism of Action, Skin Delivery, and Clinical Results

Johann W. Wiechers
JW Solutions, Gouda, The Netherlands

Anthony V. Rawlings
AVR Consulting Ltd., Northwich, Cheshire, U.K.

Nigel Lindner
Department of Research and Development, Uniqema, Gouda, The Netherlands

William J. Cunliffe
Department of Dermatology, Leeds Foundation for Dermatological Research, Leeds General Infirmary, Leeds, U.K.

INTRODUCTION

Acne is and will always remain a disturbing disease because it is highly visible as well as manifesting itself at an age when young teenagers are very concerned about their looks. However, to state that acne is only limited to adolescents (where males tend to show the more severe forms of the disease) is wrong, as especially postadolescent women are also affected by the disease (1). The primary cause of acne is an obstruction of the pilosebaceous canal. This is due to at least four pathogenic factors: (*i*) increased proliferation, cornification, and shedding of follicular epithelium (i.e., hyperkeratinization); (*ii*) increased sebum production (i.e., hyperseborrhea); (*iii*) colonization of the follicle with *Propionibacterium acnes* and *Staphylococcus aureus* (i.e., microbes); (*iv*) induction of inflammatory responses by bacterial antigens and cell signals (i.e., inflammation) (2). Earlier chapters of this book will have dealt extensively with these etiological and pathogenetical aspects of acne.

Topical treatments improving acne all affect one or more of these four main causes of acne (3). For instance, topical retinoids, of which tretinoin, isotretinoin, and adapalene are probably the most well-known examples, cause an expulsion of mature comedones, an inhibition of the formation and number of microcomedones, and an inhibition of inflammation. Benzoyl peroxide (BPO), erythromycin, clindamycin, and azelaic acid (AZA) are examples of topical antimicrobials and antibiotics, although due to the increasing development of bacterial resistance, the concentrations of the topical antibiotics clindamycin and erythromycin have been raised from 1% to 4%. AZA is a $C_{9:0}$ dicarboxylic acid with efficacy on follicular keratinization and on *P. acnes*. It seems to have some inflammatory efficacy via effects on neutrophilic granulocytes. It is used at very high concentrations (20%), although somewhat lower concentrations (15%) have recently also been shown to be effective (4). Salicylic acid, finally, has mainly a keratolytic effect. It has also a slight anti-inflammatory effect and is bacteriostatic and fungistatic at low concentrations by competitive inhibition of pantothenic acid, which is important for micro-organisms (3).

Very recently, advances in fundamental sebaceous gland research have suggested that the peroxisome proliferator-activated receptor (PPAR) might also be implicated in sebogenesis (5). PPARs are members of the nuclear hormone receptor superfamily and have been shown to be important in the regulation and catabolism of dietary fats (6), stimulation of epidermal differentiation (7,8), reduction in inflammation (9,10), and reduction in melanocyte proliferation (11,12). These activities are regulated through one or more of the three isoforms of PPARs: PPARα, PPARδ, and PPARγ. In human skin, epidermal differentiation is predominantly regulated by PPARα and to a lesser extent by PPARδ, inflammation by PPARα and some PPARγ, and melanocyte proliferation mainly via PPARγ. Using human chest sebaceous glands as seven-day cultured whole organs, Downie et al. were able to demonstrate that activators of PPARα and PPARγ inhibited the rate of sebaceous lipogenesis and reduced the synthesis of the sebum-specific lipids squalane and triacylglycerol in human sebaceous glands. They concluded that, "As suppression of sebum secretion is associated with reduced acne activity, the nuclear hormone receptors involved may open new avenues in the development of novel acne treatments" (5).

The $C_{18:1}$ dicarboxylic acid octadecenedioic acid (DCA) was recently developed as a novel building block for synthetic polymers. But the resulting polymers did not have the desired novel properties and the molecule was, therefore, tested for its antimicrobial activity against *P. acnes* because of its structural similarity to AZA. When it was found to be more active than AZA, formulations were developed with which clinical trials were performed to assess its clinical activity. Activity against acne could be demonstrated. At a later date, DCA was found to be a pan-PPAR agonist with a preference for PPARγ (13). In this chapter, the antimicrobial efficacy tests, the skin delivery of DCA-containing formulations, the results of two clinical trials, and the binding experiments to PPAR will be described, wherever possible compared with AZA. Finally, based on all the evidence collected, a rationale for the mechanism of DCA as a novel topical acne treatment as suggested by Downie et al. (5) will be presented.

OCTADECENEDIOIC ACID

DCA is the dicarboxylic version of oleic acid. Its structural formula is given in Figure 1. It cannot be made by traditional oxidative chemistry because of the presence of the double bond in the middle of the molecule, but is made via biotransformation. Normal yeasts rely on glucose and hydrocarbons such as alkanes, fatty acids, and triglycerides for their energy consumption. The hydrocarbons are taken up into the microsomes within the cells and oxidized on one end to form a fatty acid and then at the other end to form a dicarboxylic acid, generally known as dioic acid. These dioic acids are excreted from the microsome and taken up in

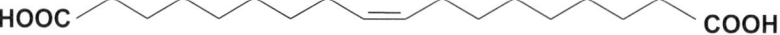

HOOC ⌒⌒⌒⌒⌒⌒ ═ ⌒⌒⌒⌒⌒ **COOH**

FIGURE 1 Structural formula of octadecenedioic acid.

the peroxisome in which β-oxidation takes place, yielding acetyl-CoA. This acetyl-CoA is transferred to the mitochondria in which it is inserted into the tricarboxylic acid cycle, yielding water, carbon dioxide, and energy in the form of ATP (Fig. 2A). A natural mutant of this specific yeast was identified, which follows the earlier-described biological pathway but in which the peroxisome is inactive. This yeast

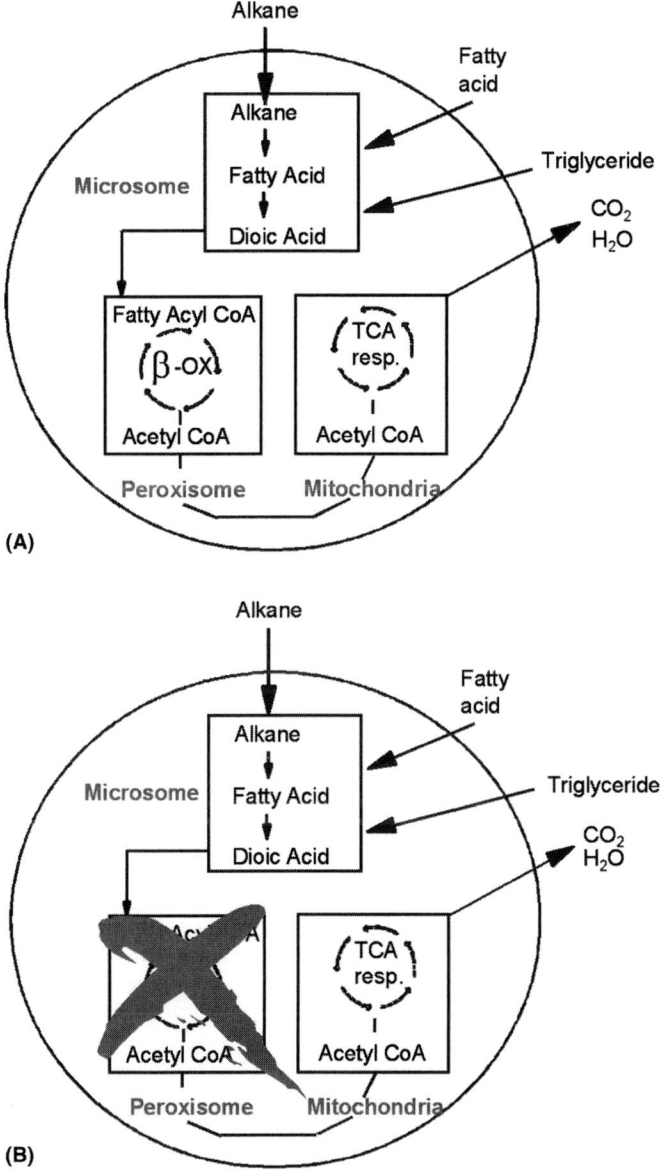

FIGURE 2 General biochemical pathways in normal yeasts (**A**) and specific mutant yeasts (**B**). *Abbreviation*: TCA, tricarboxylic acid.

will start the bioconversion of alkanes, fatty acids, and triglycerides, but cannot produce beyond the dicarboxylic acid phase (Fig. 2B). Such natural mutants can survive in nature because they can still obtain their energy via the conversion of glucose. When one feeds this natural mutant with only a very small amount of glucose to prevent it from dying and a relatively large amount of oleic acid as the fatty acid, it will convert oleic acid to DCA.

Because oleic acid is a natural product with its own distribution of chain lengths, DCA will also, similar to all other oleochemicals, have its own typical chain length distribution. DCA consists predominantly of $C_{18:1}$, $C_{18:2}$, and some C_{16} dicarboxylic acids. It is a solid with a melting point of approximately 64 to 68°C, typically in the form of flakes of a yellowish-white color. The chemical has a limited solubility in lipids such as hexane, an even lower aqueous solubility but a reasonable solubility in polar lipids such as ethyl acetate and acetone. Adding polar lipids such as propylene glycol and dipropylene glycol can enhance its solubility in aqueous media, whereas cosmetic emollients such as isostearyl alcohol and propylene glycol isostearate are typically used to dissolve it in the oil phase of formulations.

MINIMUM INHIBITORY CONCENTRATION TESTS AGAINST *PROPIONIBACTERIUM ACNES* AND *STAPHYLOCOCCUS AUREUS* USING OCTADECENEDIOIC ACID AND AZELAIC ACID

An AZA solution at pH 7.0 was added to Tryptic Soy Broth (TSB) (Baltimore Biological Laboratories, Cockeysville, Maryland, U.S.A.) at the corresponding pH to give a series of doubling agar plate dilutions ranging from 0.2 to 25 mg/mL (0.02%–2.5%). A DCA solution at pH 7.0 was similarly added to TSB agar to give the same plate dilutions.

Agar plates containing doubling dilutions of AZA or DCA, both at pH 7.0, were multipoint inoculated with 1 µL portions of bacterial cultures of *P. acnes* (ATCC 6919 and 29399), *S. aureus* (ATCC 25923 and 35556 and 29213), and *S. epidermidis* (ATCC 35859 and 31432 and 14490) at 10^4 cfu per spot. Plates were incubated at 35°C for 24 hours. Plates inoculated with *P. acnes* strains were incubated under anaerobic conditions for seven days at 35°C. The test compound-free control plates were examined at the end of the incubation for viability and signs of contamination. End-point minimum inhibitory concentration (MIC) values were determined by observing the plate containing the lowest concentration of agent that inhibited visible micro-organism growth.

The results of these experiments are summarized in Table 1. It can be clearly seen that DCA was very effective against *P. acnes* as well as *S. aureus* and *S. epidermidis*. Against *P. acnes* and *S. aureus*, DCA was more than 50-fold more active than

TABLE 1 The Minimum Inhibitory Concentration of Azelaic Acid and Octadecenedioic Acid Expressed as Percentage (% w/v) and Concentrations (mM)

Micro-organism	AZA		DCA		Ratio AZA/DCA
	%	mM	%	mM	
Propionibacterium acnes	1.25	66	0.04	1.3	52
Staphylococcus aureus	2.50	133	0.07	2.2	59
Staphylococcus epidermidis	>2.50	>133	0.31	9.9	>13

Note: The ratio of the molar concentrations (AZA/DCA) is also given.
Abbreviations: AZA, azelaic acid; DCA, octadecenedioic acid.

AZA when compared on a molar basis. Because *P. acnes* is often named to be the main causative microbial agent of acne, efficacy against this organism indicates a potential usefulness in the prevention and treatment for acne. Therefore, formulations containing AZA and DCA were prepared, which were—prior to clinical testing—studied for the skin delivery of the active ingredient.

SKIN DELIVERY OF DIFFERENT FORMULATIONS CONTAINING EITHER OCTADECENEDIOIC ACID OR AZELAIC ACID

The delivery of a functional ingredient from a topical formulation to its target site on or within skin is a crucial factor in obtaining in vivo efficacy. Skin penetration experiments were therefore performed on formulations containing either DCA or AZA. Three formulations were studied: an aqueous gel containing 10% w/w DCA, an aqueous gel containing 10% w/w AZA, and a commercial oil-in-water preparation Skinoren® (Schering, Berlin, Germany) containing 20% w/w AZA. All formulations were spiked with small quantities of radiolabeled material, either DCA or AZA. Skin penetration experiments were performed for 20 hours using Bronaugh flow-through cells (14) and pig skin dermatomed to a thickness of approximately 500 μm as the model membrane. At the end of the application time, nonpenetrated material was carefully removed, each cell dismantled, and the epidermal side of the skin membranes tape-stripped five times. The remainder of the skin was digested and counted for radioactivity. Receptor fluid collected throughout the 20-hours application period was also analyzed for radioactivity.

Figure 3 illustrates the skin delivery of the active ingredients from the three formulations. It should be noted that skin permeabilities are often log-normally distributed (15,16). Therefore, natural logarithms of each data point were taken and statistical analyses (mean values and 95% confidence limits, i.e., standard deviation)

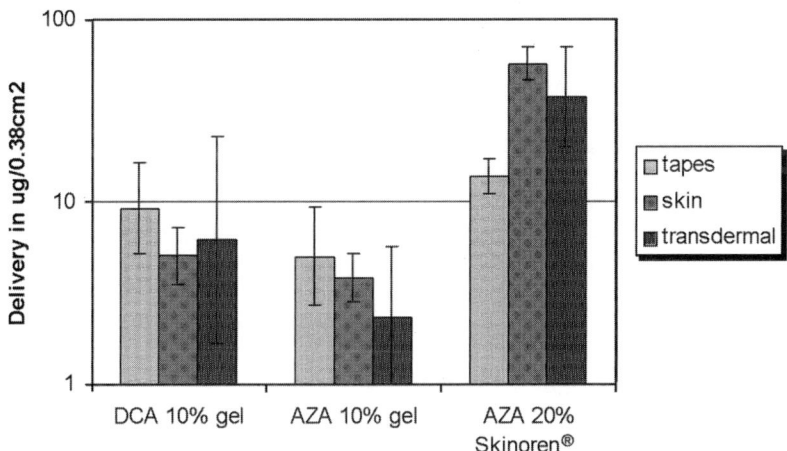

FIGURE 3 In vitro skin delivery of octadecenedioic acid and azelaic acid from aqueous gels (at 10%) or a commercially available o/w emulsion (at 20%). The data are presented as geometric mean values of absolute amounts (micrograms) delivered into and through the skin surface area available for diffusion (0.38 cm²). Please note the logarithmic Y-scale, which is necessary because of the log normal distribution of these data. *Abbreviations*: AZA, azelaic acid; DCA, octadecenedioic acid.

performed on the transformed data. This is the reason why the data in Figure 3 are presented on a logarithmic scale. Geometric mean values, which are listed in Table 2, were calculated by back transformation of the logarithmic mean values.

As was to be expected, the delivery of AZA from the marketed anti-acne preparation was by far the best. Not only did it show the highest penetration of the three formulations (absolute delivery expressed as $\mu g/0.38 \text{ cm}^2$), it also delivered more than half of the delivered AZA to the skin fraction, which is the fraction in human skin where the sebaceous glands are located. Both aqueous gels containing either DCA or AZA at 10% w/w showed a substantial lower absolute delivery. The relative distribution profiles of the two active ingredients from the three formulations were not that different (Table 2), although a relatively higher percentage of DCA penetrated transdermally (30.3% vs. 20.6% for DCA and AZA, respectively). The subdivision in deposition of delivered material in tape strips, skin, and transdermal, however, was not precise enough to predict the in vivo efficacy of these gels. Therefore, additional autoradiography experiments were performed in which skin sections were cut perpendicular to the skin surface and placed onto microscopy slides coated with photographic emulsions and left for 7 to 14 days before processing the skin sample for histological staining.

The distribution of the radiolabeled DCA and AZA was only somewhat different. For all formulations, the silver grains were concentrated at the skin surface and the stratum corneum (Fig. 4), in line with skin-delivery data presented in Table 2 and Figure 3. All three formulations showed active ingredient to be present in the upper part of some follicles, especially the infundibulum. There was no penetrant visible deep in the follicle in any of the sections viewed. It should be noted that the heavy graining adjacent to the stratum corneum, rather than directly over it, is the result of the cryostat sections which are not prefixed and shrink during staining. The only real difference in skin deposition between the two penetrants was the fact that silver grains were more evident in the viable epidermis when using AZA (Fig. 4D and H) than when DCA was the penetrant (Fig. 4F). DCA appeared to be associated only with stratum corneum and hair follicles. This can be explained by the relative higher water solubility of AZA and hence a higher solubility in the viable epidermis/dermis.

Bojar et al. (17) found the transfollicular delivery of AZA from a 20% cream to be comparable with the concentration required to inhibit the in vitro growth of *P. acnes* and *S. epidermidis* (17). In the experiments described earlier, we could confirm the transfollicular delivery of AZA (Fig. 5). DCA was more active than AZA in inhibiting the in vitro growth of *P. acnes* and *S. epidermidis* (see earlier), suggesting that lower concentrations of this lipophilic molecule would need to be transfollicularly delivered. In addition, recent transfollicular delivery research indicated that delivery to the hair follicle is improved by increasing the lipophilicity of the penetrating molecule (18,19). Relative to AZA, DCA combines a higher antimicrobial activity with a preference for transfollicular delivery. The logical next step, therefore, was to perform in vivo clinical studies.

PHASE I CLINICAL TRIAL USING OCTADECENEDIOIC ACID, AZELAIC ACID, AND BENZOYL PEROXIDE

When new chemical entities are tested on human skin, it is advisable to first conduct studies on healthy volunteers (so-called Phase I trials) prior to conducting

TABLE 2 Skin Delivery of Octadecenedioic Acid or Azelaic Acid to the Superficial Layers of the Stratum Corneum (Tapes), the Remainder of Skin (Skin), or the Receptor Fluid (Transdermal) Following Application of Three Different Formulations on Dermatomed Pig Skin in In Vitro Bronaugh Flow-Through Cells

Parameter	DCA 10% in an aqueous gel formulation		AZA 10% in an aqueous gel formulation		AZA 20% in Skinoren®, an o/w-formulation	
	Absolute delivery	Relative delivery	Absolute delivery	Relative delivery	Absolute delivery	Relative delivery
Number of cells	9		12		12	
Tapes (n = 5)	9.25	45.1	5.04	44.9	13.9	12.8
Skin (~500 µm)	5.06	24.6	3.87	34.5	57.4	52.8
Transdermal (in 20 hours)	6.22	30.3	2.31	20.6	37.4	34.4
Total delivery	20.53	100	11.23	100	108.61	100
Recovery (%)	87.9		108.6		90.1	

Note: Data are presented as geometric means of absolute amounts delivered in micrograms per 0.38 cm^2, which is the skin surface area exposed to the formulation in the penetration cell.

Abbreviations: AZA, azelaic acid; DCA, octadecenedioic acid.

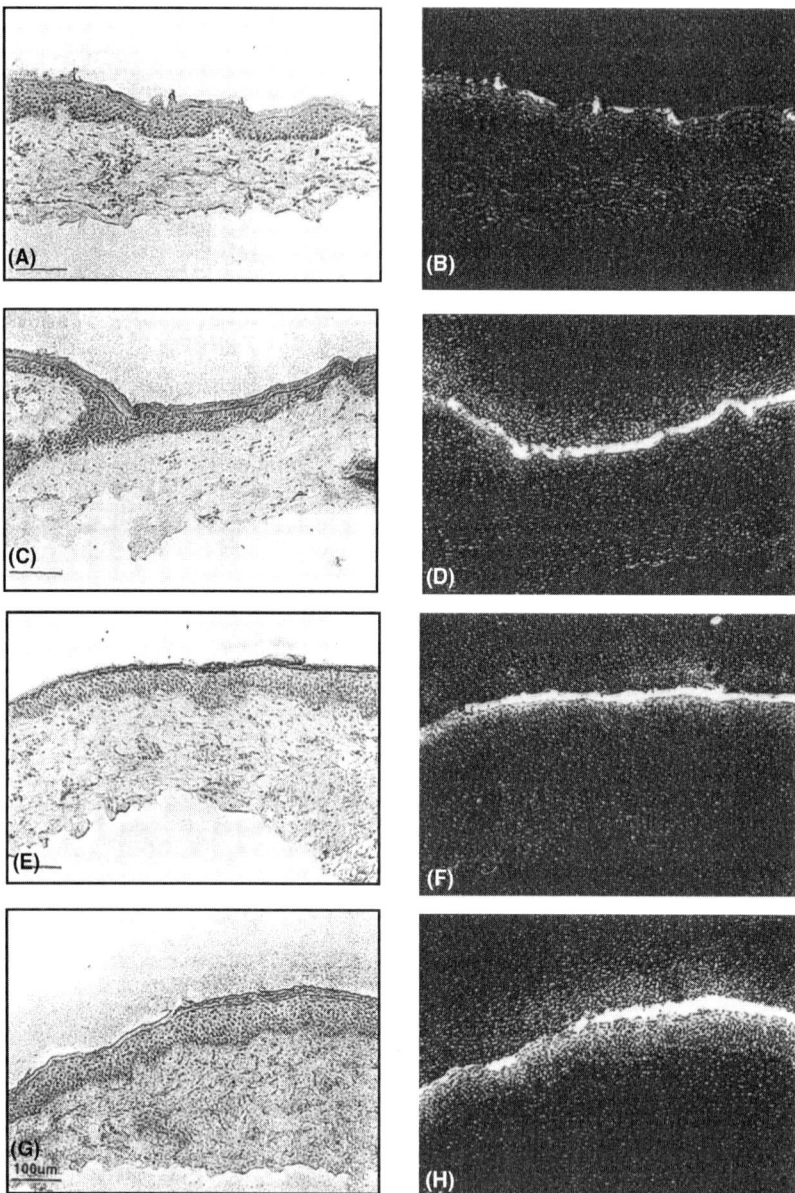

FIGURE 4 (*See color insert.*) Autoradiography of octadecenedioic acid and azelaic acid following penetration through dermatomed pig skin for 20 hours. Images show transverse sections through the upper layers of skin treated with different formulations: untreated control (**A** and **B**); Skinoren® containing 20% azelaic acid (**C** and **D**); a gel containing 10% octadecenedioic acid (**E** and **F**); a gel containing 10% azelaic acid (**G** and **H**). Stratum corneum, epidermis, and upper dermis can be seen. Bright field (**A**, **C**, **E**, and **G**) and dark field (**B**, **D**, **F**, and **H**) images were obtained using a Leitz DMRB light microscope (Leica, Milton Keynes, U.K.). The bright reflectance in each dark field picture is the stratum corneum. The scale bar in all bright field images represents 100 μm.

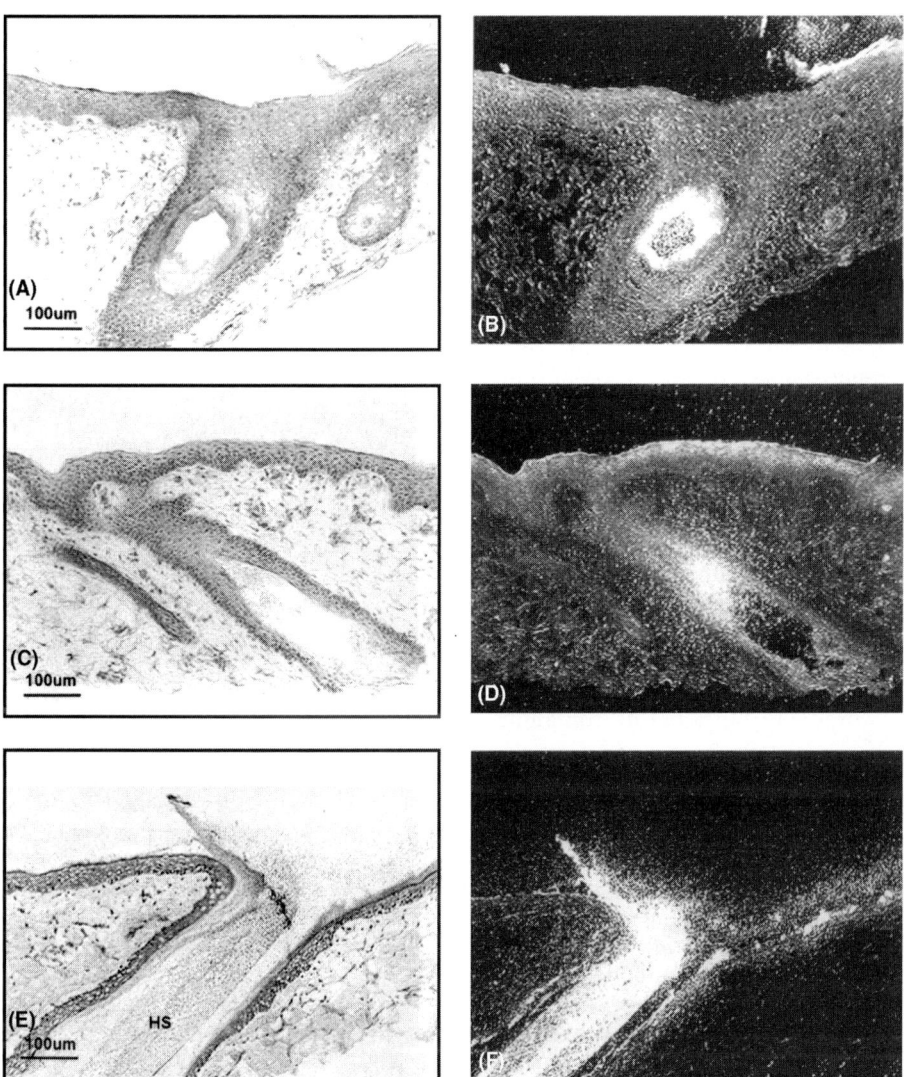

FIGURE 5 (*See color insert.*) Examples of follicular delivery following skin penetration of octadecenedioic acid from an aqueous gel containing 10% w/w octadecenedioic acid (**A** and **B**), azelaic acid from an aqueous gel containing 10% azelaic acid (**C** and **D**), and Skinoren® containing 20% azelaic acid (**E** and **F**). Images show transverse sections through the upper layers of the skin. Bright field (**A**, **C**, and **E**) and dark field (**B**, **D**, and **F**) images were obtained using a Leitz DMRB light microscope (Leica, Milton Keynes, U.K.). The bright reflectance in each dark field picture is the stratum corneum and the infundibulum. Note that the stratum corneum in (**A**) and (**B**) has been predominantly lost from this section. The scale bar in all bright field images represents 100 μm.

studies on the intended product-user population. However, this has consequences for the type of measurements that one can undertake. The objective of this Phase I trial was to compare the in vivo antimicrobial activity of topically applied DCA with that of AZA and BPO. Because acne lesions cannot be measured on healthy volunteers, the basis of this trial was to measure changes in the skin surface micro-flora count (Micrococcaceae and Propionibacteria) and skin-surface free fatty acid (FFA) levels on the faces of healthy volunteers as an indicator of potential anti-acne activity. The trial was performed as a double-blind study.

A group of 59 volunteers (37 male, 22 female) aged 16 to 35 were recruited into the study. All volunteers were medically screened to ensure their suitability to undertake the study. Their willingness to participate was documented through the completion of an informed consent form in the presence of medical staff.

Baseline levels of viable propionibacteria on the surface of the skin on the right cheek of each volunteer were determined seven days prior to commencement of the trial. The volunteers were assigned to one of five groups, as determined by previsit numbers of skin surface propionibacteria, so that each group had a similar statistical distribution of numbers of viable propionibacteria:

1. The first group ($n = 12$) received the aqueous gel containing 10% w/w DCA, which was also investigated for skin delivery.
2. The second group ($n = 12$) received the same aqueous gel formulation without the DCA (placebo).
3. The formulation of the third group ($n = 12$) was the same aqueous gel again, but this time with 10% w/w AZA.
4. The fourth group ($n = 12$) received "Panoxyl Aquagel 5," a commercially available product containing 5% BPO (Stiefel Laboratories, High Wycombe, Bucks, U.K.).
5. The fifth group ($n = 11$), finally, received Skinoren®, the commercially available product from Schering containing 20% AZA.

All volunteers were provided with a non-antimicrobial soap and instructed to wash the whole face twice daily prior to application of treatment products. Each volunteer applied one of the products to the test site (right-hand side of the face including forehead, just beyond the midline, cheek, and chin, avoiding the eyes, nostrils, and mouth) for the 21 days of duration of the trial.

The surface microbial populations (Micrococcaceae and Propionibacteria) were enumerated on the right cheek at baseline and after 3, 7, 14, and 21 days of treatment. Sebum was collected from each volunteer at baseline and after 7, 14, and 21 days of treatment, and the FFA content was determined by gas–liquid chromatography. Volunteers were also asked to maintain a daily diary and note any positive or negative effects of the treatment. Data were analyzed using parametric and nonparametric statistical tests.

The main findings of the study were as follows:

1. Of the 59 volunteers recruited into the study, only six individuals failed to complete the study (10.2% drop-out rate). The dropouts were evenly spread over the treatment groups, and there was no evidence that adverse reactions to any one treatment were responsible for noncompletion. Only those volunteers who completed the treatment were included in the subsequent statistical analysis of the results.
2. All preparations containing dicarboxylic acids (both AZA and DCA) were well tolerated. In the BPO-treated group, 92% of volunteers reported adverse events (irritancy and drying of the skin). However, the volunteers in this group were able to maintain the stipulated treatment regime throughout the study, although some were advised to use a moisturizing lotion.
3. None of the treatment regimes had any detectable effect on skin surface FFAs.

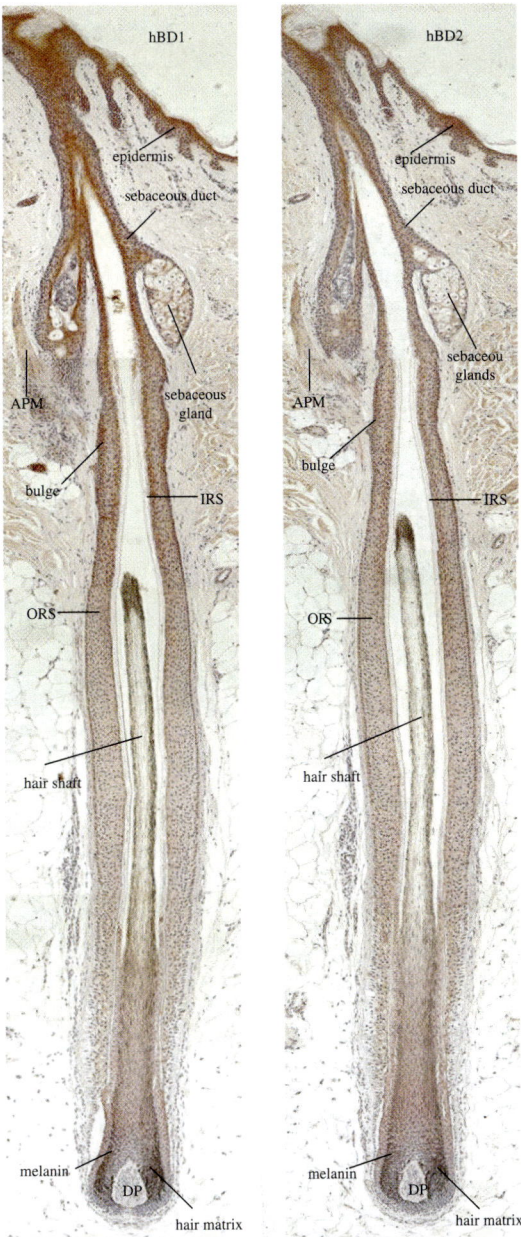

FIGURE 6.1 Human beta-defensin 1 (hBD1) and hBD2 immunoreactivity in human hair follicles. hBD1 (**A**) and hBD2 (**B**) immunoreactivity is found in the suprabasal layers of the epidermis and the distal outer root sheath (ORS) of the hair follicle. Strong basal expression is seen in the bulge area, which contains a population of epidermal stem cells. Strong β-defensin expression is also found in the sebaceous gland and duct. Weaker expression is present in the suprabasal layers of the central and proximal ORS and in the proximal inner root sheath. hBD1 and hBD2 IR are not detected in the hair matrix or the dermal papilla. *Abbreviations*: APM, arrector pili muscle; DP, dermal papilla; IRS, inner root sheath; ORS, outer root sheath. *Source*: From Ref. 9.

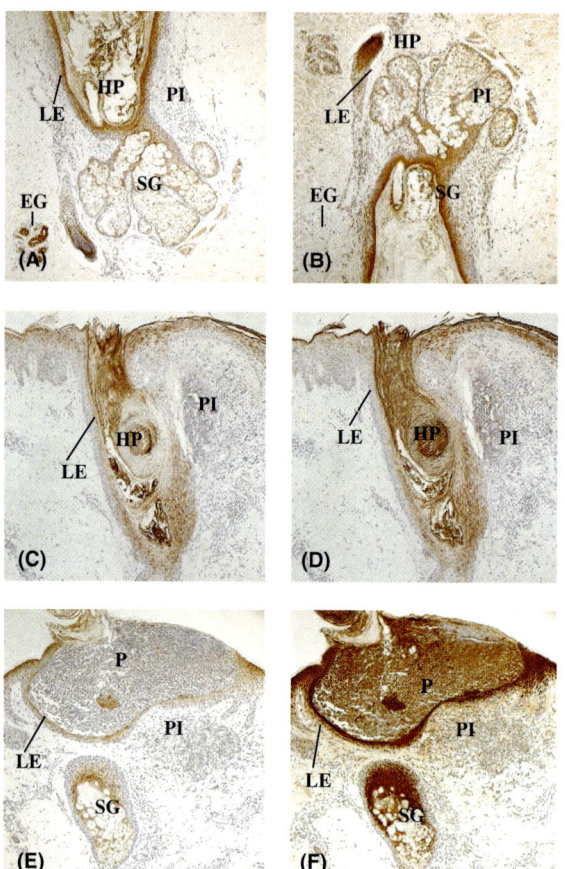

FIGURE 6.2 Human beta-defensin 1 (hBD1) and hBD2 immunoreactivity in acne lesions. (*See p. 79.*)

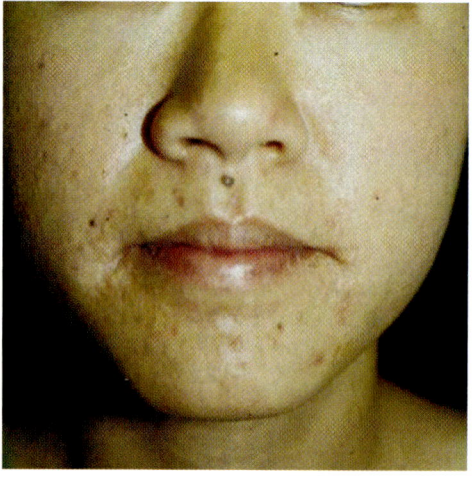

FIGURE 7.2 Adult female with acne of the lower face.

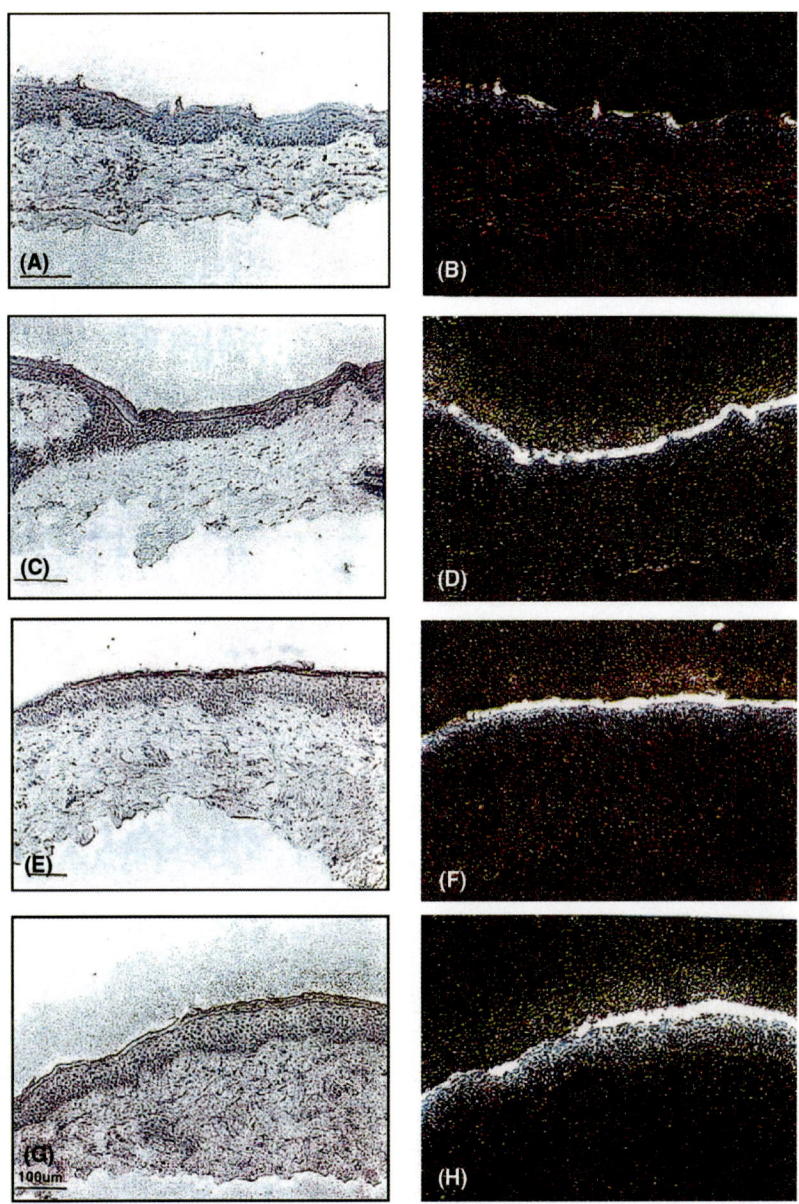

FIGURE 12.4 Autoradiography of octadecenedioic acid and azelaic acid following penetration through dermatomed pig skin for 20 hours. Images show transverse sections through the upper layers of skin treated with different formulations: untreated control (**A** and **B**); Skinoren® containing 20% azelaic acid (**C** and **D**); a gel containing 10% octadecenedioic acid (**E** and **F**); a gel containing 10% azelaic acid (**G** and **H**). Stratum corneum, epidermis, and upper dermis can be seen. Bright field (**A**, **C**, **E**, and **G**) and dark field (**B**, **D**, **F**, and **H**) images were obtained using a Leitz DMRB light microscope (Leica, Milton Keynes, U.K.). The bright reflectance in each dark field picture is the stratum corneum. The scale bar in all bright field images represents 100 μm.

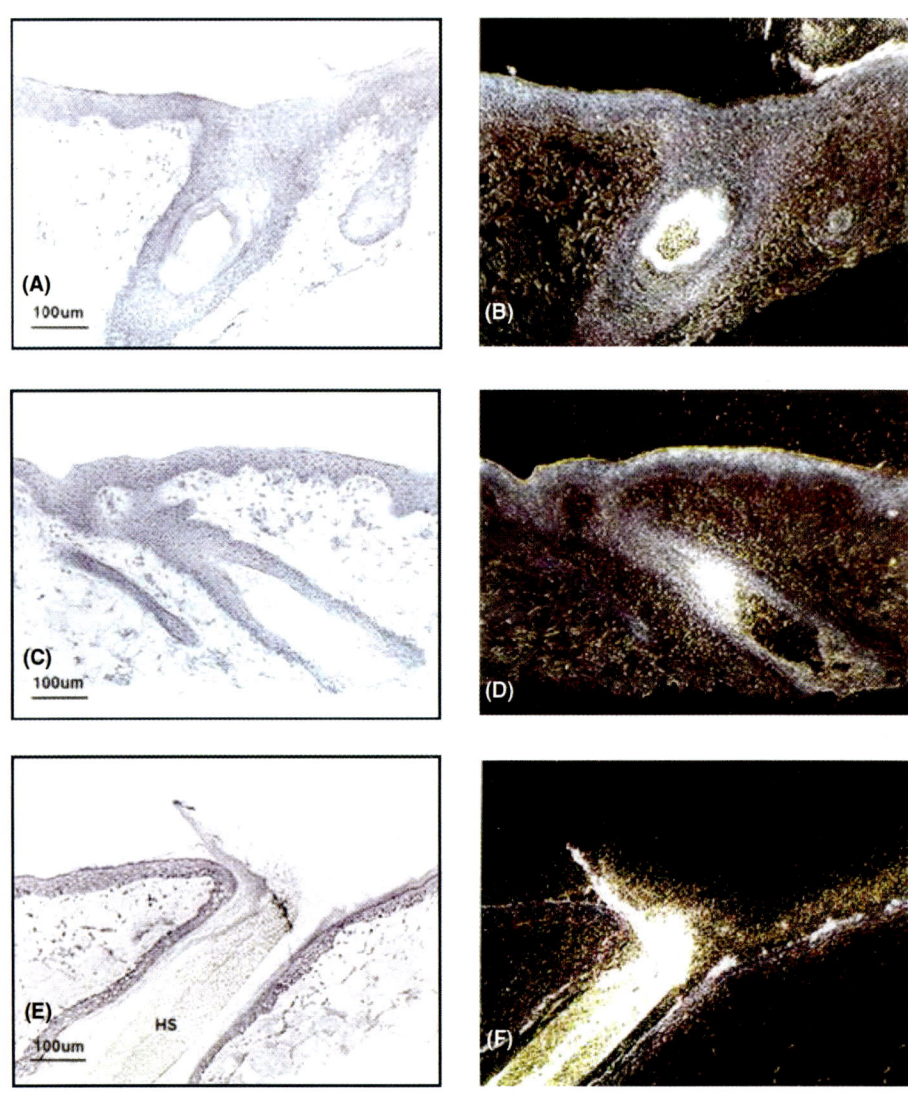

FIGURE 12.5 Examples of follicular delivery following skin penetration of octadecenedioic acid from an aqueous gel containing 10% w/w octadecenedioic acid (**A** and **B**), azelaic acid from an aqueous gel containing 10% azelaic acid (**C** and **D**), and Skinoren® containing 20% azelaic acid (**E** and **F**). Images show transverse sections through the upper layers of the skin. Bright field (**A**, **C**, and **E**) and dark field (**B**, **D**, and **F**) images were obtained using a Leitz DMRB light microscope (Leica, Milton Keynes, U.K.). The bright reflectance in each dark field picture is the stratum corneum and the infundibulum. Note that the stratum corneum in (**A**) and (**B**) has been predominantly lost from this section. The scale bar in all bright field images represents 100 μm.

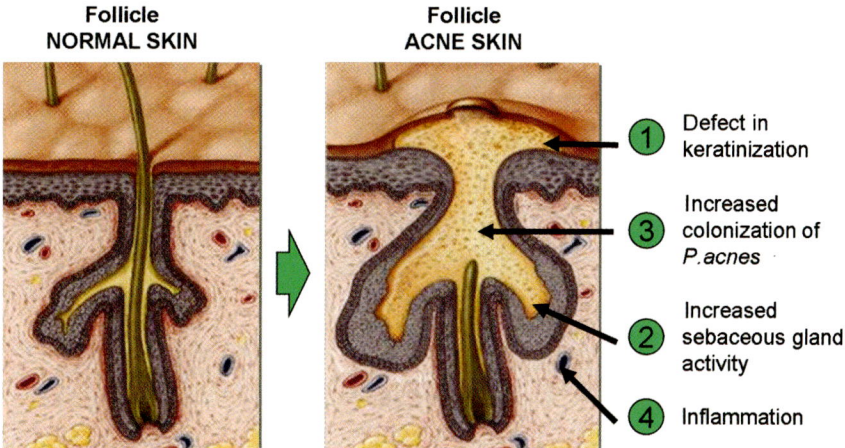

FIGURE 13.1   The reason behind acne.

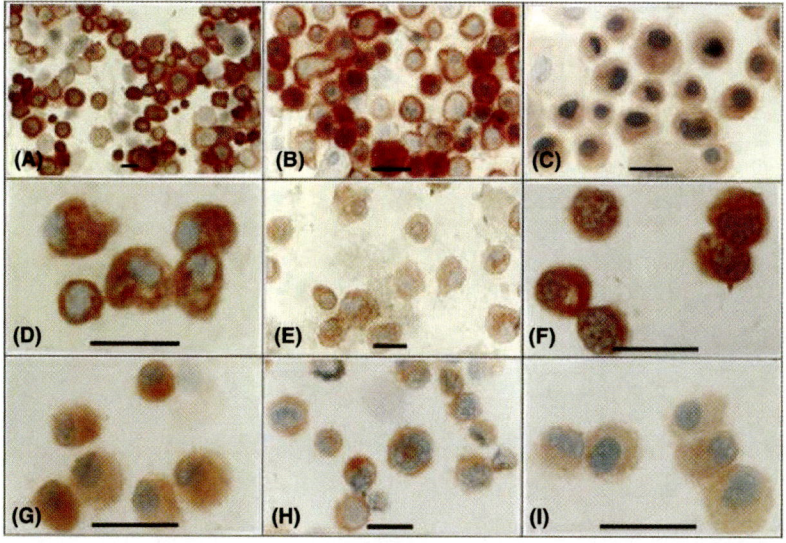

FIGURE 14.5   Immunocytochemistry using rabbit antiserum raised against human type 1 5α-reductase. (**A**) adult facial sebocytes, (**B**) neonatal foreskin keratinocytes, (**C**) adult nongenital keratinocytes (flank), (**D**) occipital dermal papilla cells, (**E**) beard dermal papilla cells, (**F**) occipital fibroblasts, (**G**) melanocytes, (**H**) dermal microvascular endothelial cells, and (**I**) chin fibroblasts. Scale bars = 50 μm. *Source*: From Ref. 8. Reproduced from Blackwell Publishing.

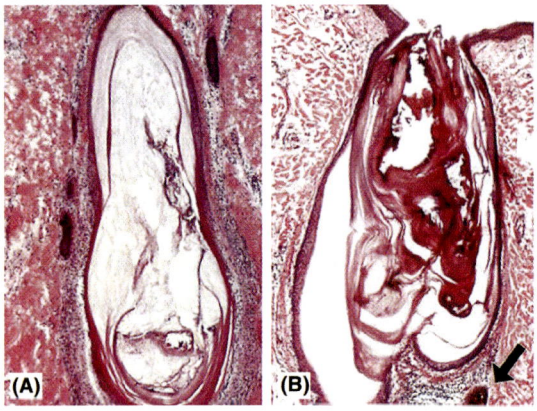

FIGURE 14.8 Immunolocalization of type 1 5α-reductase in comedones (hematoxylin and eosin). (*See p. 179.*)

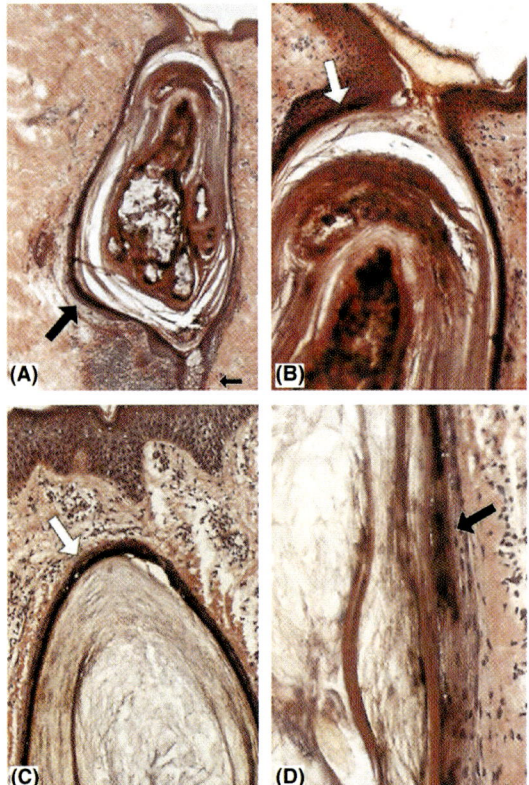

FIGURE 14.9 Immunolocalization of type 2 5α-reductase in comedones. (*See p. 180.*)

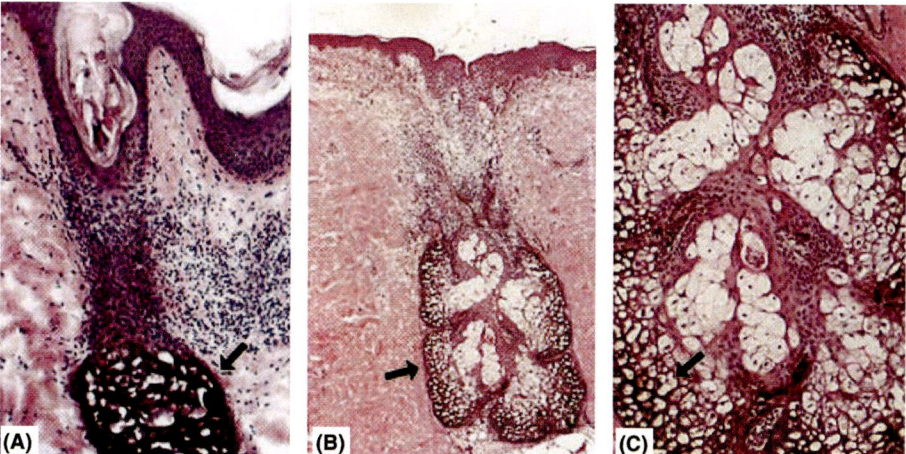

FIGURE 14.10 Immunolocalization of type 1 5α-reductase in inflammatory acne lesions. (**A**) and (**B**) Type 1 antibody localizes specifically in sebaceous glands (*arrows*) (original magnification ×17). (**C**) Localization of type 1 antibody is most predominant in basal sebocytes and more undifferentiated sebocytes in the lateral portions of the gland (*arrow*) (original magnification ×83). *Source*: From Ref. 21. Reproduced from Archives of Dermatology.

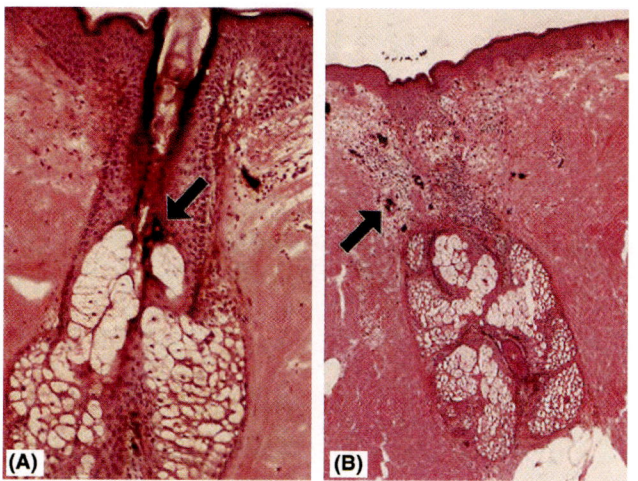

FIGURE 14.11 Immunolocalization of type 2 5α-reductase in inflammatory acne lesions. (**A**) Localization of type 2 antibody extends from the granular layer of the epidermis into the sebaceous duct (*arrow*), but not the sebaceous gland (original magnification ×17). (**B**) Type 2 antibody localizes to endothelial cells within inflammatory lesions (*arrow*) (original magnification ×17). *Source*: From Ref. 21. Reproduced from Archives of Dermatology.

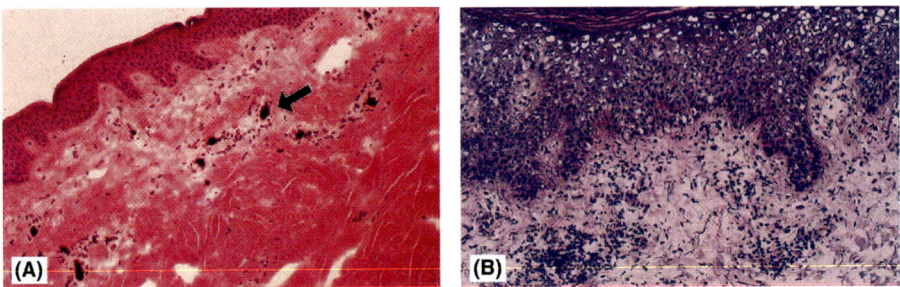

FIGURE 14.12 Type 2 reactivity in endothelial cells. (**A**) Type 2 antibody reactivity is noted in endothelial cells adjacent to an inflammatory acne lesion (*arrow*) (original magnification ×17). (**B**) No localization of type 2 antibody is noted in endothelial cells in control sections of dermatitic skin (original magnification ×41). *Source*: From Ref. 21. Reproduced from Archives of Dermatology.

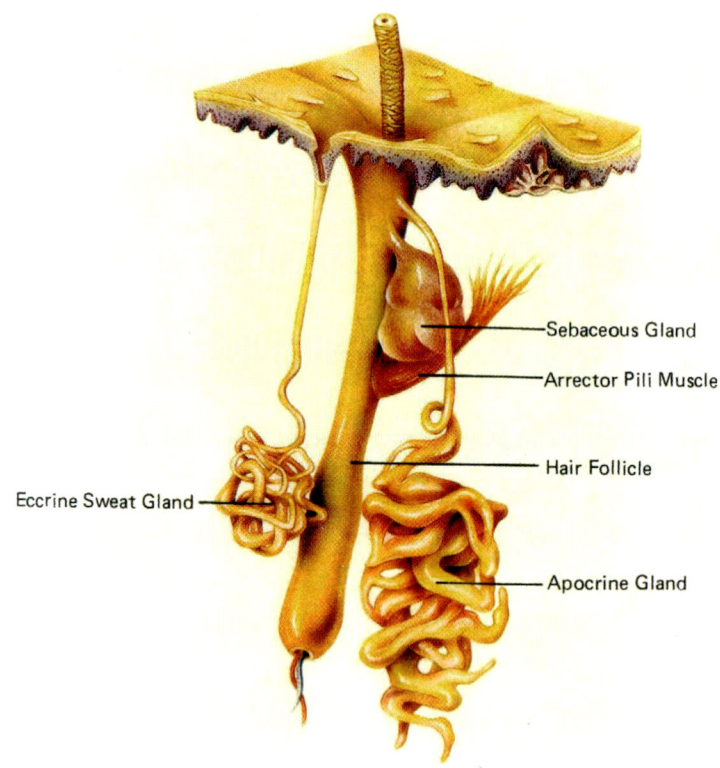

FIGURE 16.1 Schematic representation of the pilosebaceous unit and associated skin appendages. *Source*: From Ref. 70.

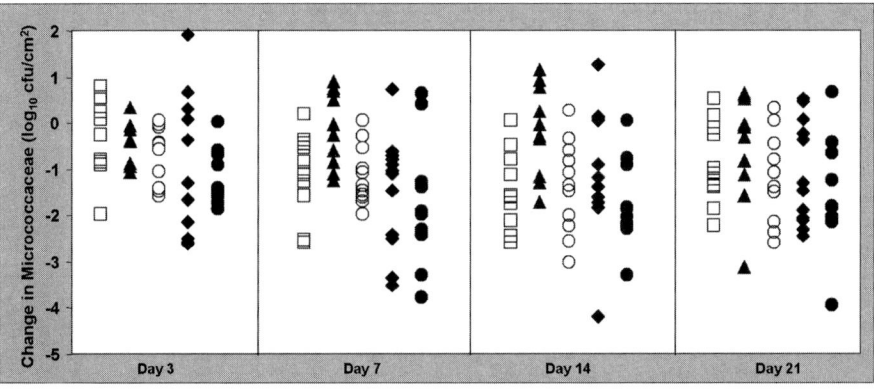

□ A: 10% DCA in gel ◆ D: 5% BPO (Panoxyl®)
▲ B: placebo gel ● E: 20% AZA (Skinoren®)
○ C: 10% AZA gel

FIGURE 6 Scatter plot of changes in Micrococcaceae count from baseline following treatment with a 10% w/w octadecenedioic acid gel (A), placebo gel (B), 10% w/w azelaic acid gel (C), 5% w/w benzoyl peroxide (Panoxyl® Aquagel 5) (D), or 20% w/w azelaic acid (Skinoren®) (E). *Abbreviations*: AZA, azelaic acid; BPO, benzoyl peroxide; DCA, octadecenedioic acid.

4. All the treatments, apart from the placebo, produced significant reductions in Micrococcaceae after one week of treatment (Fig. 6).
5. Only BPO and DCA significantly reduced the propionibacteria population (Fig. 7). Both compounds achieved reductions in propionibacteria counts in the majority of volunteers in their respective user groups.

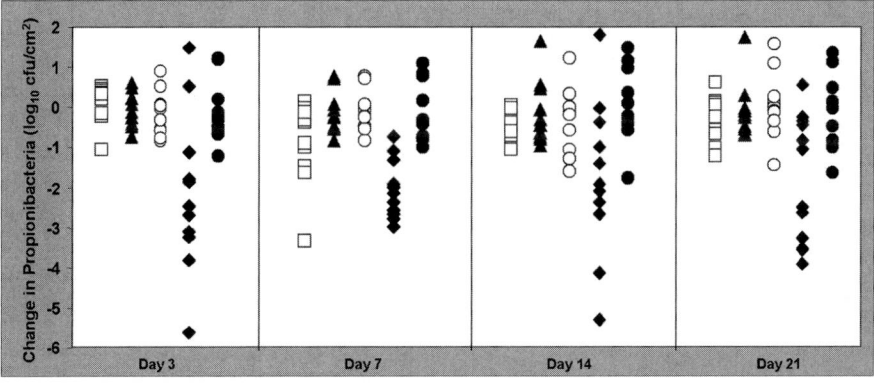

□ A: 10% DCA in gel ◆ D: 5% BPO (Panoxyl®)
▲ B: placebo gel ● E: 20% AZA (Skinore®)
○ C: 10% AZA gel

FIGURE 7 Scatter plot of the changes in propionibacteria count from baseline following treatment with a 10% w/w octadecenedioic acid gel (A), placebo gel (B), 10% w/w azelaic acid gel (C), 5% w/w benzoyl peroxide (Panoxyl® Aquagel 5) (D), or 20% w/w azelaic acid (Skinoren®) (E). *Abbreviations*: AZA, azelaic acid; BPO, benzoyl peroxide; DCA, octadecenedioic acid.

The results of this phase I trial suggested that DCA combines activity against propionibacteria with a good safety and tolerance profile. It outperformed Skinoren® in this trial. However, DCA did not produce the in vivo antimicrobial efficacy that would have been predicted from the in vitro data listed in Table 1. This suggested that the delivery of DCA from the gel formulation was not yet optimal, which was indeed confirmed in Table 2 and Figure 3.

PHASE II CLINICAL TRIAL USING OCTADECENEDIOIC ACID AND BENZOYL PEROXIDE

Although research into improving the delivery of DCA via formulation design was still ongoing, it was decided to extend the clinical investigation by examining the antibacterial activity of DCA in patients with mild-to-moderate acne, instead of healthy human volunteers, and to extend the time of the investigation to 12 weeks instead of three. As the improved delivery systems of DCA were not yet available, we continued with the DCA-containing gel formulation in this Phase II clinical trial. The objectives of the second clinical study were as follows:

1. to investigate whether the antibacterial effects of DCA against *P. acnes*, when applied to the skin of healthy volunteers over three weeks, could be reproduced when DCA was applied to the skin of patients with mild-to-moderate acne over 12 weeks;
2. to determine whether DCA demonstrated any clinical efficacy when applied to the skin of patients with mild-to-moderate acne;
3. to determine the tolerability of DCA on the skin of the patients.

Four formulations were tested in a randomized, double-blind, placebo, and active-treatment controlled trial using 60 volunteers with mild-to-moderate acne vulgaris and a clinically significant level of skin surface *P. acnes*. As in the first trial, the volunteers were medically screened to ensure their suitability to undertake the study. Their willingness to participate was documented through completion of an informed consent form in the presence of medical staff. Patients were stratified according to the number of *P. acnes* isolated from their skin at the screening visit and randomized to receive one of the following treatments: (*i*) DCA (10%) in an aqueous gel; (*ii*) DCA (2%) in an aqueous gel; (*iii*) aqueous gel without any active ingredient, the vehicle; or (*iv*) 5% BPO (Panoxyl Aquagel 5). The latter formulation was selected as the active treatment control because it is recognized as a safe, effective, nonantibiotic, and antibacterial agent and treatment for acne. Topical applications were made twice daily to the face.

Clinical grading and microbiological count was done at weeks 0, 2, 4, 6, and 12, and adverse events and product tolerability and perceptions were measured at weeks 2, 4, 6, and 12. The primary efficacy variables evaluated were the change in the number of total acne lesions from baseline and the change in the number of surface *P. acnes* from baseline. Secondary efficacy variables included the change in the number of inflamed and noninflamed acne lesions from baseline and the change in the acne grade from baseline. More details on the methodology can be found in the literature (20).

Sixty patients were recruited into the study, with 15 patients in each treatment group. Fifty-two patients completed the study without major protocol violations.

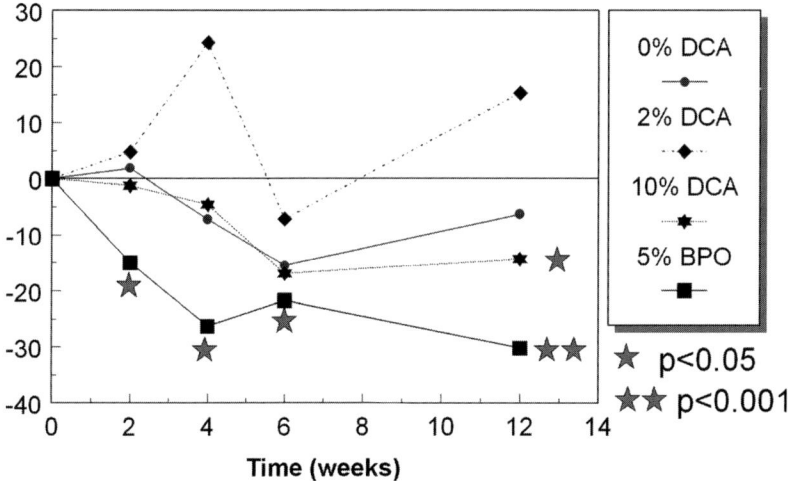

FIGURE 8 The change in total lesion count from baseline following a 12-week treatment with the aqueous vehicle [0% octadecenedioic acid (0% DCA)], the same aqueous vehicle containing 2% DCA, the same aqueous vehicle containing 10% DCA or 5% benzoyl peroxide (Panoxyl Aquagel 5). Products were applied twice daily to the face. *Abbreviations*: BPO, benzoyl peroxide; DCA, octadecenedioic acid.

Five patients withdrew due to acne exacerbation and three were lost during follow-up. The results from this second study were as follows:

1. There was a significant reduction in total acne lesions in subjects using 10% DCA ($P < 0.05$) and 5% BPO ($P < 0.001$) after 12 weeks (Fig. 8).
2. There was a significant reduction in the number of inflamed lesions in subjects using 10% DCA ($P < 0.05$), 2% DCA ($P < 0.05$), and 5% BPO ($P < 0.01$) after 12 weeks. There was a significant reduction in the number of noninflamed lesions in subjects using 5% BPO ($P < 0.05$) at week 12.
3. BPO at 5% significantly reduced *P. acnes* at weeks 2, 4, 6, and 12 ($P < 0.001$).
4. DCA at 10% significantly reduced the number of Micrococcaceae at weeks 2, 4, and 6 ($P < 0.05$) but did not significantly reduce the number of Propionibacteria.
5. Seventy-three percent of patients treated with 5% BPO and 53% of patients treated with 10% DCA had a decrease in overall acne grade at week 12.
6. Both DCA treatments were very well tolerated on the skin when compared with 5% BPO and the vehicle (Table 3).

It could therefore be concluded that DCA demonstrated a significant clinical effect against acne, as measured by the most reliable assessment method available, i.e., lesion counting. The reduction in acne lesions, in particular inflamed lesions, was not reflected by a concomitant reduction in the number of *P. acnes* on the subjects' skin. DCA compared favorably to 5% BPO in its ability to reduce acne lesions (Fig. 8) and also its tolerance profile (Table 3). The reduced antibacterial activity of DCA compared with the phase I study and the in vitro results listed in Table 1

TABLE 3   Percentage of Patients in Each Treatment Group Who Experienced Tolerance-Related Adverse Reactions Following a Twice Daily Application of the Aqueous Vehicle (Gel Vehicle), the Same Aqueous Vehicle Containing 2% Octadecenedioic Acid (2% DCA), the Same Aqueous Vehicle Containing 10% DCA, or 5% Benzoyl Peroxide (Panoxyl Aquagel 5)

Formulation	Erythema	Oiliness	Scaling	Burning
Gel vehicle	13.3	0	60	20
2% DCA	6.6	6.6	13.3	13.3
10% DCA	0	0	20	0
5% BPO	33.3	13.3	80	20

Abbreviations: DCA, octadecenedioic acid; BPO, benzoyl peroxide.

may be due to the inability of the formulation to persist on the skin and penetrate into the follicles at sufficiently high levels to exert its activity. In the meantime, new formulations have been made that deliver significantly more DCA to the skin at much lower concentrations of DCA (2%) (21), and it is expected that these new formulations will be more efficacious.

MECHANISM OF ACTION OF OCTADECENEDIOIC ACID

The clinical study using DCA clearly demonstrated an efficacy toward acne, albeit that the delivery of the active ingredient could still be improved. However, the reduction in *P. acnes* in the second study was minimal, and this is typically considered to be essential for any active ingredient to exert an anti-acne activity. Although an antimicrobial activity of DCA could not be denied (Table 1), this alone was not enough to explain its activity in patients suffering from mild-to-moderate acne. In finding an explanation for this contradiction, the data in Table 3 turned out to be of crucial importance. Whereas the vehicle alone resulted in scaling in 60% of patients, the addition of DCA reduced this percentage considerably to 13% and 20%, suggesting an anti-inflammatory side effect of DCA. A separate study did indeed suggest a slight anti-inflammatory activity, albeit statistically insignificant (data not shown). As inflammation in the human skin is regulated via the PPAR, we investigated whether DCA, an unsaturated fatty acid, did indeed bind to this receptor. After all, fatty acids are the typical ligands for these receptors.

A reporter gene assay using HeLa cells transfected with chimeric receptor genes fused to a PPAR ligand-binding domain and a reporter gene with the luciferase/luciferine system was performed. Separate cell lines were developed for PPARα, δ, and γ. A total of 2.5×10^4 cells were plated into 96-well microtiter plates with phenol red-free Dulbecco's Modified Eagles Medium (DMEM) culture media containing 6% dextran-coated, charcoal-treated fetal calf serum (DCC FCS). Cells were incubated with pharmaceutical PPAR agonists ($10^{-11} - 10^{-5}$ M), DCA ($10^{-7}-10^{-5}$ M), or pioglitazone [$10^{-8}-10^{-5}$ M; a positive control for PPARγ binding (22)] for 16 hours, and at the end of the incubation, the medium was removed and replaced with culture medium containing luciferine and a luminescent signal measured after five minutes using a Microbeta luminometer (Wallac, Turku, Finland). All experiments were performed in quadruplicate.

These experiments, the results of which are illustrated in Figure 9, showed that DCA is a pan-PPAR agonist with a greater specificity for PPARγ. As a specific PPARγ agonist, pioglitazone naturally only binds to PPARγ. Other controls for PPARα and PPARδ were included but not shown here (13).

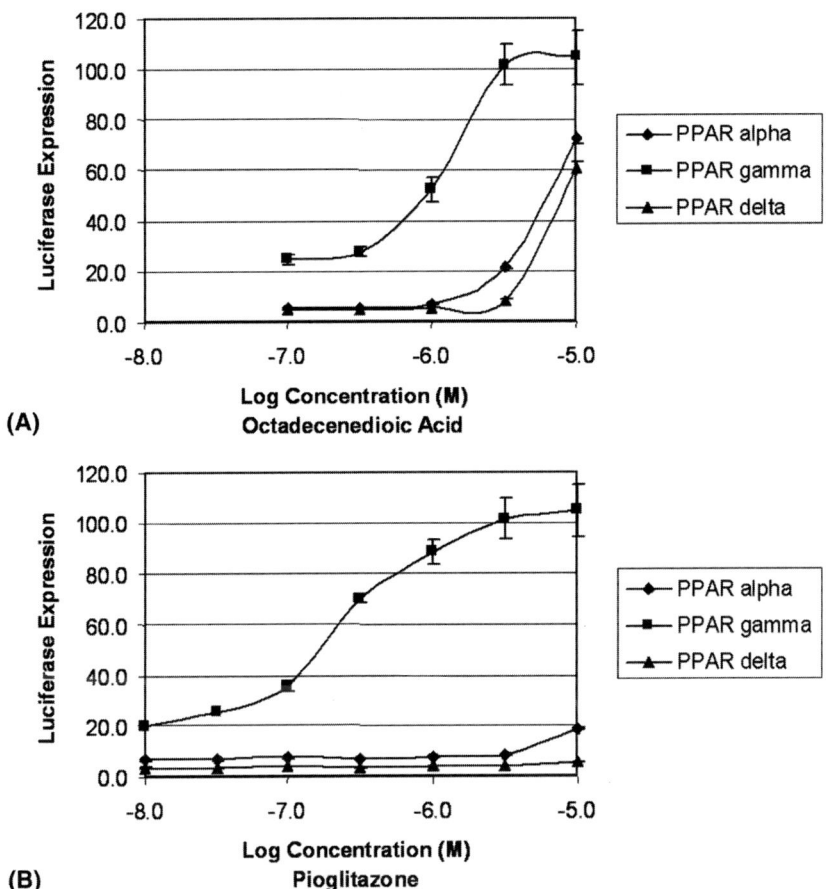

(A)

(B)

FIGURE 9 Induction of luciferase expression by octadecenedioic acid (**A**) and pioglitazone (**B**) in three separate HeLa cell lines expressing peroxisome proliferator-activated receptor α, δ, and γ separately. *Abbreviation*: PPAR, peroxisome proliferator-activated receptor.

RATIONALE FOR OCTADECENEDIOIC ACID AS A NOVEL TOPICAL ACNE TREATMENT

Acne is a common disease affecting, according to surveys, nearly one out of three teenagers, although the disease is not limited to preadolescents only. It markedly influences the quality of life and constitutes a socio-economic problem. Worldwide costs for systemic and topical acne treatment were calculated to represent 12.6% of the annual overall costs for the treatment of skin diseases (23). Its pathogenesis is multifactorial, with abnormal follicular differentiation and increased cornification, enhanced sebaceous gland activity and hyperseborrhea, bacterial hypercoloniza-tion as well as inflammation, and immunological host reactions being the major contributors (23). It is characterized by a variety of expressions and degrees depending on the distribution, type of lesions, tendency to and manifestation of scarring, start of disease in puberty, or persistence after time of physiological regression, each form requiring a different active ingredient or drug or combination thereof (24).

There are basically four modes of action for treating acne in line with the pathogenesis described earlier: most anti-acne agents have an antimicrobial activity to counteract the hypercolonization (in particular, e.g., BPO), some agents interact with the hyperkeratinization aspect of acne to fight the abnormal follicular differentiation and increased cornification (in particular, the retinoids such as tretinoin, isotretinoin, and adapalene), a few have only a moderate anti-inflammatory activity (e.g., adapalene, AZA, and BPO), whereas none have a strong sebo-suppressive effect to fight the hyperseborrhea (24). Because of the complexity of the disease, it is very difficult to differentiate between cause and effect, and as a consequence, relapses often occur because the fundamental underlying cause may not have been dealt with. As a consequence, combination therapies are popular, involving both the topical and the oral route of administration. Mammone et al. (25), for instance, proposed a combination of chemicals with antimicrobial, anti-inflammatory, and antiandrogen properties and a desquamation enhancer, resulting in a statistically significant higher reduction in noninflamed lesions relative to a 5% BPO gel, whereas there was no statistically significant additional benefit toward inflamed lesions. The downside of combination therapy, however, is that this increases the chance of side effects, as most of these products have some. AZA, for instance, causes a very strong burning and BPO results in strong scaling and erythema (24), which was confirmed in our studies (Table 3).

Here, we report the use of DCA as a novel topical treatment of acne that involves all four modes of action within a single molecule. Similar to most other anti-acne agents, DCA has an antimicrobial activity as indicated in Table 1. All three other modes of action may be produced via its binding to PPAR, as shown in Figure 9, which illustrates its capability to act as a pan-PPAR agonist. Binding to PPARγ is most pronounced, followed by that to PPARα and PPARδ. As shown by Downie et al. (5), activators of PPARα and PPARγ inhibit the rate of sebaceous lipogenesis and reduce the synthesis of the sebum-specific lipids squalane and triacylglycerol in human sebaceous glands. DCA, as a PPARγ and PPARα agonist, is therefore likely to do the same, provided it is delivered well enough. The importance of PPAR in the regulation of lipid synthesis and metabolism in human sebocytes is recognized, albeit far from clear yet. Makrantonaki and Zouboulis (26), for instance, described the stimulatory interactions between androgens and PPAR ligands, similar to the natural PPARδ/γ ligand linoleic acid, on neutral and polar lipid synthesis. Although linoleic acid is stimulating lipid synthesis in vitro in this communication (26), topical administration of 2.5% linoleic acid in a Carbopol gel formulation for one month resulted in a significant reduction (25%) in the overall size of follicular casts and microcomedones, whereas no change was found at placebo-treated sites (27). Further research will be necessary to elucidate the interrelationships between all factors involved.

DCA, however, is one of the very few molecules that has the potential to interact at all levels with acne: enhanced differentiation to prevent the increased cornification of the sebaceous duct (via PPARδ), reduction in sebum production to counteract hyperseborrhea (via PPARγ), and reduction in inflammation (PPARα). These PPAR-related effects combined with its demonstrated antimicrobial properties to overcome the hypercolonization with microbes such as *P. acnes* and *S. aureus*, make DCA a viable nonantibiotic alternative for the treatment of acne.

REFERENCES

1. Knaggs H, Wood EJ, Rizer RL, et al. Post-adolescent acne. Int J Cosmet Sci 2004; 26(1):129–138.
2. Krautheim A, Gollnick H. Transdermal penetration of topical drugs used in the treatment of acne. Clin Pharmacokinet 2003; 42:1287–1304.
3. Gollnick HPM, Krautheim A. Topical treatment of acne: Current status and future aspects. Dermatology 2003; 206:29–36.
4. Gollnick HPM, Graupe K, Zaumseil R-P.15% Azelainsaüregel in der Behandlung der Akne. Zwei doppelblinde klinische Vergleichstudien. JDDG 2004; 2:841–847.
5. Downie MMT, Sanders DA, Maier LM, et al. Peroxisome proliferator-activated receptor and farnesoid X receptor ligands differentially regulate sebaceous differentiation in human sebaceous gland organ cultures *in vitro*. Br J Dermatol 2004; 151:766–775.
6. Berger J, Moller DE. The mechanisms of action of PPARs. Annu Rev Med 2002; 53:409–435.
7. Kömüves LG, Hanley K, Lefebvre A-M, et al. Stimulation of PPARα promotes epidermal keratinocyte differentiation *in-vivo*. J Invest Dermatol 2000; 115:353–360.
8. Westergaard M, Henningsen J, Svendsen ML, et al. Modulation of keratinocyte gene expression and differentiation by PPAR—selective ligands and tetradecylthioacetic acid. J Invest Dermatol 2001; 116:702–712.
9. Kippenberger S, Loitsch SM, Grundmann-Kollmann M, et al. Activators of peroxisome proliferator-activated receptors protect human skin from ultraviolet-B-light-induced inflammation. J Invest Dermatol 2001; 117:1430–1436.
10. Sheu MY, Fowler AJ, Kao J, et al. Topical peroxisome proliferator activated receptor-α activators reduce inflammation in irritant and allergic contact dermatitis models. J Invest Dermatol 2002; 118:94–101.
11. Mössner R, Schulz U, Krüger U, et al. Agonists of peroxisome proliferator-activated receptor gamma inhibit cell growth in malignant melanoma. J Invest Dermatol 2002; 119:576–582.
12. Placha W, Gil D, Dembińska-Kieć A, et al. The effect of PPARγ on the proliferation and apoptosis of human melanoma cells. Melanoma Res 2003; 13:447–456.
13. Wiechers JW, Rawlings AV, Garcia C, et al. A new mechanism of action for skin whitening agents: Binding to the peroxisome proliferator-activated receptor (PPAR). Int J Cosmet Sci 2005; 27:123–132.
14. Bronaugh RL, Stewart RF. Methods for in vitro percutaneous absorption studies. IV. The flow-through diffusion cell. J Pharm Sci 1985; 74:69–77.
15. Williams AC, Cornwell PA, Barry BW. On the non-Gaussian distribution of human skin permeabilities. Int J Pharm 1992; 86:69–77.
16. Cornwell PA, Barry BW. Effect of penetration enhancers on the statistical distribution of human skin permeabilities. Int J Pharm 1995; 117:101–112.
17. Bojar RA, Cutcliffe AG, Graupe K, et al. Follicular concentrations of azelaic acid after a single topical application. Br J Dermatol 1993; 129:399–402.
18. Grams YY, Bouwstra JA. Penetration and distribution of three lipophilic probes *in vitro* in human skin focussing on the hair follicle. J Control Release 2002; 83:253–262.
19. Grams YY, Alaruikka S, Lashley L, et al. Permeant lipophilicity and vehicle composition influence on accumulation of dyes in hair follicles of human skin. Eur J Pharm Sci 2003; 18:329–336.
20. Burke BM, Cunliffe WJ. The assessment of acne vulgaris. The Leeds technique. Br J Dermatol 1984; 111:83–92.
21. Wiechers JW, Kelly CL, Blease TG, et al. Formulating for efficacy. Int J Cosmet Sci 2004; 26:173–182.
22. Bhagavathula N, Nerusu KC, Lal A, et al. Rosiglitazone inhibits proliferation, motility, and matrix metalloproteinase production in keratinocytes. J Invest Dermatol 2004; 122:130–139.
23. Zouboulis CC. Acne pathogenesis: New experimental findings elucidate the involvement of androgens, PPAR ligands and regulatory neuropeptides. J Invest Dermatol 2005; 124:A 48, #284.

24. Gollnick H, Schramm A. Topical drug treatment in acne. Dermatology 1998; 196:119–125.
25. Mammone T, Maes D, Gan D, et al. A multi-prong approach to the treatment of acne. J Invest Dermatol 2005; 124:A15, #086.
26. Makrantonaki E, Zouboulis CC. The effect of androgens on lipid metabolism in human sebocytes occurs in interaction with PPAR ligands. J Invest Dermatol 2005; 124:A109, #649.
27. Letawe C, Boone M, Piérard GE. Image analysis of the effect of topically applied linoleic acid on acne microcomedones. Clin Exp Dermatol 1998; 23:56–58.

The Effect of Sphingolipids as a New Therapeutic Option for Acne Treatment

Saskia K. Klee, Mike Farwick, and Peter Lersch
Degussa, Goldschmidt Personal Care, Essen, Germany

INTRODUCTION

The skin is one of the largest organs of the human body. It is a highly specialized tissue that acts as a barrier against the influences of the environment. It plays a crucial role in the protection against dehydration and the control of body temperature (1). The skin's primary role is to protect our health, but the skin's barrier is imperfect and it also has the ability to absorb external substances. Moreover, these external substances can access healthy skin via its pilosebaceous glands. Drugs have been detected in the blood stream after topical application, demonstrating transdermal delivery through the skin (2). This is desired for the treatment of many skin diseases, but this characteristic can also be a contributing factor for causing many diverse health risks.

The lipid environment of the stratum corneum is an essential factor for maintaining the skin's equilibrium. Changes in the barrier lipid composition have been directly linked to skin barrier function impairments, such as pathologically dry and rough skin (3,4). Besides protective tasks, the skin is confronted with a tremendous challenge during puberty, when the increase in circulating levels of testosterone influences the function of pilosebaceous units (PSU) and increases sebogenesis. Increased sebum levels are a major contributory factor in acnegenesis. During puberty, the pituitary gland initiates the sexual maturation process via the release of gonadotropins and the production of hormones called androgens. This process regulates the production of sebum in the sebaceous glands of both adolescent boys and girls (5). This is the time period in which most adolescents develop a more or less severe form of acne. Although superficial and non-life-threatening, acne is a disease that, if left untreated, can have serious physical and psychological consequences (6,7).

Acne is one of the most common skin diseases of human kind, affecting 80% of adolescent boys and girls during puberty (8) that may persist throughout adulthood, or it may even develop after puberty (commonly known as persistent or late onset acne, respectively) (9). Sebum hypersecretion is the first problem associated with acne-prone skin and is caused by the enzymatic hyperactivity of 5-alpha-reductase—a key enzyme that converts testosterone into dihydrotestosterone (DHT) (5). By binding to its receptor in the skin, DHT stimulates the secretion of sebum (Fig. 1). Men are more severely affected because they produce higher concentrations of androgens that regulate sebum production and enlargement of sebaceous glands (10,11).

The earliest morphological change observed in acne patients is the aberrant follicular epithelial proliferation and differentiation of the PSU that results in clinically invisible microcomedones (12–15). Due to the hormonal imbalance in

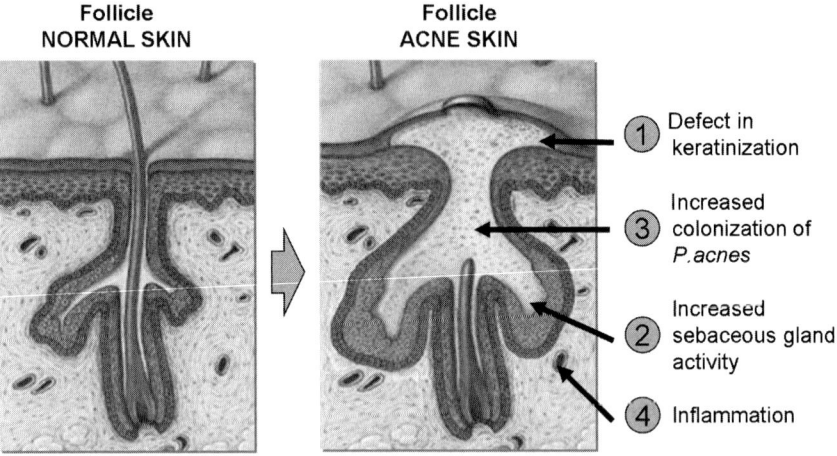

Follicle NORMAL SKIN

Follicle ACNE SKIN

1. Defect in keratinization

3. Increased colonization of *P.acnes*

2. Increased sebaceous gland activity

4. Inflammation

FIGURE 1   (*See color insert.*) The reason behind acne.

pubescent children, the sebaceous glands overproduce sebum and increase in size (sebaceous hyperplasia). In addition, the exit for sebum—the follicle opening—is obstructed due to an abnormal keratinization of the infundibular epithelium. The horny layer becomes thicker, resulting in the accumulation of corneocytes in the pilosebaceous duct (16,17), and the sebum secretion is hindered. Then the visible comedone, which is a noninflammatory lesion, becomes clinically apparent (Fig. 1).

The skin flora comprises corynebacteria such as *Propionibacterium acnes*, which are lipophilic bacteria and preferentially occupy the sebum-enriched follicles. High sebum concentration and microscopically small keratinous material lead to a change of the follicular milieu with consecutive proliferation of semi-anaerobic bacteria, like *P. acnes* (18). The bacteria secrete a lipase that hydrolyses sebum triglycerides to glycerol and free fatty acids, which have proinflammatory and comedogenic properties (19,20). The overproduction of sebum is an ideal condition for the proliferation of the bacterial flora. Consequently, the concentration of free sterol levels in the intercorneocytic comedone lipids is further reduced, which leads to an increased corneocyte adhesion and, consequently, to a retention hyperkeratosis (21). In addition, sebocytes themselves are able to synthesize free fatty acids in the absence of bacterial colonization (22), and express the inflammatory cytokine interleukin (IL)-1-alpha by an intrinsic mechanism (18). These, together with bacterial cell wall products, set up the inflammatory process. The inflammatory acne lesions, pustules, and papules are then generated.

Depending on the degree of deregulated sebum production, hyperkeratosis, bacterial colonization, and inflammation, acne occurs with increasing severity. The most common form is acne vulgaris, which does not have to be seen by a dermatologist in 70% of cases. More severe forms of acne, like acne conglobata, or forms that induce nodules and pseudocysts need intensive medical care because the formed abscesses coalesce and dissect under the skin to produce highly inflamed sinus tracts (12–15). Mild and temporary acne forms occur after hormonal changes in women (23), that is, after giving birth or during menstruation. Newborn children may also show slight signs of acne, which are explained by a temporary androgen overproduction of the adrenal gland (24). Furthermore, acne symptoms may be induced by cosmetics, medication, and occupational influences (25). Many genetic studies have been performed, and the pathogenesis of acne is well- documented in twins (26); however, further research is needed to investigate the genetic effects.

As the pathogenesis of acne is multifactorial (Fig. 1), the treatment of acne is diverse. Therapies target: (*i*) sebum production, (*ii*) hyperkeratinization, (*iii*) *P. acnes*, and (*iv*) the inflammatory response. Hormonal treatment to regulate sebum production can be applied to young women by the intake of contraceptives. Tretinoin and isotretinoin belong to a family of vitamin A derivatives, and are essential for both the maintenance of epithelial differentiation and the reduction of the hyperproliferation of keratinocytes (27,28). Benzoyl peroxide (BPO) acts antimicrobially and shows weak comedolytic activity (29). However, the comedolytic and keratolytic activities of salicylic acid have been shown to be superior to BPO by increased reduction of the total number of acne lesions (30). Multiple antibiotics (tetracycline, erythromycin, and clindamycin) are applied both orally and topically to reduce the number of bacteria. In addition, peeling treatments using, for example, alpha-hydroxy acids (mainly glycolic acid) are used to shed off old cells from the most upper layer of the skin. Recently, Zouboulis (31) has demonstrated that the total lipid level in sebum, especially the proinflammatory lipids, was reduced by a specific lipoxygenase inhibitor, suggesting that the down regulation of acne-related inflammatory signals is the future therapy. Also, scientists at the Annual Meeting of the Society of Dermopharmacy have proposed a change of paradigm from antibacterial to anti-inflammatory treatment (32). Along these lines, the third-generation retinoid, adapalene, is able to inhibit indirectly the release of cytokines from monocytes and macrophages and thereby suppresses an inflammatory response (33). As a result, other agents that possess anti-inflammatory effects may be a useful adjunct to the anti-acne armory.

SPHINGOID BASES—A MAJOR COMPONENT OF HUMAN SKIN

The membranes of all eukaryotic cells contain numerous classes of glycerolipids and sphingolipids. In the past decade, the long-neglected ceramides have become one of the most attractive lipid molecules in molecular cell biology, because of their involvement in essential structures (stratum corneum) and processes (cell signaling). Long-chain ceramides are among the most hydrophobic molecules in nature; they are totally insoluble in water and they hardly mix with phospholipids in membranes, giving rise to ceramide-enriched domains. Most natural ceramides have a long *N*-acyl chain comprising 16–22 C atoms, but short *N*-acyl chain ceramides with two to six C atoms also exist in nature. These molecules have been extensively used in experimentation, because they can be dispersed easily in water.

Ceramides play major roles in maintaining the epidermal barrier (34). Depletion of ceramides, associated with disrupted barrier function in the epidermis, leads to the clinical manifestation of dryness and inflammation. Besides their contribution to the structural integrity of a cell, ceramides are sphingoid-based signaling molecules that regulate cell cycle arrest, proliferation, differentiation, and apoptosis (35,36). There are specific structural and stereochemical requirements for the production of biological responses by the activation of specific biochemical targets. Endogenous levels of ceramides are regulated by a balance between its de novo synthesis and the rate of its breakdown to the corresponding sphingoid bases.

The core structures are sphingoid bases and constitute a large group of structurally diverse, biologically important long-chain amino alcohols, possessing a 2-amino-1,3-diol moiety. The most common member of this group found in nature is (2S,3R)-D-erythro-2-amino-1,3-octadec-4E-ene-diol, dubbed sphingosine. Another member is phytosphingosine (PS), typically consisting of an 18-carbon chain that incorporates a 2-amino-1,3,4-triol moiety at one end. It is a bioactive lipid that displays various physiological activities and it also occurs widely in animals, plants, and yeasts (2).

PS is present in human skin, but only in low concentrations, since it is an enzymatic breakdown product of ceramides. It comprises about 40% of the epidermal sphingoid bases and plays an important part in regulating the micro-flora of the skin, since it mediates a wide variety of activities, such as stimulating the biosynthesis of new PS-based ceramides by keratinocytes. Furthermore, it acts as a potent anti-inflammatory antagonist to a number of inflammatory cytokines, which are expressed by epidermal keratinocytes.

Both PS and sphingosine originate from sphinganine as a common precursor either by action of a desaturase introducing a (4E)-double bond to yield sphingosine or by action of a hydroxylase that adds a third hydroxy group to the C-4 of dihydroceramide to yield PS. The metabolic pathway starts from ceramides, and sphingoid bases are released upon amidolysis of the core structures. Both have shown to exert potent growth-suppressive effects in various cell types. Since PS and its derivatives are available only in a limited amount from natural sources, there is a continuing interest in developing efficient synthesis routes.

CURRENT SYNTHESIS ROUTES FOR SPHINGOID BASES

Sphingolipids are natural substances. More than 300 kinds of sphingolipids are known, displaying a wide variety of biological activities. However, access to sphingolipids is not very straightforward. Although these compounds are widespread in nature, it is difficult to isolate substantial quantities because the concentration of sphingolipids in natural products is very low. Because sphingolipids have a very specific and complex three-dimensional structure, they are not easy to synthesize via chemical routes. Chemical routes to sphingoid bases are usually an economical challenge because their synthesis involves multiple protection and deprotection steps, as well as low yields due to necessary purification steps because of unwanted side products.

Economically, sphingolipids can be produced only in large quantities in a biotechnological process. Large quantities of the sphingoid-based PS and ceramides are being produced via fermentation for the personal care industry. Through enzymatic modification and/or organic chemistry, fatty acids can be added to the building block to create ceramides. Degussa has developed a patented biofermentation process for the large-scale production of PS. The process utilizes a natural, non-GM yeast and the product is chemically identical to PS, which is naturally present in the human skin because of the same stereochemical D-erythro configuration. Because of this, a wide range of sphingolipids including ceramides and sphingoid bases such as PS are nowadays commercially available.

PS serves also as a starting material for a better and more efficient way to produce the naturally occurring D-erythro-sphingosine. Sphingosine and its most prominent derivative sphingosine-1-phosphate (S1P) have been initially described as intermediates in the metabolic pathway of long-chain sphingoid bases. Now, it is widely accepted that S1P is a unique bioactive lipid messenger and is involved in a variety of cellular functions, including vascular maturation, angionesis, tumor necrosis factor-alpha signaling, regulation of cell motility, and in signal transduction pathways of platelet-derived growth factor. The addition of sphingosine has been claimed, for example, to suppress significantly DNA synthesis in human keratinocytes, and can regulate proliferation and survival intracellularly. Also, it serves as a ligand for G protein-coupled receptors of the Edg-I subfamily extracellularly. The effect of Sphingosine and its derivatives are specific and depend on the presence of the Δ4-double bond.

Today, 50 years after the report describing the preparation of racemic D-erythro-sphingosine (37), an efficient, cost-effective, and regio-/stereoselective synthesis has been developed, starting from the commercially available and cheap D-ribo-PS (38). As shown in Figure 2, first attempts were undertaken to generate 5 directly from 2; however, the used reaction conditions resulted in the formation of 7 which easily transformed into 8. The alternative route via 9–12 resulted in 5 with high yield (82%). However, further examination of a direct transformation from 2 to 5 resulted in the successful reaction conditions h. Subsequent reactions via 13 and 6 resulted in the desired regio- and stereo-selectively correct product 14. Finally, D-erythro-sphingosine was generated in high yield (70%) over seven steps.

PHYTOSPHINGOSINE POSSESSES MANY PROPERTIES THAT ARE USEFUL FOR THE TREATMENT OF ACNE

Firstly, PS possesses antimicrobial activity (39). The skin's microflora is very diverse; however, they exist in a healthy equilibrium. This balance is partly due to the free fatty acids that are released by the bacterial breakdown of triglycerides, having a limiting action on numbers of microorganisms. However, more importantly, is the liberation of free sphingoid bases, which show growth inhibitory activity against gram-positive bacteria, yeast, and moulds. It is suggested that by topical application of PS, the growth of undesirable microorganisms will be inhibited.

To examine the antimicrobial activity of PS, solutions of various PS-concentrations were prepared (39). The final PS test solutions contained 0.83% ethanol, 1.5% Tween 80, and 267–1066 mg/L PS. As described by Bibel et al. (40), ethanol inhibits the growth of microorganisms by itself. In our studies, however, we have used an ethanol concentration that is far below the inhibitory level. Table 1 shows the determined minimal inhibitory concentration of PS for different microorganisms.

Second, PS affects inflammation. The outcome of several different gene expression studies (41) on cultured primary human keratinocytes was as follows:

1. The expression of proinflammatory chemokines like IL-8, CXCL2, and endothelin-1 was significantly down regulated.
2. The regulation of various genes involved in cellular reactive oxygen species (ROS) metabolism was observed, indicating that these compounds may substantially modulate the skin's capacity to handle ROS, and thus also encounter inflammation.

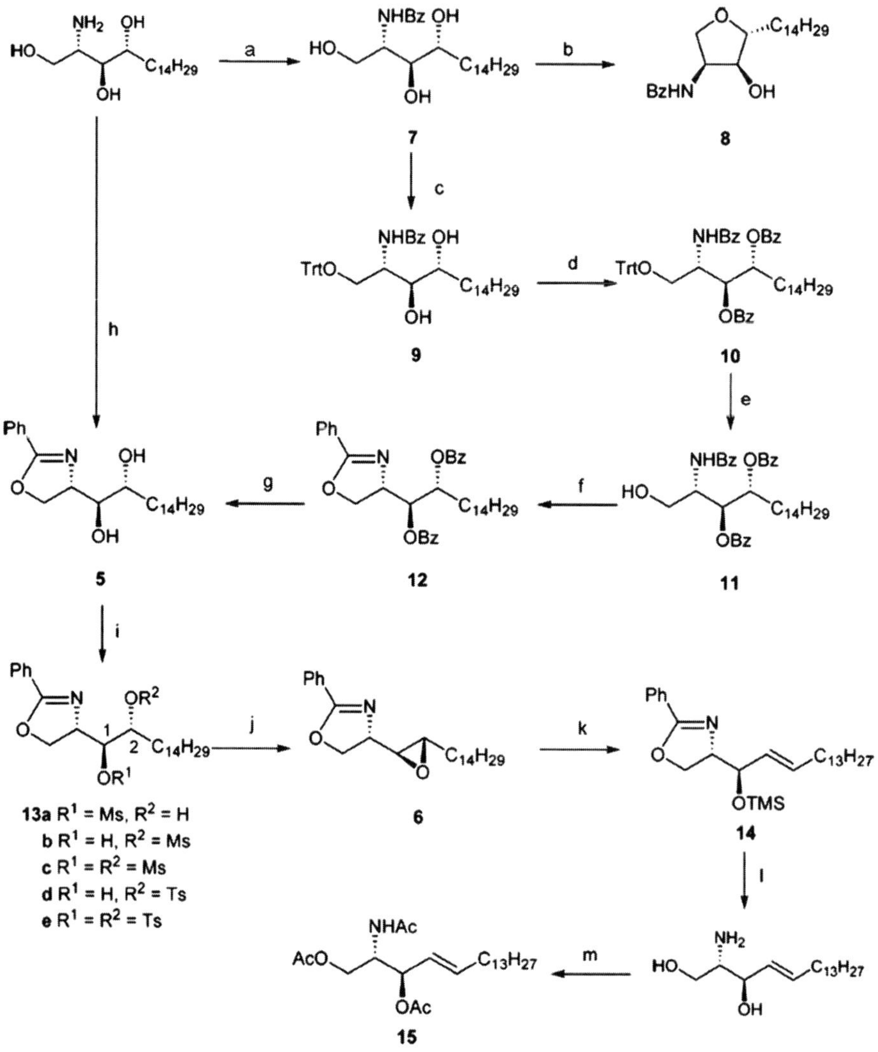

FIGURE 2 Reagents and conditions: (a) BzCl, TEA, THF, RT, 30 min, 99%; (b) TsCl, pyridine, 0 → 20°C, 18 hr, 80%; (c) TrtCl, TEA, EtOAc, 80°C, 2.5 hr, 99%; (d) BzCl, TEA, EtOAc, RT, 16 hr, 99%; (e) BF$_3$, OEt$_2$, MeOH/toluene (1:1, v/v), RT, 1.5 hr, 99%; (f) MsCl, TEA, DCM, 0 → 20°C, 18 hr, 86%; (g) K$_2$CO$_3$, MeOH, DCM, 40°C, 18 hr, 99%; (h) ethyl benzimidate hydrochloride, DCM, 40°C, 48 hr, 95%; (i) MsCl or TsCl, pyridine/DCM (3:2, v/v), DMAP (5%), 69% (13b), 75% (13d); (j) tBuOK, THF, 0°C, 1 hr, 99%; (k) TMSI, DBN, acetonitrile, 40 → 86°C, 94%; (l) (*i*) 2 N HCl, THF, RT, 18 hr and (*ii*) NaOH, MeOH, 100°C, 2 hr, 79%; (M) Ac$_2$O, pyridine, RT, 2 hr, 99%. *Source*: From Ref. 38.

3. The expression of differentiation markers like loricrin, involucrin, transglutaminase1, and filaggrin was induced after treatment with PS. This leads to a shift from proliferation to differentiation and thus reduces the symptoms of hyperkeratinization.

TABLE 1 In Vitro Determination of Minimal Inhibitory Concentration Values

Microorganism	Undesirable phenomena	Phytosphingosine (g/L)
Staphylococcus aureus	Atopic eczema, infections, sores	0.20
Corynebacterium xerosis	Axillary odor	0.16
Micrococcus luteus	Axillary odor	0.20
Propionibacterium acnes	Acne, oily skin	0.20
Escherichia coli	Wound infections, sores	0.40
Pseudomonas aerigunosa	Wound infections, sores	0.10
Candida albicans	Yeast infection	0.012
Microsporum canis	Fungal infection	0.06

Note: Concentration of phytosphingosine (g/L) required for complete growth inhibition within one hour.
Source: From Ref. 39.

Along this line, experiments with reconstituted human epidermis (SkinEthic™) (42) were performed. The reconstituted human epidermis consists of a three-dimensional, multilayered keratinocyte structure grown on an air–liquid interphase, without any other cell type. Inflammatory conditions were simulated by the topical application of a 0.35% sodium dodecyl sulphate (SDS) solution for 40 minutes. Afterward, an O/W formulation containing 0.2% PS and a placebo formulation without PS were applied to the treated and untreated skin model for 28 hours. For the determination of general viability effects, an XTT assay was performed and the total protein amount was assigned using a Bradford test. Additionally, potential cytotoxicity of the sample was excluded by the measurement of lactate dehydrogenase release. The IL-1 amount was quantified using an ELISA-kit. The results demonstrated that IL-1 was down regulated on the protein level after treatment with PS. Under unstressed conditions, the release of IL-1 was decreased by 52% 24 hours after the topical application of 0.2% PS out of a basic cream formulation. The incubation of the reconstituted human epidermis with SDS prior to the experiment led to a 3.4, -fold increase in IL-1 secretion (12.8–42.9 pg/mL), mimicking an inflamed skin status. Under these conditions, the application of PS even decreased the release of IL-1 by 69%.

Additional benefits may be derived from the effect of topical PS, as it is known to act as a precursor to ceramides, and PS-based ceramides are reduced in the skin of acne subjects. It has been demonstrated by electrospray-ionization-mass spectroscopy on extracts of the lipid phase of cultured keratinocytes (43) that PS can be taken up efficiently by the cells. Furthermore, PS can be metabolized and converted to glucosylceramides, which are the precursors of the different barrier ceramides. In our experiments (43), the level of PS -derived barrier ceramides was increased, too. This indicates that the depleted PS-ceramide reservoirs that occur during acne can be filled up by the topical application of PS. However, the level of PS-derived ceramides was not increased by the upregulation of gene expression. Genes that are involved in the ceramide synthesis pathway, like fatty acid synthase, serine palmitoyl transferase, or UDP-glucose ceramide glycosyltransferase did not show a significantly increased expression profile (41).

Nevertheless, the best way to demonstrate the efficacy of PS is in a clinical study (44). Volunteers with moderate, inflamed acne on the face participated in a half-face study. Objective criteria for the studies were based on "Echelle d'évaluation clinique des lesions d'acné"/ECLA/Clinical evaluation of acne injuries: the number of comedones, the number of pustules, and the number of papules.

The evaluated products were applied on one-half of the face. The evaluated products included the commonly used compound BPO as the benchmark ingredient against acne. Since the combination of BPO and PS in a formulation has been shown to be unstable (chemical interaction between the active ingredients), the two compounds have to be separated from each other. Therefore, a two-chamber dispenser was used. The following trial combinations were chosen:

- Placebo versus 0.2% PS (15 volunteers aged 10–50 years)
- 4% BPO versus 0.2% PS + 4% BPO formulated in a two-chamber dispenser (30 volunteers aged 15–25 years)

The consultations of the volunteers with the dermatologist were on day 0, day 30, and day 60. Neither PS nor BPO caused cutaneous intolerance throughout the study period. However, PS had a strong effect on diminishing the number of papules, pustules, but not comedones. After 60 days of treatment with 0.2% PS, papules and pustules were decreased by 89% (Table 2). In addition, PS is perfectly tolerated by the skin and shows a very good action against inflammatory superficial acne. Despite a good cutaneous acceptance, the antibacterial potential of BPO was only able to decrease the observed papules and pustules, and comedones by 32% and 22% (Table 2), respectively, after 60 days of treatment. However, the combination of 0.2% PS with 4% BPO resulted in a synergistic effect. Already, after 30 days of treatment, the number of papules plus pustules and comedones were diminished to 60% and 43%, respectively, compared with 25% and −6% (" − " corresponds to an increase!) respectively, with PS only, or to 10% and 15% with BPO only (Table 2). Although PS was not able to prevent the formation of comedones, it was able to at least control the number of comedones that were induced by the placebo formulation alone.

Subjective efficacy was clear: the skin was less inflamed, and the volunteers noticed clearly a rapid improvement in the inflammatory lesions and a diminution of comedones. In most cases, the effect was noticed after one week of treatment. The use of PS resulted in a softening and "comfort" of the skin, which the volunteers had lost when they developed acne. Both PS and the combination product (PS and BPO) were considered to have the following characteristics: easy to use, good cosmetic quality, good cosmetic acceptability with ease of use, and nongreasy appearance. Even make-up could still be applied without problems.

TABLE 2 A Clinical Study on the Reduction of Comedones, and Papules and Pustules[a]

	Placebo	PS	BPO	PS + BPO
Reduction of comedones (%)				
Day 30	−43	−6	15	43
Day 60	−43	−6	22	72
Reduction of papules and pustules (%)				
Day 30	0	25	10	60
Day 60	0	89	32	88

[a]Determined by "Echelle d'évaluation clinique des lesions d'acné"/ECLA/Clinical evaluation of acne injuries.
Abbreviations: BPO, benzoyl peroxide, PS, phytosphingosine.
Source: From Ref. 44.

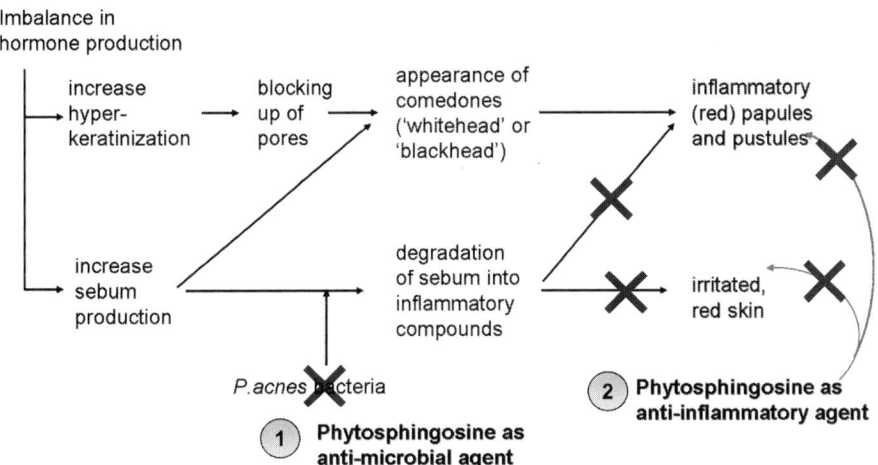

FIGURE 3 The strong antimicrobial and anti-inflammatory properties of phytosphingosine work synergistically on acne.

Taken together, the effects as an anti-inflammatory and a bacteriostatic agent could be the reasons for the reduction of comedone formation compared with placebo (Fig. 3).

CONCLUSIONS

Acne is a common dermatological diagnosis that affects boys and girls during puberty and may persist throughout adulthood. Anti-acne therapies target: (*i*) the enhanced sebum production, (*ii*) the enhanced hyperkeratinization, (*iii*) the increased *P. acnes* colonization, and (*iv*) the inflammatory response. In addition, there is increasing evidence for the need of the treatment of the non-lesional sites to prevent comedogenesis and to improve skin barrier function. On the basis of the latest scientific findings, agents that possess anti-inflammatory effects are highly interesting because they seem to represent a useful adjunct to the established anti-acne armory.

PS is naturally occurring in human skin since it is an enzymatic breakdown product of ceramides. It comprises about 40% of the epidermal sphingoid bases and plays an important part in regulating the microflora of the skin. A commercial bio-fermentation process for PS has been established and is based on a non-GM yeast. PS obtained via this route is chemically identical to the material found in human skin because of the same stereochemical D-erythro configuration. This unique configuration is crucial for optimal performance since only the right three-dimensional structure makes favorable interactions with any stereoselective cellular targets.

Starting from PS, an economical and efficient chemical route for another sphingoid base, sphingosine, has been developed. The skin-identical sphingosine is generated by a seven-step chemical reaction cascade in high yield and represents a bioactive sphingoid base with yet unexplored profiles but should potentially be also an effective molecule to treat the blemished skin. First study results do point is this direction.

PS has been proven to be a clinically useful adjunct for the treatment of acne. The use of PS resulted in a softening and comfort of the skin, which the volunteers had lost when they developed acne. Both PS and a combination product of PS and BPO were considered to be effective treatments and offer qualities such as good cosmetic acceptability with ease of use and non-greasy appearance.

Taken together, the effects of PS as an anti-inflammatory and a bacteriostatic agent could be considered a new effective way to treat acne-prone skin and might find its way into a number of skin products designed for this specific purpose.

ACKNOWLEDGMENT

The authors wish to thank Dr. Kees Korevaar for his helpful contribution to the manuscript.

REFERENCES

1. Rawlings AV, Harding CR. Moisturization and skin barrier function. Dermatol Ther 2004; 17(suppl 1):43–48.
2. Van Hoogendalem EJ. Transdermal absorption of topical anti-acne agents in man; review of clinical pharmacokinetic data. J Eur Acad Dermatol Venereo 1998; 11(suppl 1):13–19; discussion 28–29.
3. Wertz PW, Swartzendruber DC, Madison KC, Downing DT. Composition and morphology of epidermal cyst lipids. J Invest Dermatol 1987; 89:419–425.
4. Williams ML, Elias PM. The extracellular matrix of stratum corneum: role of lipids in normal and pathological function. Rev Ther Drug Carrier Syst 1987; 3:95–122.
5. Thiboutot D, Knaggs H, Gilliland K, et al. Activity of 5-alpha-reductase and 17-beta-hydroxysteroid dehydrogenase in the infrainfundibulum of subjects with and without acne vulgaris. Dermatology 1998; 196:38–42.
6. Clark SM, Goulden V, Finlay AY, et al. The psychological and social impact of acne: a comparison study using three acne disability questionnaires (Abstract). Br J Dermatol 1997; 137(suppl 50):41.
7. Gupta MA, Johnson AM, Gupta AK. The development of an acne quality of life scale: reliability, validity, and relation to subjective acne severity in mild to moderate acne vulgaris. Acta Derm Venereol 1998 (Stockhausen); 78:451–456.
8. Kligman AM. An overview of acne. J Invest Dermatol 1974; 62:268–287.
9. White GM. Recent findings in the epidemiology, classification and subtypes of acne vulgaris. J Am Acad Dermatol 1998; 39:534–537.
10. Schmidt JB, Spona J, Huber J. Androgen receptor in hirsutism and acne. Gynecol Obstet Invest 1986; 22:206–211.
11. Henze C, Hinney B, Wuttke W. Incidence of increased androgen levels in patients suffering from acne. Dermatology 1998; 196:53–54.
12. Cunliffe WJ, Gollnick H. Acne diagnosis and management. In: Martin Dunitz. London: Taylor & Francis Group, 2001.
13. Zouboulis CC. Human skin: an independent peripheral endocrine organ. Horm Res 2000; 54:230–242.
14. Plewig G, Kligman AM. Acne and Rosacea. 3rd Completely Revised and Enlarged ed. Berlin: Springer-Verlag, 2000:581–582.
15. Gollnick HP, Zouboulis CC, Akamatsu H, et al. Pathogenesis and pathogenesis related treatment of acne. J Dermatol 1991; 18:489–499.
16. Knaggs HE, Holland DB, Morris C, et al. Quantification of cellular proliferation in acne using the monoclonal antibody Ki-67. J Invest Dermatol 1994; 102:89–92.
17. Thiboutot DM, Knaggs H, Gilliland K, et al. Activity of type I 5-alpha-reductase is greater in the follicular infundibulum compared with the epidermis. Br J Dermatol 1997; 136:166–171.
18. Zouboulis CC, Xia L, Akamatsu H, et al. The human sebocyte culture model provides new insight into development and management of seborrhoea and acne. Dermatology 1998; 196:21–31.

19. Holland KT, Greenman J, Cunliffe WJ. Growth of cutaneous propionibacteria on synthetic medium: growth yields and enzyme production. J Appl Bacteriol 1979; 47:383–394.
20. Shalita AR, Lee WL. Inflammatory acne. Dermatol Clin 1983; 1:361–364.
21. Melnik B, Plewig G. New biochemical aspects of lipids in the pathogenesis of abnormal follicular keratinisation in acne vulgaris (Article in German). Z Hautkr 1988; 63:591–596.
22. Fujie T, Shikiji T, Uchida N, et al. Culture of cells derived from the human sebaceous gland under serum-free conditions without a biological feeder layer or specific matices. Arch Dermatol Res 1996; 288:703–708.
23. http://www.medizininfo.de/hautundhaar (accessed April 2005).
24. Jansen T, Burgdorf W, Plewig G. Pathogenesis and treatment of acne in childhood. Pediatr Dermatol 1997; 14:7–21.
25. Humbert P. Induced Acne (Article in French). Rev Prat 2002; 52:838–840.
26. Friedman GD. Twin studies of disease heritage based on medical records: application to acne vulgaris. Acta Genet Med Gemellol 1984; 33:487–495.
27. Gollnick H. Current concepts of the pathogenesis of acne. Drugs 2003; 63:1579–1596.
28. Törmä H. Interaction of isotretinoin with endogenous retinoids. J Am Acad Dermatol 2001; 45(suppl 5):143–149.
29. White GM. Acne therapy. Dis Mon 1999; 45:301–330.
30. Zander E, Weisman S. Treatment of acne vulgaris with salicylic acid. Clin Ther 1992; 14:247–253.
31. Zouboulis CC. Exploration of retinoid activity and the role of inflammation in acne: issues affecting the future directions for acne therapy. J Eur Acad Dermatol Venereol 2001; 15(suppl 3):63–67.
32. Müller-Bohn T. Neue Chancen in der Dermatologie. Deutsche Apotheker Zeitung 2004; 144:1967–1974.
33. Vega B, Ferret C, Jomard A, et al. Regulation of Toll-like receptor 2 expression by adapalene: implications for the treatment of inflammatory acne. Poster P0156, International Investigative Dermatology Meeting, Miami Beach, FL, April 30–May 4, 2003.
34. Elias PM. Structural lipids, barrier function, and desquamation. J Invest Dermatol 1983; 80:44s–49s.
35. Harris IR, Farrell AM, Grunfeld C, Holleran WM, Elias PM, Feingold KR. Permeability barrier disruption coordinately regulates mRNA levels for key enzymes of cholesterol, fatty acid, and ceramide synthesis in the epidermis. J Invest Dermatol 1997; 109(6):783–787.
36. Geilen CC, Wieder T, Orfanos CE. Ceramide signalling: regulatory role in cell proliferation, differentiation and apoptosis in human epidermis. Arch Dermatol Res 1997; 289(10):559–566.
37. Shapiro D, Segal K. The synthesis of sphingosine. J Am Chem Soc 1954; 76: 5896–5895.
38. van den Berg RJBH, Korevaar CGN, Overkleeft HS, et al. Effective, high-yield, and stereospecific total synthesis of D-erythro-(2R,3S)-sphingosine from D-ribo-(2S,3S,4R)-phytosphingosine. J Org Chem 2004; 69:5699–5704.
39. Inhibition of bacterial growth by phytosphingosine: An in-vitro antimicrobial study, Degussa AG (unpublished data).
40. Bibel, DJ, Aly, R, Shienfield, HR. Antimicrobial activity of sphingosines. J Invest Dermatol 2000; 98(3):269–273.
41. DNA-Chip analysis of changes in the gene expression patterns of keratinocytes after incubation with phytosphingosine, Degussa AG (unpublished data).
42. Influence on the application of phytosphingosine on reconstituted epidermis, Degussa AG (unpublished data).
43. Analysis of changes in the lipid composition of keratinocytes after incubation with phytosphingosine, Degussa AG (unpublished data).
44. Phytosphingosine clinical study on acne: determination of the effectiveness of phytosphingosine to enhance or complement existing acne therapies, Degussa AG (unpublished data).

5α-Reductase and Its Inhibitors

Rainer Voegeli
Department of Research and Development, Pentapharm Ltd., Basel, Switzerland

Christos C. Zouboulis
Departments of Dermatology and Immunology, Dessau Medical Center, Dessau, Germany

Peter Elsner
Department of Dermatology and Allergology, Friedrich-Schiller-University Jena, Jena, Germany

Thomas Schreier
Department of Research and Development, Pentapharm Ltd., Basel, Switzerland

INTRODUCTION

5α-dihydrotestosterone (DHT) exerts a 2 to 10 times stronger androgen activity than testosterone. Thus, this steroid hormone was supposed to play a more important role than testosterone in many androgen-dependent diseases such as acne, hirsutism, androgenetic alopecia, benign prostatic hyperplasia, and prostate carcinoma. DHT is converted from testosterone by the enzyme 5α-reductase. There are two isoenzymes of 5α-reductase (types 1 and 2) that differ in their localization within the body and even in the skin. Activity of the type 1 isoenzyme predominates in sebaceous glands, where it may be involved in regulation of sebum production. Therefore, specific inhibition of type 1 5α-reductase may represent a therapeutic approach to acne. This review refers to the features both of 5α-reductases and of their inhibitors.

ANDROGEN METABOLISM IN THE SKIN

The androgenic provoked stimulation of sebum production plays a crucial role in the pathogenesis of acne. Although numerous factors contribute to the development of acne, the requirement for androgens is absolute (1). Thiboutot et al. (2) and Fritsch et al. (3) demonstrated that human skin is indeed a steroidogenic tissue. The skin functions as an independent peripheral endocrine organ (4) expressing all the enzymes necessary for androgen synthesis and catabolism. It can synthesize cholesterol from acetate and can further metabolize steroids such as dehydroepiandrosterone sulfate into potent androgens such as testosterone and DHT. DHT itself further induces enzymes such as 3α-hydroxysteroid dehydrogenase and 17β-hydroxysteroid dehydrogenase (5).

The skin compartment responsible for both the initiation of steroidogenesis and the local production of potent androgens seems to be the sebaceous gland. Therefore, selective local interruption of this pathway can be of therapeutic benefit in androgen-mediated diseases of the skin and allows for effective treatments (3).

Further details on the androgen metabolism in the skin are explicitly described in Chapter 7.

5α-REDUCTASE
Historical Background
It was not until 1954 that a series of 5α-reduced steroids, produced from the incubation of androst-4-ene-3,17-dione with rabbit liver homogenate, was recognized by paper chromatography. Two years later, DHT was first identified as the major metabolite of the incubation of testosterone with rat liver homogenate. Both independent experiments indicated the presence of 5α-reductase in the liver tissues of rabbits and rats. Since then, this membrane-bound enzyme has been demonstrated to be present in many other organs and androgen-sensitive tissues of mammalian species (6). Subsequent investigations revealed that the enzyme catalyzes the reduction of a variety of steroids, while nicotinamide adenine dinucleotide phosphate-oxidase (NADPH) is needed as an essential cofactor (Fig. 1) (7).

The realization that 5α-reductase plays an important role in androgen metabolism began in the early 1960s, when in bioassays, DHT was demonstrated to be a more potent androgen than testosterone in the prostate. Further studies revealed that administration of radiolabeled testosterone led to an accumulation of DHT in the nuclei of ventral prostate cells. Moreover, DHT was shown to bind preferentially to the specific nuclear androgen receptor in target organs. The androgen receptor is a member of the steroid-thyroid-retinoid family of transcription regulatory factors. The DHT-receptor complex interacts with specific portions of the genome to regulate gene activities. Developmental studies revealed that 5α-reductase activity in mammalian embryos was high in the primordia of the prostate and external genitalia prior to their virilization but very low in Wolffian duct structures, suggesting that the enzyme was crucial for the development of the normal male phenotype during embryogenesis. Taken together, these data implied that conversion of testosterone to DHT by 5α-reductase was a critical step in male sexual differentiation and focused attention on the role of 5α-reductase in androgen physiology and pathophysiology (7).

Studies in the 1970s and 1980s revealed that the skin, in addition to the prostate, is rich in 5α-reductase. In this respect, it appeared very likely that 5α-reductase functions as an autocrine mediator in both the skin growth and skin differentiation (8). In 1976, the biochemical properties of 5α-reductase were investigated in cell-free extracts of fibroblasts cultured from genital and nongenital skin of healthy subjects and patients with male hermaphroditism. In these experiments, two types of 5α-reductase activities were distinguished: one detectable mainly in genital skin with an optimal pH of about 5.5 and another with an optimal pH between six

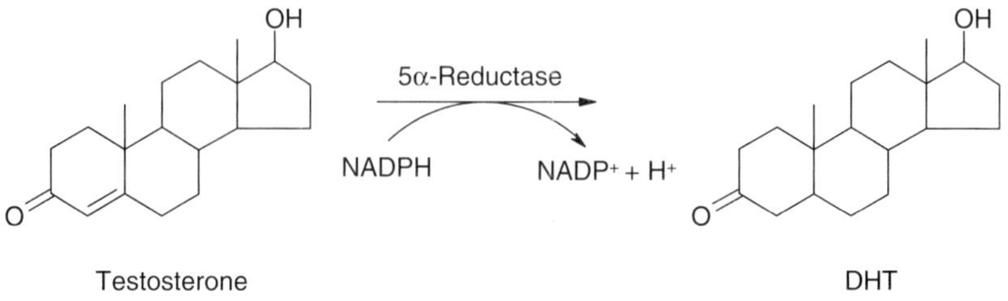

FIGURE 1   Reduction of steroids to 5α-steroids by 5α-reductase.

and nine in all fibroblasts, cultured from normal and mutant skin taken from both genital and nongenital areas. Patients with congenital 5α-reductase deficiency seemed to lack the former enzyme only (9). In contrast to type-2 isoenzyme, no human pathology with a deficiency or mutation of the type 1 isoenzyme has been identified so far (10).

In the following, attention has been focused on molecular biological approaches to identifying and isolating 5α-reductase. In 1989, a cDNA encoding a rat liver 5α-reductase was isolated and used to identify a single mRNA species in both liver and prostate of the rat. When this rat 5α-reductase cDNA was used to screen cDNA libraries constructed from human prostate mRNA, a corresponding cDNA was isolated in 1990. However, when the human cDNA was expressed in COS cells, the 5α-reductase activity produced was highest at the physiological pH values, and not at 5.5 as deduced from earlier biochemical studies. Moreover, the enzyme showed different inhibitor specificity than expected. As the gene encoding this cDNA was also normal in 5α-reductase-deficient individuals, it was again suggested in 1991 that there must be at least 2 isoforms of human 5α-reductase (11), as already proposed by Moore and Wilson (12) by biochemical means in 1976. Later on, a second 5α-reductase gene was also isolated from a human prostate genomic library. This gene encoded a protein with 50% homology to the former one. Accordingly, these enzymes were designated as type 1 and type 2 5α-reductase, respectively, in the order in which they were cloned (11).

Physiological Role

5α-reductase is the key enzyme in androgen metabolism. Altered enzyme function and/or regulation are responsible for numerous human pathologies. In humans, the normal activity of 5α-reductases routinely maintains testosterone-mediated biological functions, such as anabolic actions (muscle-mass increase, penis enlargement, scrotum enlargement, and vocal cords enlargement), spermatogenesis (male sex drive and performance), and DHT-mediated effects, such as increased facial and body hair, scalp hair recession, acne, and prostate enlargement (6).

The deficiency of 5α-reductase in males results in incomplete differentiation of the external genitalia at birth. At puberty, patients have normal-to-elevated levels of testosterone in plasma, and virilization occurs, but the prostate remains small and there is no acne. Male pseudohermaphroditism is accompanied by low levels of DHT. However, females with 5α-reductase deficiency appear to have no clinical signs, however, the enzyme also metabolizes other 4-ene-3-oxosteroids, such as progesterone and corticosterone. Abnormally, high 5α-reductase activity in humans results in excessively high DHT levels in peripheral tissues, which is implicated in the pathogenesis of prostate carcinoma, benign prostatic hyperplasia, acne, hirsutism, and androgenetic alopecia (6).

The exact physiological role of type 2 5α-reductase in tissues other than prostate and accessories of the external genitalia remains unknown, since these organs do not appear to be affected by the genetic absence of this isoenzyme or by its pharmacological inhibition and the women concerned have normal sexual development and are fertile. The physiological reasons and the factors that mediate this temporal pattern of expression are not known. However, given the role of androgens in 5α-reductase regulation, it is intriguing to speculate that the expression of one gene may influence the timing or expression level of the other: type 2 isoenzyme had a priming effect on tissues, such as the prostate, skin and scalp, on which type 1 isoenzyme will act later in life (13).

The androgen control of sebum production and the role of type 1 5α-reductase in the pathogenesis of acne are confirmed by the following data and clinical observations:

1. Male castrates produce less sebum than normal males and they do not have acne unless testosterone is given.
2. Androgen administration also results in a significant increase in sebum production in women.
3. Human sebaceous glands are rich in type 1 5α-reductase activity.
4. Sebum production is not detectable in subjects with complete androgen insensitivity (13).
5. Adult males with type 2 5α-reductase deficiency have sebum production scores identical to normal age-matched males.
6. Males with benign prostatic hyperplasia treated with Finasteride (5 mg/day for one year) did not show decreased sebum production, although the serum 5α-DHT level was lowered (14).

Biochemical Characterization

Both types of human 5α-reductases are hydrophobic, microsomal enzymes with a molecular mass of approximately 29 kDa (Table 1). Type 1 isoenzyme, composed of 259 amino acids, has an optimal pH of 6.5 to 8.0, whereas type 2 isoenzyme is composed of 254 amino acids and has an optimal pH of 5.5 (Fig. 2). The determinants of androgen binding are encoded at the ends of the molecule, while those of NADPH binding are encoded in the carboxyl terminal half of the enzyme. Both isoenzymes have similar substrate preferences for gene structures (9). An average of 37% of the amino acids have side chains commonly found buried in the hydrophobic interior of globular proteins. These hydrophobic residues are distributed throughout the enzyme and do not give rise to clear-cut transmembrane regions in hydropathy plots. This structural feature suggests the 5α-reductase isoenzymes are intrinsic membrane proteins deeply embedded in the lipid bilayer (15).

The enzymes have never been fully biochemically characterized (11), as the isolation and purification have been difficult due to the insolubility and, generally, the rather low activity of these membrane-bound proteins. Since X-ray patterns are still to be determined (16), only indirect information is available on the

TABLE 1 Properties of Human Type 1 and Type 2 5α-Reductases

Properties	Type 1	Type 2
pH optimum	6.5–8.0	5.0–5.5
Amino acids	259	254
Molecular mass	29,494 Da	28,389 Da
Base pairs	2100	2437
Gene	SRD5A1	SRD5A2
Locus	Chromosome 5p15	Chromosome 2p23
Mutations	None	Multiples
Homology human/human	50%	50%
Homology human/rat	61%	75%
Homology human/cynomolgus	93%	95%
General localization	Peripheral skin	Prostate, male external genitalia

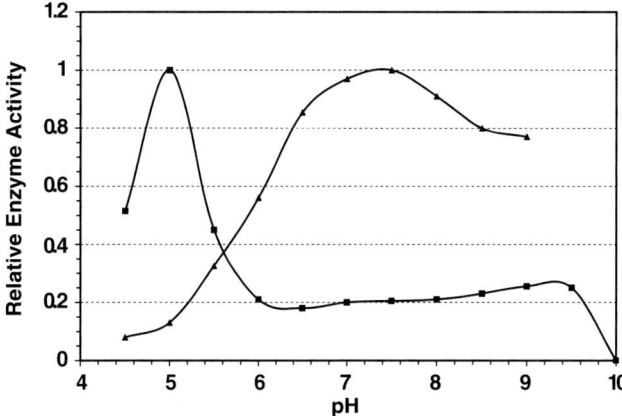

FIGURE 2 Activities of human recombinant type 1 and type 2 5α-reductase expressed in CHO cells. The activities were determined over the indicated pH range in the presence of 1 to −1.5 μM [^{14}C] testosterone and have been normalized to the highest value in each data set. They consequently are represented as relative enzyme activities. ▲ = type 1 isoenzyme (50 pmol min^{-1} mg^{-1}), ■ = type 2 isoenzyme (15 pmol min^{-1} mg^{-1}). *Source*: Adapted from Ref. 19.

three-dimensional structures of their binding sites. To circumvent these difficulties, expression-cloning strategies have been used to isolate cDNA (17).

Genetically, the type 1 isoenzyme is encoded by the SRD5A1 gene on the short arm of chromosome 5 (band p15), while the type 2 isoenzyme by the SRD5A2 gene on chromosome 2 (band p23). Both gene structures are similar in that each contains five exons separated by four introns (14).

Western blot studies of human cell cultures (sebocytes, keratinocytes, fibroblasts, dermal microvascular endothelial cells, and melanocytes) by Chen et al. (8) show two closely lying bands of type 1 5α-reductase in the range of 21 to 27 kDa, possibly indicating the existence of heterogeneous proteins. This finding is supported by a study of Lopez-Solache (18) that reveals the presence of two forms of mRNA species for rat type 1 5α-reductase. Possible explanations of the two bands could be:

1. partial protein denaturation during the process of extraction or isolation,
2. the existence of the enzyme in two states, activated or inactivated, through either phosphorylation, dephosphorylation (8), or proteolytic cleavage of a zymogen, and
3. alternative splicing of mRNA.

Species Variation

Intraspecies and interspecies comparisons of the amino acid sequences between type 1 and type 2 isoenzymes show only moderate homologies, suggesting differing structure, functions, and/or regulations. Homology between the human type 1 and type 2 5α-reductases is approximately 50% (Fig. 3). The type 1 human and rat isoenzymes have approximately 61% amino acid sequence identity, while the two corresponding type 2 5α-reductases are 75% homologous (Table 1). The considerable differences of the enzymes concerning protein structure, functional characteristics,

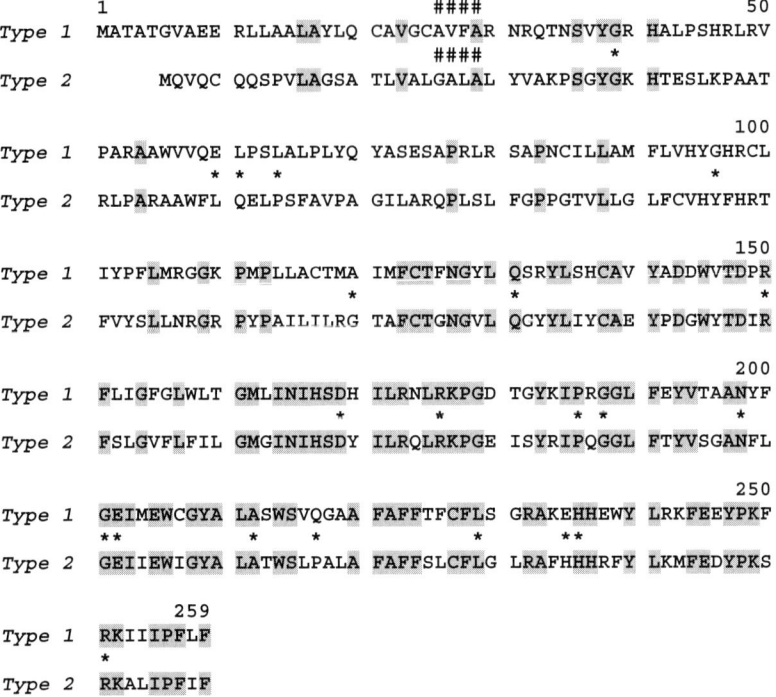

```
        1                              ####                          50
Type 1  MATATGVAEE RLLAALAYLQ CAVGCAVFAR NRQTNSVYGR HALPSHRLRV
                                       ####                *
Type 2     MQVQC QQSPVLAGSA TLVALGALAL YVAKPSGYGK HTESLKPAAT

                                                                    100
Type 1  PARAAWVVQE LPSLALPLYQ YASESAPRLR SAPNCILLAM FLVHYGHRCL
                     *    *    *                                   *
Type 2  RLPARAAWFL QELPSFAVPA GILARQPLSL FGPPGTVLLG LFCVHYFHRT

                                                                    150
Type 1  IYPFLMRGGK PMPLLACTMA IMFCTFNGYL QSRYLSHCAV YADDWVTDPR
                        *                    *                     *
Type 2  FVYSLLNRGR PYPAILILRG TAFCTGNGVL QGCYYLIYCAE YPDGWYTDIR

                                                                    200
Type 1  FLIGFGLWLT GMLINIHSDH ILRNLRKPGD TGYKIPRGGL FEYVTAANYF
                        *         *          *  *                  *
Type 2  FSLGVFLFIL GMGINIHSDY ILRQLRKPGE ISYRIPQGGL FTYVSGANFL

                                                                    250
Type 1  GEIMEWCGYA LASWSVQGAA FAFFTFCFLS GRAKEHHEWY LRKFEEYPKF
         * *           *    *              *          * *
Type 2  GEIIEWIGYA LATWSLPALA FAFFSLCFLG LRAFHHHRFY LKMFEDYPKS

                259
Type 1  RKIIIPFLF
         *
Type 2  RKALIPFIF
```

FIGURE 3   Amino acid sequences of human type 1 and type 2 5α-reductase. Shaded amino acids represent homologous items. Asterisks above the sequence stand for amino acid positions of naturally occurring mutants in type 2 isoenzyme deficient patients. Hash keys above the sequence denote the tetrapeptide sequence implicated in Finasteride binding. *Source*: Adapted from Ref. 19.

and tissue distribution would seem to make the rat a poor choice as a model for comparative in vivo pharmacological assessment of novel human 5α-reductase inhibitors. For example, rat type 1 isoenzyme is at least 50-fold more susceptible to inhibition by Finasteride than its human counterpart and the activities of both type 1 and type 2 5α-reductases can be monitored in rat prostate, while activity of the type 2 isoenzyme predominates in tissue from the mature human organ (19).

In the Cynomolgus monkey, 5α-reductases are highly homologous to their human protein analogs, sharing about 93% (type 1) and 95% (type 2) amino acid sequence identity. The results of inhibition studies indicate that the monkey isoenzymes are comparable on a molecular level to their respective human counterparts, supporting the relevance and use of the Cynomolgus monkey as a pharmacological model for in vivo evaluation of 5α-reductase inhibitors (19).

Enzymatic Activity and Specificity

5α-reductase, or more precisely NADPH: 4-ene-3-oxosteroid 5-oxidoreductase (EC 1.3.99.5), is a NADPH-dependent enzyme that selectively and irreversibly catalyzes the reduction of the 4,5-double bond of 4-ene-3-oxosteroids (e.g., testosterone,

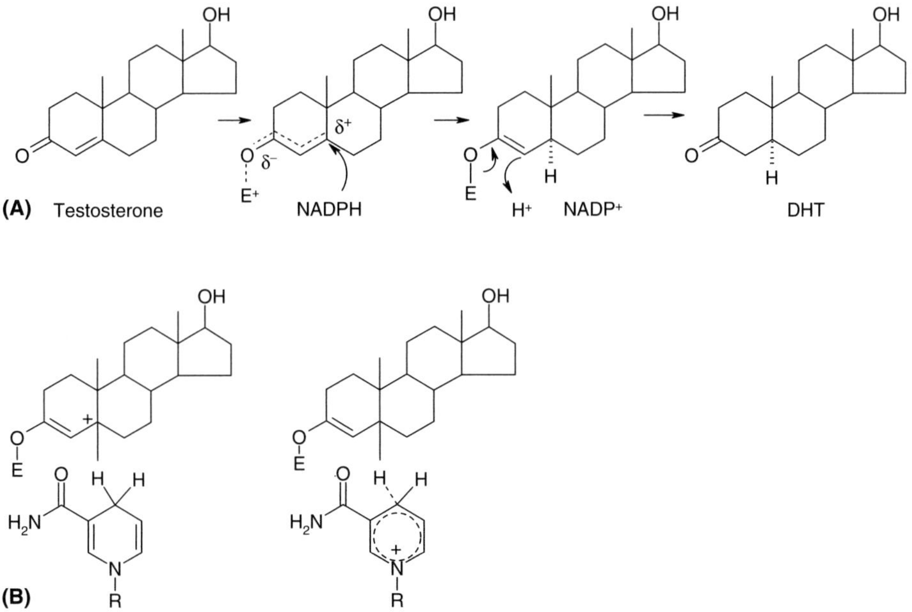

FIGURE 4 (A) Proposed mechanism of the catalysis of testosterone to DHT by 5α-reductase. (B) Substrate-like transition state (*Left*) and product-like transition state (*Right*). *Source*: Adapted from Ref. 16.

progesterone, and androstenedione) into the corresponding 5α-3-oxosteroids (DHT, 5α-dihydroprogesterone, and 5α-androstanedione) (13).

The proposed mechanism (Fig. 4A) of testosterone reduction to DHT by 5α-reductase catalysis involves, as a key step, the activation of the 4-en-3-on moiety of testosterone by the interaction of the carbonyl group with an electrophilic residue E^+ of the active site, followed by hydride transfer from NADPH to the position 5 (16). This leads to enolate formation at C-3, C-4, which presumably is stabilized by E^+ at the active site. The process may be viewed alternatively as activation of the enone by E^+ leading to a positively polarized species, which accepts a hydride from NADPH at C-5. Enzyme mediated tautomerism then leads to DHT with release of $NADP^+$ (5). Thus, it is possible to postulate two different transition states: the "substrate-like" transition state in which the C-5 has not yet changed its sp^2 hybridization and the "product-like" transition state, in which the C-5 has assumed the final sp^3 hybridization (Fig. 4B) (16).

The differences in primary sequences result in unique functional characteristics of the two isoenzymes. It has been proposed that the two isoenzymes have different roles in androgen metabolism (13).

5α-reductases have apparent K_m values in the micro- to nanomolar range for steroid substrates (Table 2) (20). The relative affinity of $\Delta^{4(5)}$-steroids for type 1 isoenzyme is:

20α−hydroxyprogesterone $\longrightarrow$ progesterone $\longrightarrow$ androstenedione
$\longrightarrow$ testosterone $\longrightarrow$ corticosterone

TABLE 2 Substrate Preference of Recombinant Steroid 5α-Reductase Isoenzymes

	Type 1			Type 2		
Steroid substrate	K_m (µM)	V_{max} (pmol min^{-1} mg^{-1})	V_{max}/K_m (pmol min^{-1} mg^{-1} µM^{-1})	K_m (µM)	V_{max} (pmol min^{-1} mg^{-1})	V_{max}/K_m (pmol min^{-1} mg^{-1} µM^{-1})
Testosterone	3.5–5.2	220	40–60	0.7	88	115
Androstenedione	1.0	395	390	0.8	90	110
Progesterone	0.3	370	1230	0.3	80	260
20α-Hydroxyprogesterone	0.2	570	2850	0.4	85	240
Corticosterone	18	210	12	4	42	11

Note: Type 1 and type 2 5α-reductase activities were determined at pH 7.5 (50 mM sodium phosphate) and pH 5.0 (50 mM sodium citrate), respectively. 1 mM glucose-6-phosphate and 0.5 U/mL glucose-6-phosphate dehydrogenase was included as a cofactor regenerating system (NADP$^+$ to NADPH). Experiments were conducted using recombinant type 1 (0.05–0.10 mg protein per assay) and type 2 (0.02–0.15 mg protein per assay) isoenzymes expressed in CHO cells. Standard errors for all values were less than 20% of the indicated entries.

Source: Adapted from Ref. 19.

and for the type 2 isoenzyme:

progesterone $\longrightarrow$ 20α$-$hydroxyprogesterone $\longrightarrow$ testosterone

$\longrightarrow$ androstenedione $\longrightarrow$ corticosterone

The conversion of testosterone to DHT amplifies the androgenic signal through four mechanisms:

1. DHT, unlike testosterone, cannot be aromatized to estrogen, thus its effect remains purely androgenic (14).
2. DHT binds to the human androgen receptor with a several-fold higher affinity than testosterone does (14). It has also been suggested that the DHT/androgen receptor complex has a higher affinity for the acceptor site in the nuclear chromatin (5).
3. The DHT/androgen receptor complex appears to be more stable (14).
4. Both the 5α-reductase genes are adjusted by DHT via a feed-forward regulation (13).

Although testosterone and DHT share the same androgen receptor, it is not surprising that the two androgens exert varying physiological effects.

Localization, Distribution, and Cutaneous Enzymatic Activity
General
The specific localization and activity of type 1 isoenzyme in sebaceous glands makes this isoenzyme a potential therapeutic target for the treatment of acne. For this reason, it becomes important to understand where and how the two isoenzymes of 5α-reductase act in the skin (21).

Type 1 5α-reductase is present, above all, in the skin, whereas type 2 is predominantly located in the prostate and in genital skin (9). Both the isoenzymes are expressed in the liver. In humans type 1 is not detectable in the fetus but is permanently expressed in skin and scalp from the time of puberty (13).

Cutaneous Distribution
In humans, the cutaneous distribution of type 1 isoenzyme was identified immunohistochemically to be localized predominantly within sebaceous glands (8). The enzymatic activity is significantly higher, on the one hand in sebaceous glands of the face and scalp compared to nonacne-prone areas, and on the other hand in sebaceous glands in men than women (14). Type 1 isoenzyme was also found in epidermis, eccrine sweat glands, apocrine sweat glands (in normal ones as well as in people with osmidrosis), hair follicles (outer root sheath cells, dermal papilla cells, matrix cells), endothelial cells of small vessels, and in Schwann cells of cutaneous myelinated nerves (8).

Within hair follicles, type 2 isoenzyme was localized by prominent immunostaining in the inner layer of outer root sheaths, inner root sheaths, and the infundibulum, as well as in sebaceous ducts. Regional studies showed the type 2 mRNA present in beard dermal papilla, but absent from occipital scalp and axillary dermal papilla. The type 2 isoenzyme in beard dermal papilla has a three-times higher activity than the type 1 5α-reductase present in the occipital scalp and axillary dermal papilla. The specific activity of 5α-reductase in the hair dermal papilla exceeded those in other hair follicle compartments (connective tissue sheaths and outer root sheaths) by a factor of at least 14 in the scalp and at least 80 in the beard. The beard dermal papilla cells appeared to generate more DHT than those from nonbalding scalp hair follicles. However, the individual freshly isolated intact dermal papilla was shown to possess considerably different levels of ex vivo enzyme activities (14).

Taken together, while the type 1 5α-reductase has been definitely demonstrated in sebaceous glands, the isoenzyme distribution in hair follicle is less well defined, probably due to

1. local and temporal variation of enzyme activity,
2. utilization of different polyclonal/monoclonal antibodies, and
3. inadequate assessment of enough specimens.

More evidence is needed to better define the existence of the type 1 isoenzyme in hair follicles and the precise localization of the type 2 isoenzyme within the hair follicles (in outer root sheaths or in dermal papilla) (14).

In the following sections we refer extensively to three eminent publications demonstrating the localization of 5α-reductase in cells, in sebaceous follicles, and its enzymatic activity in epidermal and infrainfundibular keratinocytes.

Subcellular Localization and Expression of Type 1 5α-Reductase

Chen et al. (8) examined cutaneous expression and subcellular localization of type 1 5α-reductase in vitro by using human cell cultures (sebocytes, keratinocytes, fibroblasts, dermal microvascular endothelial cells, hair dermal papilla cells, and melanocytes) with immunocytochemistry, western and northern blot studies.

With immunocytochemistry it was shown that type 1 5α-reductase is located in the cytoplasm of all examined cultured skin cell types and not in the nucleus as described by some authors. The expression could be broadly divided into three groups, in the order of decreasing intensity (Fig. 5):

1. adult facial sebocytes and neonatal foreskin keratinocytes,
2. adult nongenital keratinocytes (flank), occipital dermal papilla cells, occipital fibroblasts, and
3. beard dermal papilla cells, melanocytes, dermal microvascular endothelial cells, and chin fibroblasts.

Moreover, among sebocytes, the smaller, less differentiated sebocytes were more strongly stained than the larger, differentiated ones (Fig. 6).

Further findings of the study were:

1. The most abundant expression of type 1 5α-reductase is in neonatal foreskin keratinocytes, followed by adult facial sebocytes.
2. The strongest expression of type 1 5α-reductase among skin cells from adult subjects is in facial sebocytes.
3. The expression of type 1 5α-reductase in fibroblasts and keratinocytes is subject to regional variance.
4. Type 1 5α-reductase is present in dermal papilla cells of both beard and occipital hair cells, whereas it is expressed more strongly in the latter.
5. Type 1 5α-reductase is expressed in cultured melanocytes. The significance of this interesting finding remains unknown.

The strongest expression of type 1 5α-reductase in sebocytes among adult skin cells examined confirmed the previous hypothesis of the authors that the sebaceous

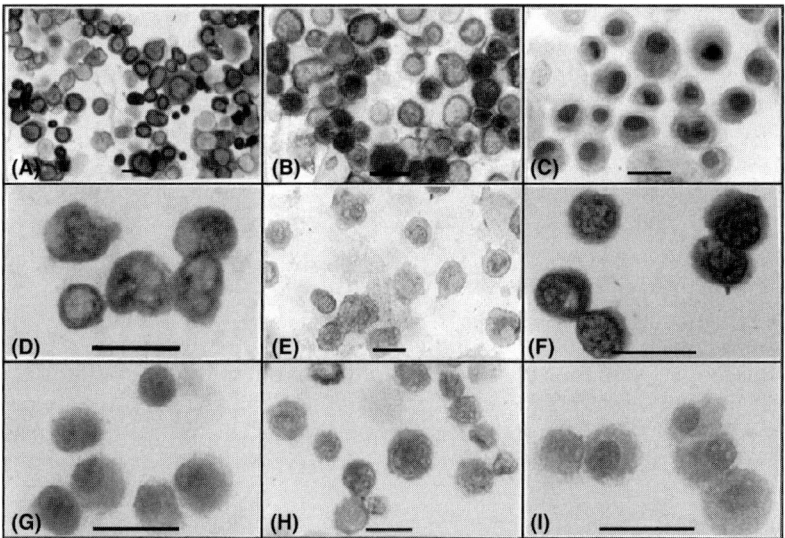

FIGURE 5 (*See color insert.*) Immunocytochemistry using rabbit antiserum raised against human type 1 5α-reductase. (**A**) adult facial sebocytes, (**B**) neonatal foreskin keratinocytes, (**C**) adult nongenital keratinocytes (flank), (**D**) occipital dermal papilla cells, (**E**) beard dermal papilla cells, (**F**) occipital fibroblasts, (**G**) melanocytes, (**H**) dermal microvascular endothelial cells, and (**I**) chin fibroblasts. Scale bars = 50 μm. *Source*: From Ref. 8. Reproduced from Blackwell Publishing.

gland would be the main source of high concentration of tissue active androgens in the pilosebaceous unit.

The authors suggest in examining further, whether the expression of type 1 5α-reductase in keratinocytes decreases with aging or not, and the role of androgens in the physiological function of epidermis, such as maintenance of the integrity of skin barrier (8). Lately, testosterone has been shown to perturb epidermal permeability barrier homeostasis (22).

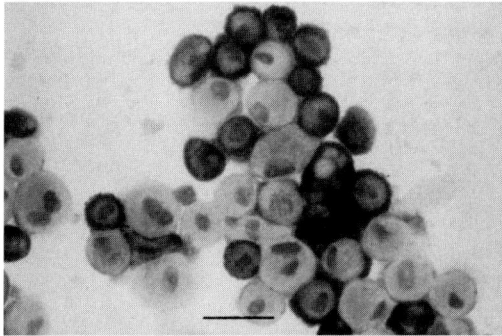

FIGURE 6 Immunocytochemistry of adult facial sebocytes from the fourth passage in culture. The smaller, less differentiated sebocytes are more strongly stained with type 1 5α-reductase antibody as compared with larger, well-differentiated ones. Scale bar = 50 μm. *Source*: From Ref. 8. Reproduced from Blackwell Publishing.

Immunolocalization of 5α-Reductases in Sebaceous Follicles

Thiboutot et al. (21) determined immunohistochemically (hematoxylin-eosin staining) the distribution of 5α-reductase isoenzymes within sebaceous follicles and terminal hair follicles in acne lesions and normal skin. Higher levels of type 1 isoenzyme are detected in sebaceous glands derived from acne-prone areas of skin, such as the face, compared to the glands from other areas, such as the legs or arms. This seems to correlate with the finding that the stimulatory effect of DHT on cell proliferation is more prominent on facial than on nonfacial sebocytes, as shown by Akamatsu et al. (23).

5α-Reductase Localization in Sebaceous Follicles of Normal Skin

In subjects with clinically normal skin, the majority of follicles contained a mild degree of hyperkeratosis. Monoclonal antibodies to type 1 5α-reductase specifically localized to the sebaceous glands of sebaceous follicles from normal skin (Fig. 7A). Reactivity was most pronounced at the periphery of the gland, that is, at the area of undifferentiated sebocytes in concomitance with the data by Chen et al. (8), but was noted throughout the sebaceous gland in most sections. No localization within hair follicles was noted (21).

Antibodies to type 2 5α-reductase localized to the companion layer (innermost layer of the outer root sheath) of sebaceous follicles and sebaceous ducts (Fig. 7B). Immunoreactivity was also noted in the granular layer of the epidermis and in the sheath of myelinated cutaneous nerves (not shown). No staining within sebaceous glands was observed with type 2 antibody (21).

5α-Reductase Localization in Acne Lesions

The pattern of immunoreactivity in acne lesions was similar to that observed in normal sebaceous follicles. In sections of closed (Fig. 8A) and open comedones (Fig. 8B), type 1 immunoreactivity was noted only in remnants of sebaceous

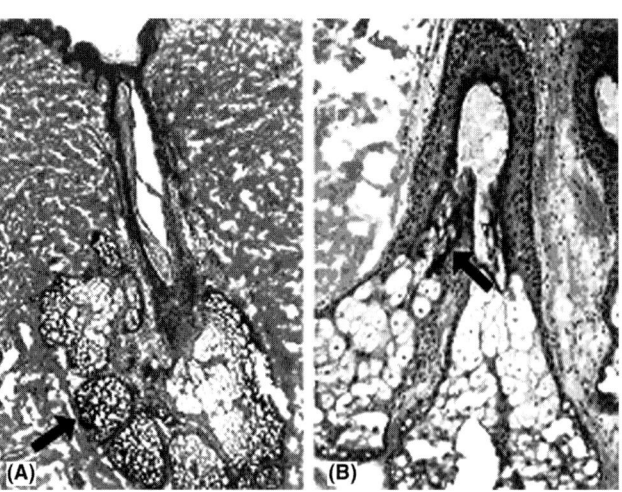

FIGURE 7 Immunolocalization of 5α-reductase in sebaceous follicles from the back of a subject without acne. (**A**) Skin incubated with antibody to type 1 5α-reductase reveals specific localization within sebaceous glands (*arrow*) (original magnification ×17). (**B**) Skin incubated with an antibody to type 2 5α-reductase reveals localization within the follicle and sebaceous duct (*arrow*), but not within the sebaceous gland (original magnification ×42). *Source*: From Ref. 21. Reproduced from Archives of Dermatology.

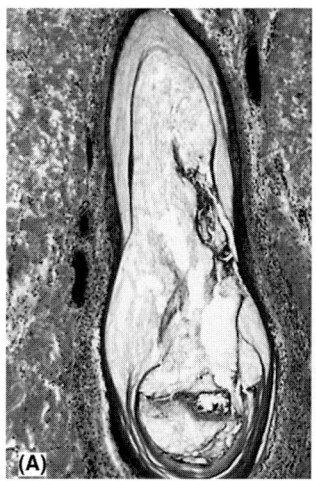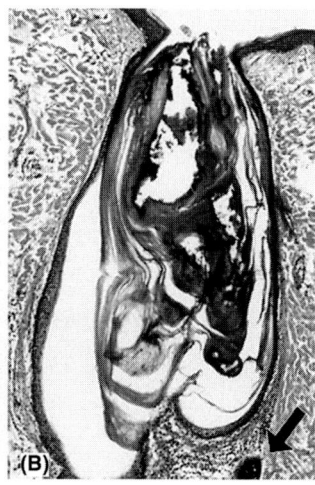

FIGURE 8 (*See color insert.*) Immunolocalization of type 1 5α-reductase in comedones (hematoxylin and eosin). (**A**) Sections of closed comedones and (**B**) of open comedones reveal no localization of type 1 antibody within the comedone (original magnification ×17). Of note is type 1 antibody localization in a sebaceous gland adjacent to an open comedone (*arrow*). *Source*: From Ref. 21. Reproduced from Archives of Dermatology.

glands and not within follicles. Type 2 antibody localized within the walls of both open and closed comedones, but not in the adjacent sebaceous gland, and extended into keratinized cells contained within the lumen (Fig. 9). In inflammatory lesions, type 1 immunoreactivity was noted specifically in sebaceous glands and not in follicles or any other epidermal or dermal structures (Fig. 10A and B). Immunoreactivity was most pronounced within basal sebocytes and least evident in highly differentiated sebocytes in proximity to sebaceous ducts (Fig. 10C). Localization of type 2 antibody was observed within the granular layer of the epidermis, the companion layer of the follicle, and the sebaceous duct, but not in the sebaceous gland (Fig. 11A). Type 2 immunoreactivity was noted in endothelial cells adjacent to an inflammatory acne lesion (Figs. 11B and 12A) but not in endothelial cells in control sections of dermatitic skin (Fig. 12B).

An interesting observation is the localization of the type 2 isoenzyme of 5α-reductase in the walls of both open and closed comedones and in endothelial cells surrounding inflammatory acne lesions. This localization parallels are seen in similar regions of normal follicles. The significance of the localization of the type 2 isoenzyme within the walls of the open and closed comedones or endothelial cells in inflammatory acne lesions remains unknown. It has been suggested that androgens may play a role in the follicular hyperkeratinization seen in acne. Although a cause-and-effect relationship between androgens and follicular hyperkeratinization cannot be drawn from immunohistochemical findings, localization of 5α-reductase within the comedonal wall provides a rationale for research in this area (21).

Enzymatic Activity of 5α-Reductase in Epidermal and Infrainfundibular Keratinocytes

Thiboutot et al. (24) determined the activity of 5α-reductase in keratinocytes excised and cultured from the infrainfundibulum and the epidermis of the forehead, using (1,2-^{3}H) testosterone as substrate.

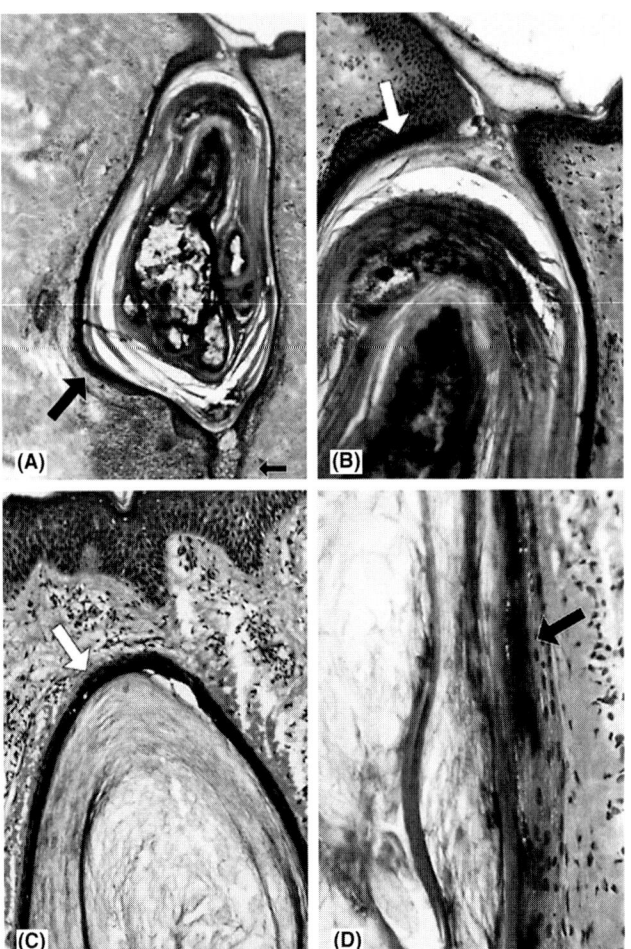

FIGURE 9 (*See color insert.*) Immunolocalization of type 2 5α-reductase in comedones. (**A**) Open comedone: type 2 antibody localizes within the comedone wall (*large arrow*) but not in the adjacent sebaceous gland (*small arrow*) (original magnification ×17). (**B**) Open comedone: type 2 antibody localizes in the granular layer of the epidermis extending into the wall of the comedone (*arrow*) (original magnification ×41). (**C**) Closed comedone: type 2 antibody localizes within the comedone wall (*arrow*) (original magnification ×41). (**D**) Closed comedone: type 2 antibody localization extends into fully keratinized cells within the lumen of the comedone (*arrow*) (original magnification ×83). *Source*: From Ref. 21. Reproduced from Archives of Dermatology.

Overall, the mean activity of 5α-reductase was not significantly different in the acne subjects compared to the nonacne subjects (Table 3). The mean enzyme activities in the acne groups were, however, slightly higher than in the groups without acne. When grouped by sex, males demonstrated significantly higher 5α-reductase activity in infrainfundibular keratinocytes compared to females. The activity of 5α-reductase was significantly higher in infrainfundibular keratinocytes compared to epidermal keratinocytes in all subject groups.

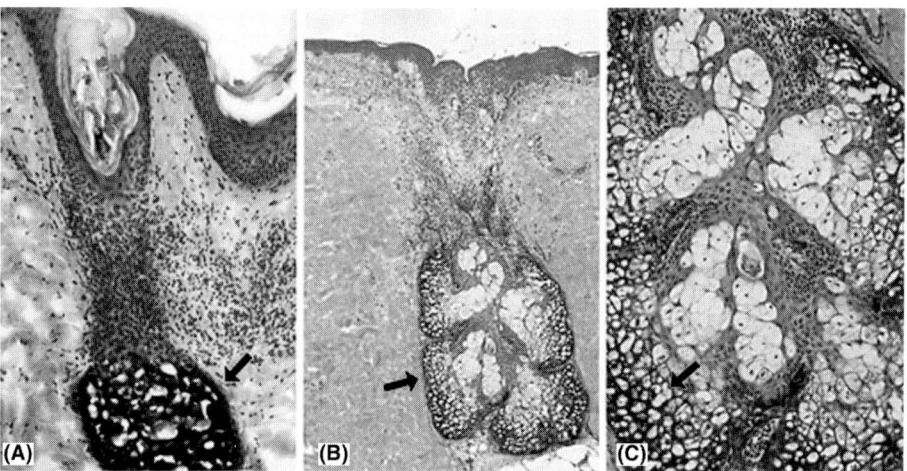

FIGURE 10 (*See color insert.*) Immunolocalization of type 1 5α-reductase in inflammatory acne lesions. (**A**) and (**B**) Type 1 antibody localizes specifically in sebaceous glands (*arrows*) (original magnification ×17). (**C**) localization of type 1 antibody is most predominant in basal sebocytes and more undifferentiated sebocytes in the lateral portions of the gland (*arrow*) (original magnification ×83). *Source*: From Ref. 21. Reproduced from Archives of Dermatology.

The activity of type 1 5α-reductase exhibits regional differences in isolated sebaceous glands. Increased activity of 5α-reductase could result in increased local concentrations of DHT, which may influence follicular keratinization. Although the data showed a tendency for a slight increase in enzyme activity in the acne group, these differences were not statistically significant.

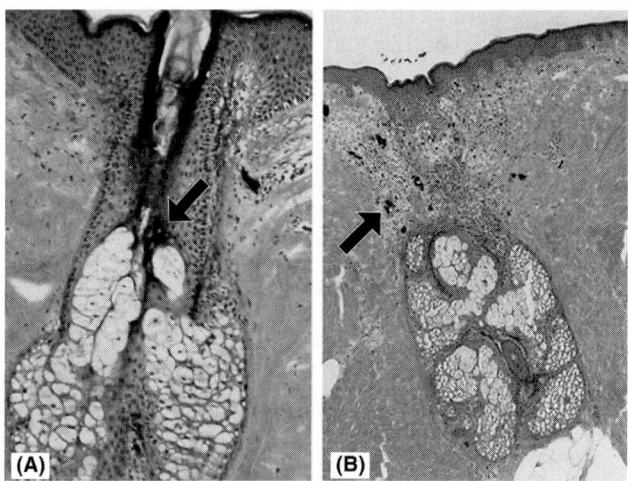

FIGURE 11 (*See color insert.*) Immunolocalization of type 2 5α-reductase in inflammatory acne lesions. (**A**) Localization of type 2 antibody extends from the granular layer of the epidermis into the sebaceous duct (*arrow*), but not the sebaceous gland (original magnification ×17). (**B**) Type 2 antibody localizes to endothelial cells within inflammatory lesions (*arrow*) (original magnification ×17). *Source*: From Ref. 21. Reproduced from Archives of Dermatology.

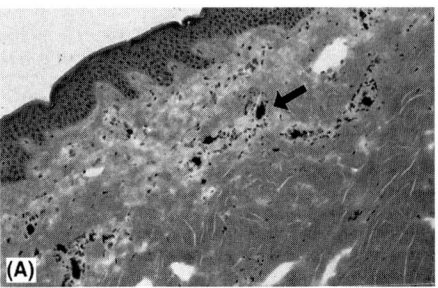 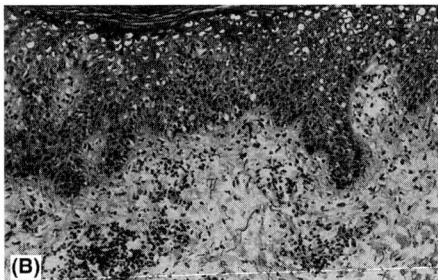

FIGURE 12   (*See color insert.*) Type 2 reactivity in endothelial cells. (**A**) Type 2 antibody reactivity is noted in endothelial cells adjacent to an inflammatory acne lesion (*arrow*) (original magnification ×17). (**B**) No localization of type 2 antibody is noted in endothelial cells in control sections of dermatitic skin (original magnification ×41). *Source*: From Ref. 21. Reproduced from Archives of Dermatology.

These observations lead to the following interpretations:

1. Androgens may not be as important in follicular keratinization as inflammatory signals and peroxisome proliferator-activated receptors (PPAR) regulation of lipids.
2. The differences observed in enzyme activities between acne and nonacne groups may approach significance if the sample sizes were larger (24).

Discussion

Although the study designed by Thiboutot et al. (24) could be optimized, generally, one would expect a more pronounced difference in enzymatic activity of 5α-reductase when comparing acne subjects with nonacne subjects. Open questions in this context could pertain to the mechanism of the regulation of enzymatic activity: do the 5α-reductases exist as zymogens to be proteolytically activated, or are there any endogenous inhibitors? Riboflavin, detected at high levels in the follicular duct, is suggested to play a certain role as an endogenous 5α-reductase inhibitor (25).

TABLE 3   Activity of 5α-Reductase in Keratinocytes

Subjects	Age (years)	n	Keratinocytes	Mean activity ($\pm$ SEM) (pmol min^{-1} mg^{-1}protein)
Acne, female	31 $\pm$ 5	7	Infrainfundibular	1.11 $\pm$ 0.32
		6	Epidermal	0.50 $\pm$ 0.13
Nonacne, female	33 $\pm$ 7	10	Infrainfundibular	1.01 $\pm$ 0.19
		10	Epidermal	0.68 $\pm$ 0.14
Acne, male	26 $\pm$ 7	6	Infrainfundibular	2.35 $\pm$ 0.83
		6	Epidermal	0.68 $\pm$ 0.16
Nonacne, male	34 $\pm$ 7	8	Infrainfundibular	1.37 $\pm$ 0.30
		7	Epidermal	0.48 $\pm$ 0.15

Source: From Ref. 24.

5α-REDUCTASE INHIBITORS
General
During the past three decades, research has focused on understanding the biological functions and effects of 5α-reductases and their 5α-reduced metabolites in order to obtain compounds able to block androgenic action through the inhibition of 5α-reductases (13). A high degree of selectivity is important to ensure that no other enzyme is affected and that no interactions exist with steroid receptors (10). Development of specific 5α-reductase inhibitors began in 1983, soon after DHT was reported to be the major androgen acting in the periphery. Great progress has since been made and continuing interests grow in designing and developing more potent and specific 5α-reductase inhibitors. DHT, being 2 to 10 times stronger than testosterone in androgen activity, was supposed to play a more important role than testosterone in many androgen-dependent diseases (14). Approximately 70% to 80% of serum DHT in men is produced by the type 2 isoenzyme, and 20% to 30% by the type 1 isoenzyme (21).

Since sebum production is regulated by DHT, inhibitors of type 1 5α-reductase may, therefore, form a new therapeutic class of agents designed to treat acne. It is expected that 5α-reductase inhibitors will produce fewer side effects than the presently available hormonal therapies. Inhibition of type 1 isoenzyme may represent a means of blocking the local production of DHT within the sebaceous glands. This inhibition, in turn, may reduce sebum production and improve acne (21).

5α-reductase inhibitors can be classified according to their

1. chemical structures (steroidal/nonsteroidal),
2. type of inhibitor activity (competitive/noncompetitive/uncompetitive), and
3. specificity (type 1/type 2/dual inhibitors).

Notice that the mentioned inhibition constant values (K_i values) and IC_{50} values vary, depending on the species (e.g., human versus rat), the cells (primary cultures versus cell lines), and the tissue origin (e.g., testis versus prostate) examined.

In the following, a number of 5α-reductase inhibitors are highlighted. Due to the vast quantity of corresponding papers we are far from a position to claim a complete listing of all published inhibitors. However, we focus mainly on essential structural requirements for inhibitors, on characterized inhibitors for human type 1 isoenzyme, and on inhibitors that stand in clinical testing phase or that are already commercially available.

Structural Requirements for Inhibitors
The design of most synthetic 5α-reductase inhibitors is based on the transition state inhibitor paradigm, a concept that states that the affinity for the enzyme should be greater for molecules that mimic the transition state of the enzymatic process (Fig. 4B) (16). Molecular modeling studies suggest that there is a requirement for

1. Groups to mimic the steroid A ring, in particular, the C-3 carbonyl group (Fig. 13) (26). It is concluded that any steroid-derived structure, possessing a C-3 polar group, should exhibit 5α-reductase inhibitory activity, whereas other structural factors determine the extent of the inhibition (27).

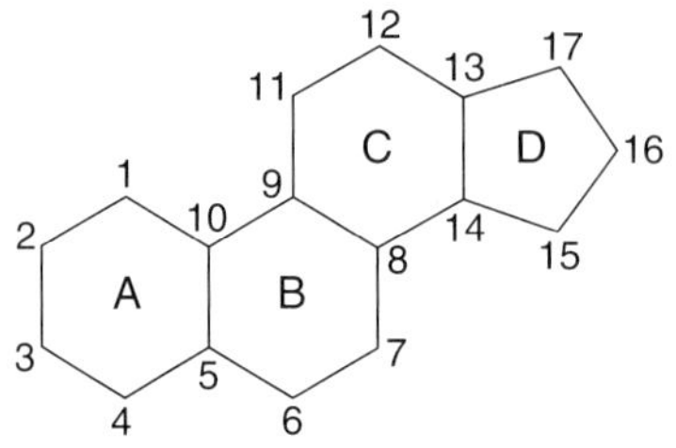

FIGURE 13   Numbering of C-atoms and designation of the steroidal tetracyclic ring system.

2. The space below the steroidal plane area about C-3, C-4, C-5, and C-6. This area should be sterically hindered, since the NADPH moiety requires access to the Δ4 site (26).
3. The area of the active site of the enzyme about the C-17 position of the steroid substrate, which appears to lack hydrogen bonding groups and is unrestricted (26).

In most synthetic and natural steroids, loss of the C-19 methyl group reduces the potency of the steroid to be recognized by 5α-reductase. Appropriate substitution at C-17 is, therefore, of particular importance in inhibitor design (5). That the C-17 hydroxyl group is not essential for inhibition is supported by inhibitors where the D-ring has been altered to a six-membered lactam resulting in potent activity. The volume of space occupied by the C-17 side chain of inhibitors is extensive. Therefore, it is postulated that the entry/exit to the active site of 5α-reductase results from this position (26) by lodging the C-17 side chains in specific cavities of the enzyme (28). A further postulation is that the increased inhibitory activity is associated with the lengthening of side chains. It is also proposed that the two isoenzymes possibly vary in the positioning of the reducing NADPH moiety (26).

Steroidal Inhibitors
Azasteroids
The first generation of synthetic inhibitors were steroids with a nitrogen atom located at different positions of the steroidal structure. Because of this characteristic, they are designated as azasteroids (Figs. 14A–C) (10). The presence of the nitrogen atom in the steroid structure increases the nucleophilicity of the carbonyl group at

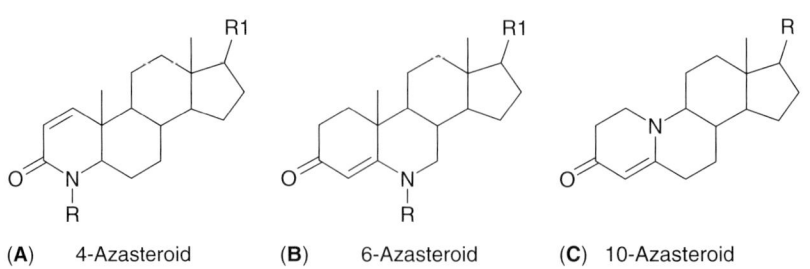

(A)   4-Azasteroid   **(B)**   6-Azasteroid   **(C)**   10-Azasteroid

FIGURE 14   Basic structure of azasteroids: (A) 4-azasteroid, (B) 6-azasteroid, and (C) 10-azasteroid.

C-3 and, thus, favors the interaction with an electrophilic residue in the active site. In general, azasteroids interact with the enzyme NADPH complex and are competitive with respect to testosterone (16).

4-Azasteroids are mimics of the "product-like" transition state, whereas 6-azasteroids and 10-azasteroids, which have an enone structure in the A ring, are mimics of the "substrate-like" transition state (Fig. 4B). 4- and 6-azasteroids are generally more rigid structures than 10-azasteroids, and thus may be more suitable for developing models of the 5α-reductase active site (16).

4-Azasteroid Derivatives

4-Azasteroids have been studied extensively (6). Hundreds of substituted 4-azasteroids have been published and patented since the early 1980s, especially from Merck, Glaxo, and Pharmacia (29). Among these inhibitors, Finasteride (MK906) (Fig. 15A) was the first and, for the last decade, the only available active ingredient in systemic drugs, (Proscar and Propecia, Merck) approved for clinical use. Finasteride is a specific competitive type 2 5α-reductase inhibitor ($IC_{50 \; type \; 2} = 9.4 \, nM$, $IC_{50 \; type \; 1} = 313 \, nm$) (10) and has been shown to be effective for the treatment of benign prostatic hyperplasia (Proscar) and androgenetic alopecia (Propecia), respectively (14). In humans Finasteride decreases prostatic DHT levels by 70% to 90% and reduces prostate size, while testosterone tissue levels remain constant (5). In males with benign prostatic hyperplasia treated with Finasteride, there was no reduction of sebum production, which may be related to the possibility that 5α-reductase in the sebaceous gland remains unaffected by the drug (30). The corresponding amino acid sequences proposed to be involved in the Finasteride/human 5α-reductase

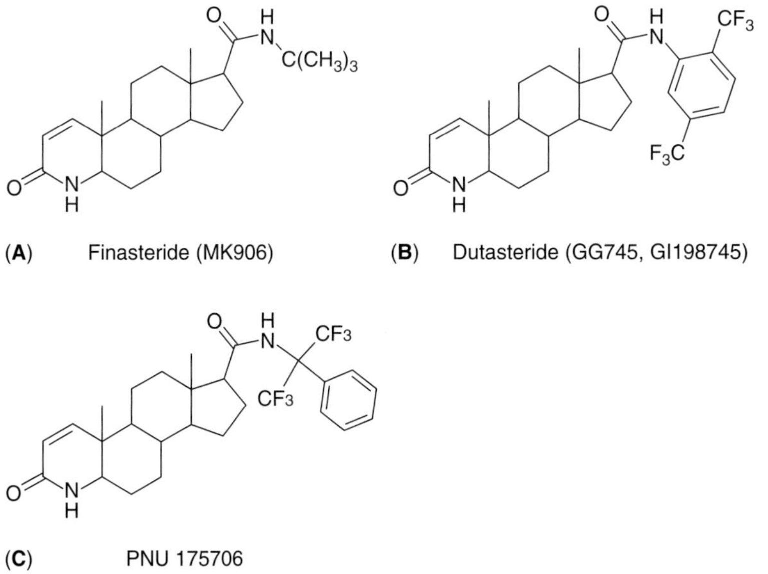

(A) Finasteride (MK906) **(B)** Dutasteride (GG745, GI198745)

(C) PNU 175706

FIGURE 15 4-Azasteroids: **(A)** finasteride (MK906), **(B)** dutasteride (GG745, GI198745), and **(C)** PNU 175706.

interaction are Ala_{26}-Val_{27}-Phe_{28}-Ala_{29} for type 1 isoenzyme and Gly_{21}-Ala_{22}-Leu_{23}-Ala_{24} for type 2 isoenzyme (Fig. 3) (19).

On the other hand, Dutasteride (GI198745, GG745) (Fig. 15B), one of the most potent dual inhibitors to date, is the first active ingredient in a drug (Avodart, GlaxoSmithKline) that inhibits both the isoenzymes (16). Avodart received Food and Drug Administration (FDA) approval in 2002 and was launched in 2003 so that after a monopoly for a decade as the only available 5α-reductase inhibitor, Finasteride will be joined by a second (20). This dual 5α-reductase inhibitor shows a greater inhibition of type 1 isoenzyme compared with Finasteride and is also potent against type 2 isoenzyme ($IC_{50\ type\ 1} = 2.4$ nM, $IC_{50\ type\ 2} = 0.5$ nm) (29). Biochemically, Dutasteride achieves greater and more rapid DHT suppression compared with Finasteride. It is reported to reduce circulating DHT levels by 90%. Clinically, it appears to be at least as good in terms of improving symptoms of benign prostatic hyperplasia. However, until these two drugs are formally compared, the true benefits of additional type 1 isoenzyme inhibition are unknown (20).

PNU 157706 (Pharmacia & Upjohn) (Fig. 15C) is highly potent in inhibiting human recombinant type 1 and 2 5α-reductase, showing IC_{50} values of 3.9 and 1.8 nM, respectively. PNU 157706 was shown to have no binding affinity for the rat prostate androgen receptor and to be devoid of any antiandrogen activity (31).

4-Methyl-4-Azasteroids

In contrast to 4-azasteroid derivatives, compounds with 4-methyl-4-aza functionality are generally more potent to type 1 5α-reductase (6). Experimental data showed that azasteroid derivatives containing groups larger than methyl result in poorer inhibition due to the restricted access of NADPH (32).

After the launch of Proscar in the early nineties, Merck has continued the research efforts and conducted clinical trials for at least three further compounds MK963, MK434, and MK386 for the treatment of acne, alopecia, and hirsutism (16), but will probably not bring any of these to the market. MK386 (Fig. 16A) is a selective inhibitor of human type 1 5α-reductase with an IC_{50} of 20 nM. A fourteen-day oral application with MK386 resulted in a dose-dependent suppression of serum and sebum DHT, without affecting semen DHT concentrations. Serum DHT concentrations were reduced 22% by a daily dose of 50 mg MK386, with no significant change in serum testosterone. Sebum DHT was reduced by 55% and 35% by doses of 50 and 20 mg, respectively (33). However, due a certain degree of hepatic toxicity in men the development of MK386 was stopped (10). A further development is L-751788 (Fig. 16B), which differs from Merck's other 5α-reductase inhibitors by having a substituent on C-16 than on C-17. This makes it more selective for type 1 isoenzyme.

The dual inhibitor 4-MA (Fig. 16C) (Merck) has been studied extensively and progressed to clinical trials for the treatment of benign prostatic hyperplasia. It showed a high activity for both isoenzymes ($IC_{50} = 8.5$ nM) (16) and a very low affinity for the androgen receptor and was thus not expected to produce undesirable antiandrogenic effects. However, 4-MA was subsequently shown to be an inhibitor of 3β-hydroxysteroid dehydrogenase, another steroid metabolizing enzyme, and to cause hepatoxicity, like MK386 (15).

Turosteride (FCE 26073, GlaxoSmithKline) (Fig. 16D), a promising new drug currently in clinical studies, is a selective inhibitor of type 2 isoenzyme (29).

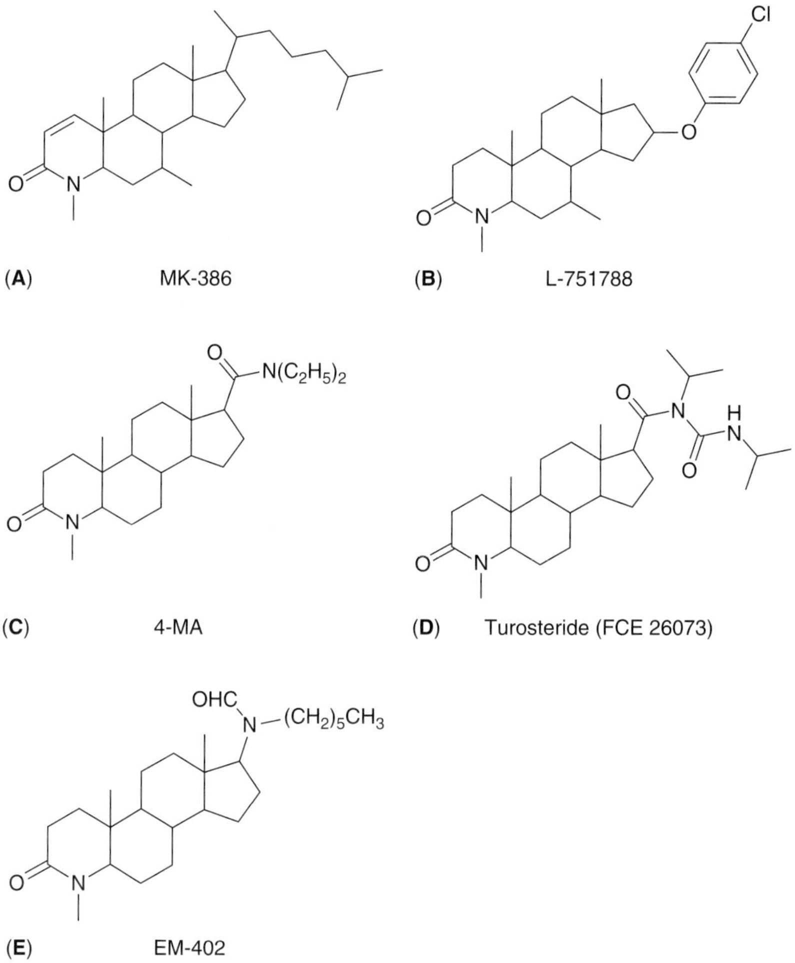

FIGURE 16 4-Methyl-4-azasteroids: (**A**) MK-386, (**B**) L-751788, (**C**) 4-MA, (**D**) turosteride (FCE 26073), and (**E**) EM-402.

Turosteride caused inhibition of the human enzyme with IC_{50} values of 53 nM and does not show relevant binding affinity to prostate androgen receptor.

EM-402 strongly inhibits human type 1 5α-reductase ($IC_{50} = 7.3$ nM) and shows low potency on the type 2 isoenzyme in transfected cells in vitro. Topically applied EM-402 (Fig. 16E) exerts a potent local antiandrogenic effect without any systemic action in the hamster. EM-402 decreased the size of flank organs of hamsters and also of the underlying sebaceous glands. Twice daily applications for four weeks at doses of 30, 100, and 300 μg reduce the size of the sebaceous glands by 38%, 42%, and 59%, respectively. Comparable results were observed on the sebaceous glands of the ears. In addition, a concentration-dependent inhibition of 5α-reductase activity of 47% to 80% in the flank organs and ears, respectively, were observed. EM-402 had no effect on prostatic and seminal vesicle weights (34).

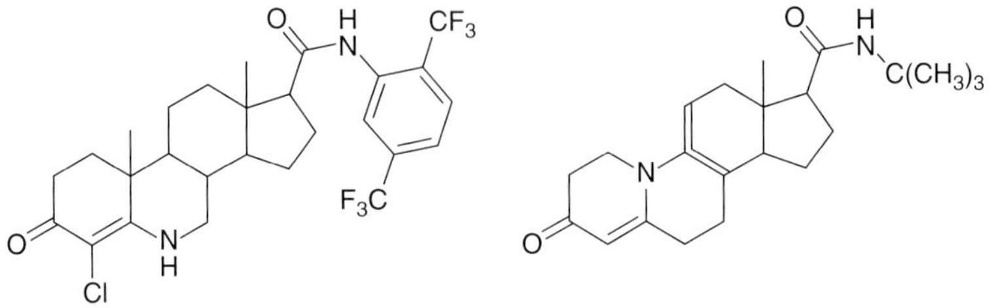

(**A**) Aryl substituted 6-azasteroid   (**B**) *t*-Butyl substituted 10-azasteroid

FIGURE 17   6- and 10-azasteroid derivatives: (**A**) aryl substituted 6-azasteroid and (**B**) *t*-butyl substituted 10-azasteroid.

6- and 10-Azasteroids

6- and 10-azasteroids 5α-reductase inhibitors have been synthesized showing different degree of 5α-reductase inhibition and different selectivity, some of them are under investigation for clinical application (10).

The presence of the nitrogen atom at position 10, conjugated with the carbonyl at C-3 (Fig. 14C), is an essential feature for good inhibition since, providing an increase of the negative partial charge on the oxygen, it probably determines a strong interaction with an electrophilic residue in the enzyme active site (35).

Among 6-azasteroids, the aryl substituted derivative (Fig. 17A) is a potent dual inhibitor of both isoenzymes and 17β-N-(t-butyl)carbamoyl substituted 10-azasteroid (Fig. 17B) displayed an inhibitory potency against type 2 5α-reductase with that of Finasteride ($IC_{50} = 10$–122 nM, depending on the isomer), and was more active against type 1 isoenzyme ($IC_{50} = 127$ nM) (16).

4-Oxa- and 4-Thiasteroids

A series of irreversible inhibitors related to 4-azasteroids but with a different heteroatom at the C-4 position (sulphur and oxygen) has also been reported by Merck (29).

Pregnatriene Derivatives

Flores et al. (5) synthesized novel pregnadiene-dione and pregnatriene-dione derivatives (Fig. 18A and B). The trienones showed consistently higher 5α-reductase inhibitory activity than the corresponding dienones. Unfortunately, there is no hint on the enzyme specificity. It is believed that the trienones inactivate the enzyme by an irreversible Michael type addition of the nucleophilic portion of the enzyme to the

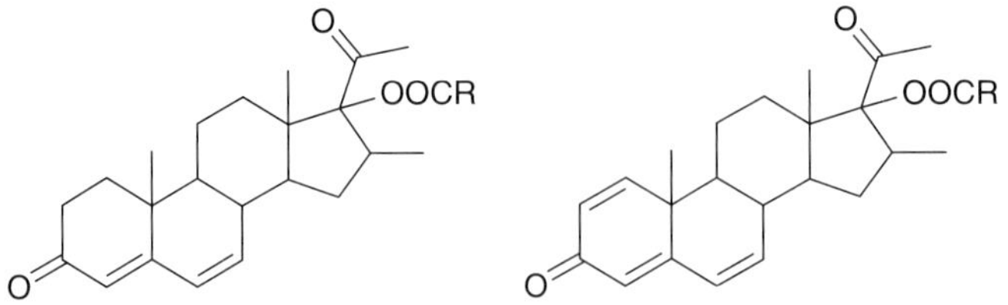

(**A**)   Pregnadiene-diones   (**B**)   Pregnatriene-diones

FIGURE 18   Pregnatriene derivatives: (**A**) pregnadiene-diones and (**B**) pregnatriene-diones.

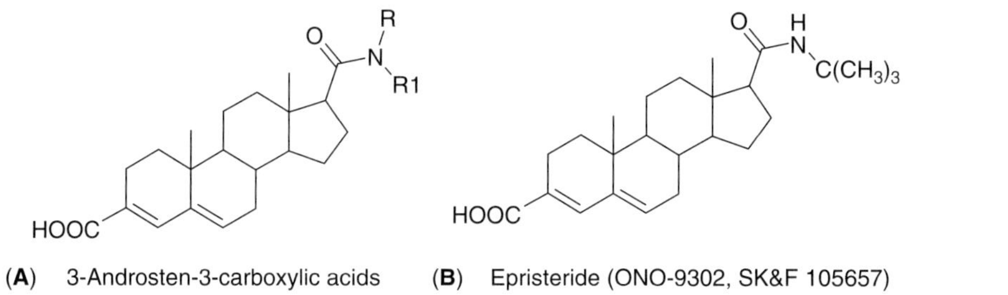

(A) 3-Androsten-3-carboxylic acids   **(B)** Epristeride (ONO-9302, SK&F 105657)

FIGURE 19 Steroidal carboxylic acids: **(A)** 3-androsten-3-carboxylic acids and **(B)** epristeride (ONO-9302, SK&F 105657).

conjugated double bond of the steroid. The trienones having a more coplanar structure react faster with the enzyme and thus show a higher inhibitory activity.

Steroidal Carboxylic Acids

A number of 3-androsten-3-carboxylic acids (Fig. 19A) were designed to mimic the putative enzyme bound enolate intermediate. Because of favorable electrostatic interactions between the carboxylate and the positively charged oxidized cofactor, the acrylate preferentially binds in a ternary complex with enzyme and NADP$^+$, which leads to the observed uncompetitive kinetic (6).

Epristeride (ONO-9302, SK&F 105657, GlaxoSmithKline) (Fig. 19B) is an uncompetitive, potent selective 5α-reductase type 2 inhibitor and is under phase III clinical testing for the treatment of benign prostatic hyperplasia (36). Epristeride has exhibited the ability to lower serum DHT levels by 50% (5).

Steroidal Oxime Inhibitors

Novel steroidal oxime inhibitors (Fig. 20) show an excellent inhibitor activity toward both types of the human 5α-reductases (5).

Nonsteroidal Inhibitors

Benzoquinoline Derivatives

In the field of nonsteroidal inhibitors, the most interesting molecules are the group of benzoquinolinone and benzo[c]quinolizinone derivatives. Benzoquinolinone derivatives have been designed starting from the related parent 4-azasteroids and the benzo[c]quinolizinone derivatives from 10-azasteroids. They are very potent inhibitors of human 5α-reductases with, in most cases, higher activity against the type 1 isoenzyme. Some compounds are dual inhibitors (35).

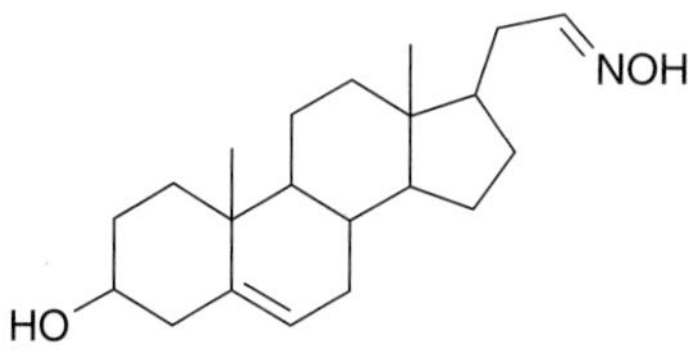

FIGURE 20 Steroidal oxime.

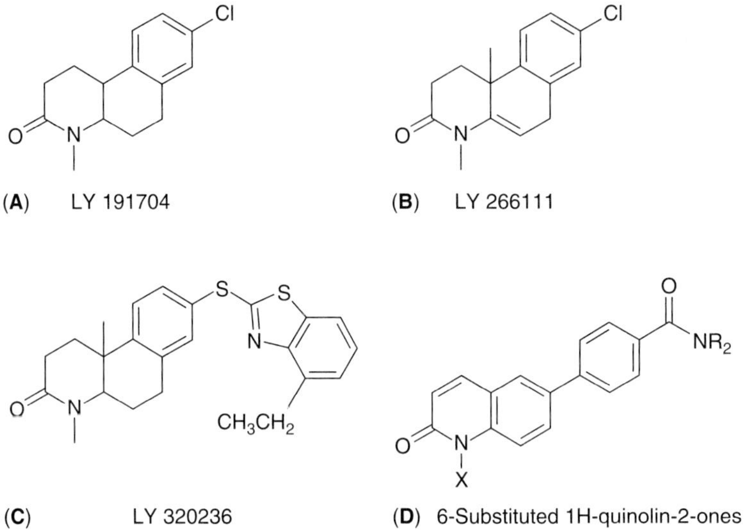

FIGURE 21 Benzoquinolinone derivatives: (**A**) LY 191704, (**B**) LY 266111, (**C**) LY 320236, and (**D**) 6-substituted 1H-quinolin-2-ones.

Benzoquinolinone Derivatives

Among the benzoquinolinones LY 191704 and LY 266111 (Eli Lilly) (Fig. 21A and B) possess an ideal 4-*N*-methyl, 8-chloro, *trans*, angular hydrogen arrangement (6) leading to a high inhibition potency against type 1 isoenzyme (29). Analysis on human 5α-reductases expressed from transfected cDNAs in simian COS cells indicate that LY 191704 is a specific noncompetitive inhibitor of the human type 1 isoenzyme with an IC$_{50}$ of 8 nM (37). LY 266111 showed a corresponding IC$_{50}$ of 9 nM on recombinant CHO cells (35). These benzoquinolinone derivatives demonstrated that potent inhibition of the type 1 5α-reductase could be realized by a compact rigid tricyclic nucleus that does not require the full steroid ring system (6).

LY 320236 (Eli Lilly) (Fig. 21C) is a potent dual inhibitor with differing modes of activity against the two human 5α-reductase isoenzymes. LY 320236 inhibits 5α-reductase activity in human scalp skin competitively ($K_{i\ type\ 1}$ = 28.7 nM) and prostatic homogenates noncompetitively ($K_{i\ type\ 2}$ = 10.6 nM) (38). LY 320236 is currently under phase 1 clinical trials against prostate cancer.

6-Substituted 1H-Quinolin-2-ones

Another interesting class of nonsteroidal compounds are the 6-substituted 1H-quinolin-2-ones (Fig. 21D) (39).

1H-Benzoquinolizine-3-one Derivatives

The 1H-benzoquinolizine-3-one derivatives are selective inhibitors of human type 1 5α-reductase. IC$_{50}$ of AS-97004 (Ares Serono) (Fig. 22) determined on recombinant CHO cells accounts for approximately 300 nM.

Serono's antiacne program focused on the preclinical lead compound AS-601811. Phase 1 trials began in the second quarter of 2001. The agent was orally bioavailable in rodents and dogs and generally well tolerated in animal models. At doses up to 15 mgkg^{-1}d^{-1} no toxicity was observed at 15 days after dosing.

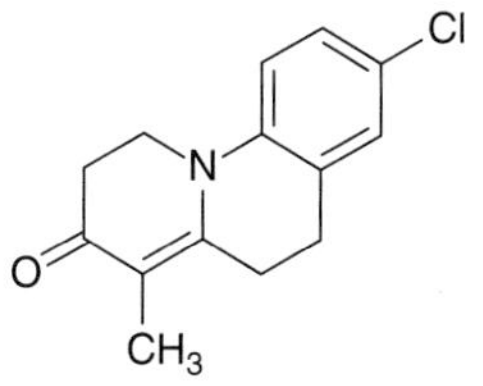

AS 97004

FIGURE 22 1H-Benzoquinolizine-3-one derivative: AS 97004.

Phenylethyl Cyclohex-1-ene Carboxylic Acids

A novel approach to the synthesis of conformationally flexible nonsteroidal mimics of Epristeride is cyclohex-1-ene carboxylic acids (Fig. 23A). The compounds turned out to be good inhibitors of type 2 isoenzyme (e.g., R = CON(*i*-propyl)$_2$, IC$_{50}$ = 760 nM). Type 1 isoenzyme was only slightly inhibited. The compounds were tested for inhibition of human 5α-reductase isoenzymes, using prostatic tissue for type 2 and DU 145 cells for type 1 isoenzyme. This cell line, deriving from brain metastases of an epithelial human prostate adenocarcinoma, has been demonstrated to express only type 1 isoenzyme and has been recently used to test inhibitors toward this 5α-reductase isoform (40).

Biphenyl-4-Carboxylic Acids

It was recently demonstrated that in the class of A-C ring steroidmimetics the biphenyl-4-carboxylic acids were appropriate 5α-reductase inhibitors. As a consequence of structure-activity studies, 3,4-dihydro-naphtalene-2-carboxylic acids and naphthalene-2-carboxylic acids (Figs 23B and C), which are structurally based on the steroidal inhibitor Epristeride, were synthesized and evaluated for 5α-reductase inhibitory activity. Human prostate homogenates and the DU 145 cell line served as enzyme sources.

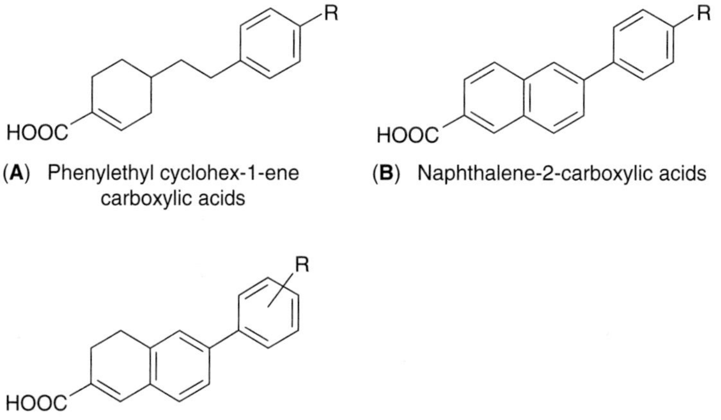

(A) Phenylethyl cyclohex-1-ene carboxylic acids

(B) Naphthalene-2-carboxylic acids

(C) 3,4-Dihydro-naphtalene-2-carboxylic acids

FIGURE 23 Cyclic carboxylic acids: **(A)** phenylethyl cyclohex-1-ene carboxylic acids, **(B)** naphthalene-2-carboxylic acids, and **(C)** 3,4-dihydro-naphthalene-2-carboxylic acids.

Apparently, the 3,4-dihydronaphtalene-2-carboxylic and naphthalene-2-carboxylic acid moiety mimicking the steroidal A-B ring is appropriate for generating potent transition state analogs of the steroidal substrate testosterone and androsterone. The most potent inhibitors of the human enzymes show IC_{50} values in the nM range. These naphthalene derivatives exceeded similarly substituted 1H-quinolin-2-ones in their inhibitory activities. This was to be expected, since in the class of biphenyl type inhibitors, a benzoic acid moiety is superior to a 2-pyridone structure as a steroidal A ring mimetic.

The strong influence of the type and the position of the substituents at the 6-phenyl group as well as the absence or presence of a double bond in 1 position on the activity of the compounds are remarkable. The big difference in their inhibitory activities toward type 1 and type 2 isoenzyme in the case of single compounds demonstrates that they are appropriate to elaborate the structural requirements for a selective or a dual inhibition of type 1 or type 2 isoenzyme inhibition (39).

Indolizine- and Indol-Butanoic Acids

FR146687 (Fujisawa Pharmaceutical) (Fig. 24A) shows a noncompetitive inhibition of both isoenzymes in vitro and has no inhibitory effects on other steroid oxido-reductases (41).

FK143 (Fujisawa Pharmaceutical) (Fig. 24B) was shown to inhibit both types of human 5α-reductase equally. The mode of inhibition against both the isoenzymes is noncompetitive. The inhibition constants for the human type 1 and type 2 isoenzymes were 27 and 20 nM, respectively. Species selectivity between human and rat on the inhibitory activity of FK143 was not found for both the isoenzymes. No other inhibitory effects were shown to other oxidoreductases (42). After a single oral administration of FK143 (100–500 mg) on healthy volunteers, DHT plasma concentrations decreased to about 65% of a predose value (43).

Cations

Zinc has long been used in dermatology and is reported to reduce sebum secretion. Metal ions have numerous roles in protein function, especially at the active site of enzymes. They could be complexed to a substrate or modify the structure of the protein. The two types of human 5α-reductases were transfected into SW-13 cells, a human adrenal carcinoma cell line, containing negligible endogeneous

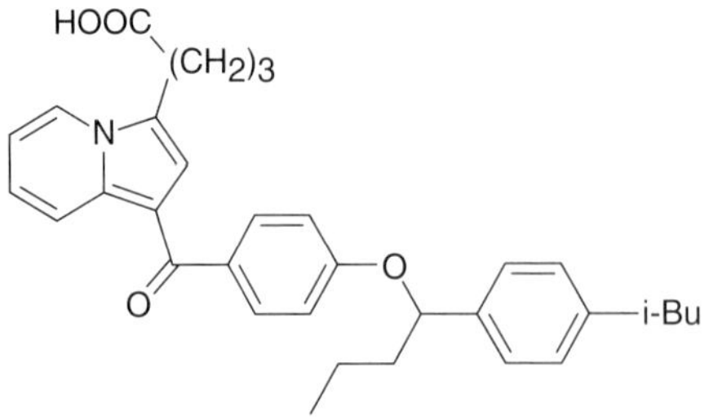

(A)   FR 146687 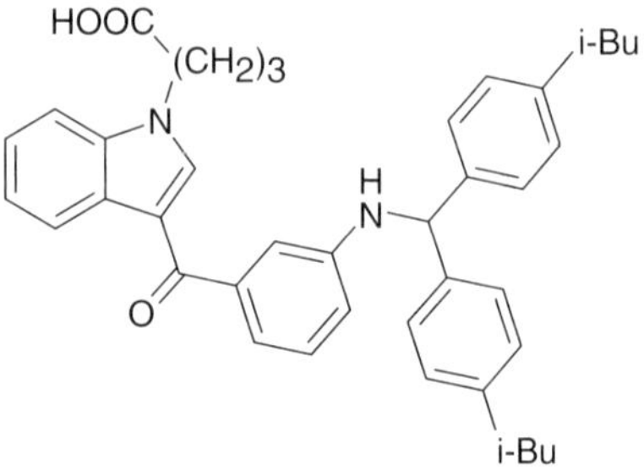   (B)   FK 143

FIGURE 24   Indolizine- and indol-butanoic acids: (A) FR 146687 and (B) FK 143.

TABLE 4 Inhibition Constants of Various Salts for Type 1 and Type 2 Human 5α-Reductase Activities

Compounds	$K_{i \text{ Type 1}}$ (μM)	$K_{i \text{ Type 2}}$ (μM)
$CuCl_2$	3.47 ± 0.43	11.0 ± 1.42
$CdCl_2$	0.61 ± 0.01	n.i.
$ZnCl_2$	1.51 ± 0.21	n.i.
$NiCl_2$	176 ± 26	$>10,000$
$FeCl_3$	250 ± 15	n.i.
$MnCl_2$	>1000	$>10,000$
$MgCl_2$	n.i.	n.i.
$CaCl_2$	n.i.	n.i.
LiCl	n.i.	n.i.

Note: Transfected SW13 human adrenal carcinoma cells were homogenized and incubated with 200 nM [^{14}C]androstenedione in the presence of 50 mM sodium phosphate buffer, pH 7.5, and 400 mM NADPH. K_i values were determined by the Cornish-Bowden method and are expressed as mean $\pm$ SD. "n.i." indicates that no significant inhibition was observed.
Source: Adapted from Ref. 44.

5α-reductase activity. The expressed 5α-reductases were analyzed for their sensitivity to heavy metal ions using 0.2 μM (^{14}C)androstenedione as a substrate.

The addition of $CuCl_2$, $CdCl_2$, and $ZnCl_2$ led to a potent inhibition of type 1 isoenzyme, with K_i values of 3.47, 0.61, and 1.51 μM, respectively (Table 4). $NiCl_2$ and $FeCl_3$ exerted weaker inhibition, with K_i values of 176 and 250 μM. $MnCl_2$, $MgCl_2$, $CaCl_2$, and LiCl, however, did not significantly inhibit either type 1 or type 2 5α-reductase activities. It is somewhat surprising that type 2 5α-reductase was not inhibited by $ZnCl_2$ or $CdCl_2$, as it contains a triple stretch of histidine residues at amino acid positions 229 to 231, and thus is more likely to bind zinc and its analogs than is type 1. Of the cations studied, only $CuCl_2$ significantly inhibited type 2 5α-reductase activity with a K_i value of 11 μM.

Anions only showed a moderate influence on the type 1 isoenzyme inhibition. $ZnSO_4$ has an effect similar to $ZnCl_2$, whereas $Zn(CH_3COO)_2$ showed a slightly decreased inhibition (44).

Phytochemical Inhibitors

Phytotherapeutics are generally well accepted by consumers and, therefore, received considerable attention from the pharmaceutical industry. However, a limiting factor for the use and effectiveness of phytotherapy is the lack of standardization of most of these products.

The berries of saw palmetto (*Serenoa repens*), a small palm native to the south east United States, possess a dual 5α-reductase inhibition activity, due to their high content of phytosterols (β-sitosterol (Fig. 25A), stigmasterol (Fig. 25B), lupeol (Fig. 25C), lupenone (Fig. 25D), and cycloartenol (Fig. 25E). Saw palmetto was used by native Americans as herbal treatment for enuresis, nocturia, atrophy of testes, impotence, inflammation of the prostate, and low libido in men. Standardized lipophilic saw palmetto extracts are commercially available: e.g., Regu®-Seb (Pentapharm) for topical treatment of seborrheic skin conditions and Permixon® (Pierre Fabre Medicament) for systemic application to treat benign prostatic hyperplasia. A 90-day topical treatment of a Regu®-Seb, containing emulsion lead to a statistically significant decrease of 46% ($p < 0.01$) in severity of seborrheic skin conditions

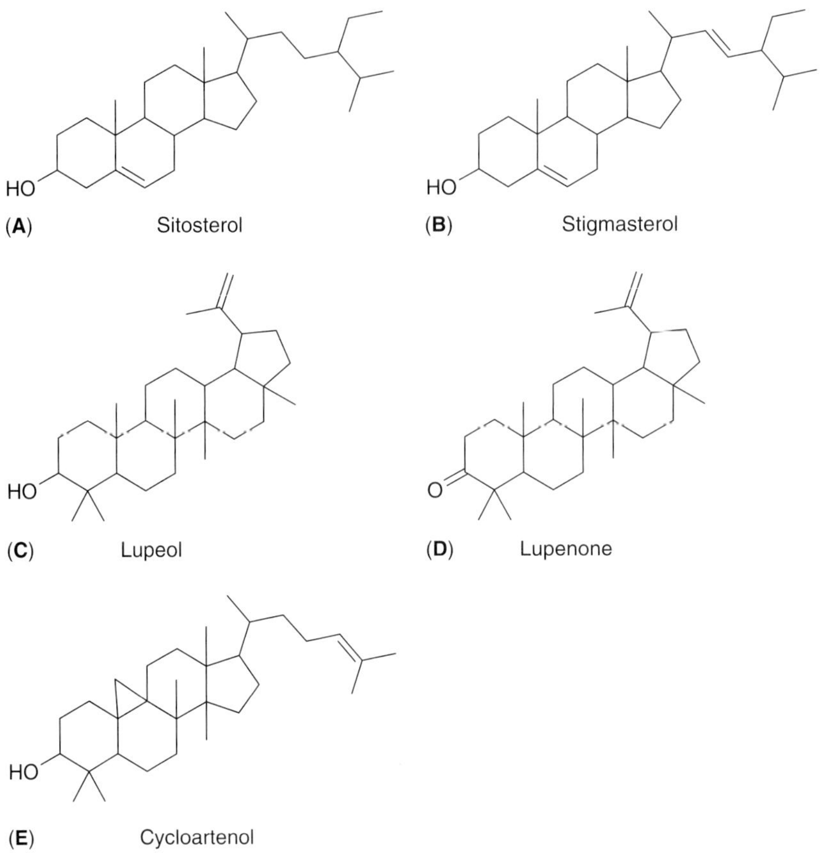

(A)   Sitosterol   **(B)**   Stigmasterol

(C)   Lupeol   **(D)**   Lupenone

(E)   Cycloartenol

FIGURE 25   Phytosterols: **(A)** β-sitosterol, **(B)** stigmasterol, **(C)** lupeol, **(D)** lupenone, and **(E)** cycloartenol.

(Fig. 26). Permixon® was launched in Europe in 1984 but has no FDA approval. The lipido-sterol extract markedly inhibits both the human isoenzymes. Type 1 isoenzyme is noncompetitively ($K_i = 7.2$ µg/mL) and type 2 isoenzyme uncompetitively ($K_i = 4.9$ µg/mL) inhibited (45).

Further dual phytotherapeutic 5α-reductase inhibitors include, among other extracts of *Pygeum africanum, Artocarpus incisus* (14), *Thuja orientalis, Laminaria saccharina, Arnica Montana, Cinchona succirubra, Eugenia caryophyllata, Humulus lupulus, Hypericum perforatum, Mentha piperata, Rosmarinus officinalis, Salvia officinalis* and *Thymus officinalis* (46); furthermore, diterpens (29), flavins (25), and isoflavonoids such as genistein (Fig. 27A) and daidzein (Fig. 27B), lignans, resveratrol (Fig. 28) (14), curcumin (Fig. 29) ($IC_{50 \text{ type } 1} = 3$ µM, $IC_{50 \text{ type } 2} = 5$ µM) (47), and certain polyunsaturated fatty acids. The relative inhibitory potencies of unsaturated fatty acids are, in decreasing order: γ-linolenic acid (Fig. 30A), α-linolenic acid (Fig. 30B), linoleic acid (Fig. 30C), palmitoleic acid (Fig. 30D), oleic acid (Fig. 30E), and myristoleic acid (Fig. 30F). Other unsaturated fatty acids such as undecylenic acid, erucic acid, and nervonic acid, are inactive (48).

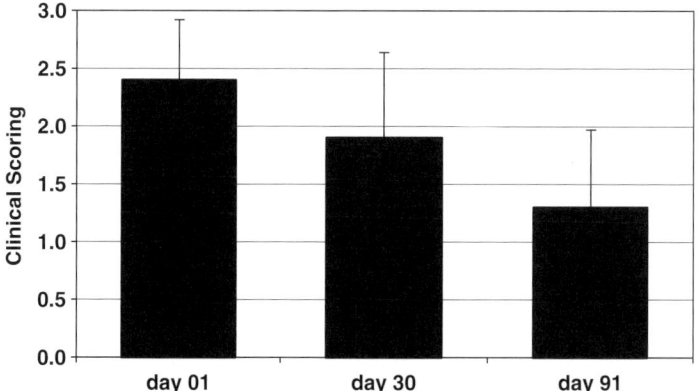

FIGURE 26 Efficacy of topically applied Regu®-Seb on seborrheic skin conditions. Score: 0 = no clinical relevant seborrheic skin, <3 comedones, 1 = slightly seborrheic skin, 3–10 comedones, 2 = easily visible seborrheic skin, 10 −30 comedones, 3 = obviously seborrheic skin, >30 comedones, 4 = extensive seborrhoea covering the whole face, >30 comedones.

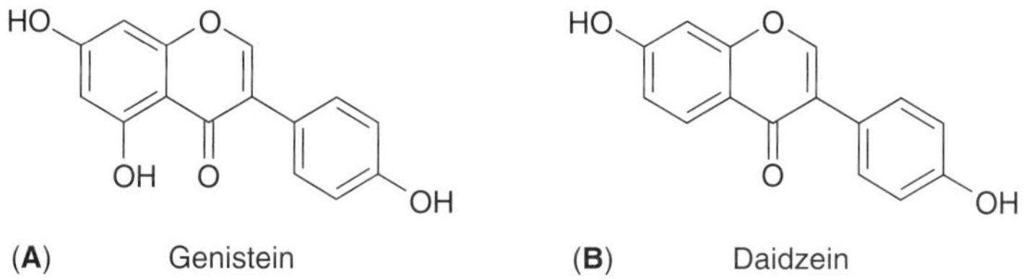

(**A**) Genistein (**B**) Daidzein

FIGURE 27 Isoflavonoids: (**A**) genistein and (**B**) daidzein.

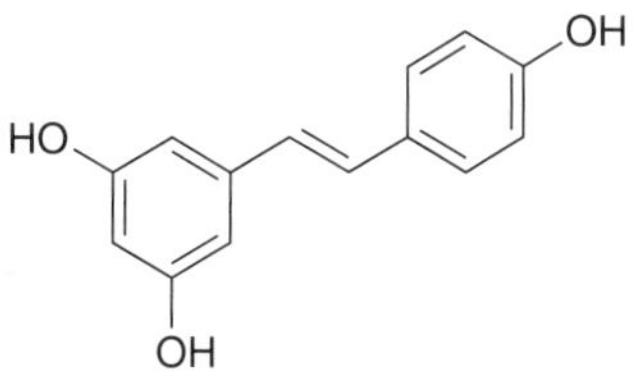

FIGURE 28 Resveratrol.

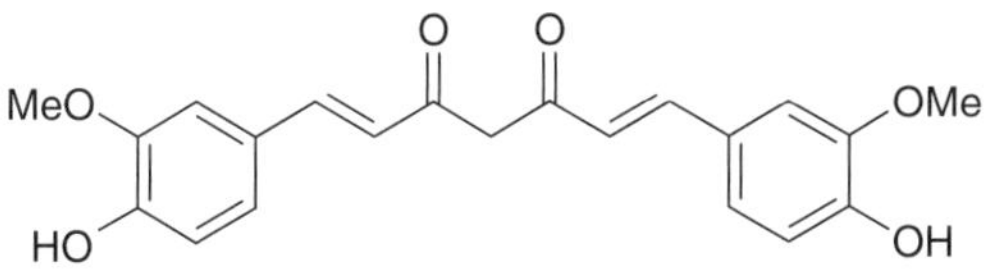

FIGURE 29 Curcumin.

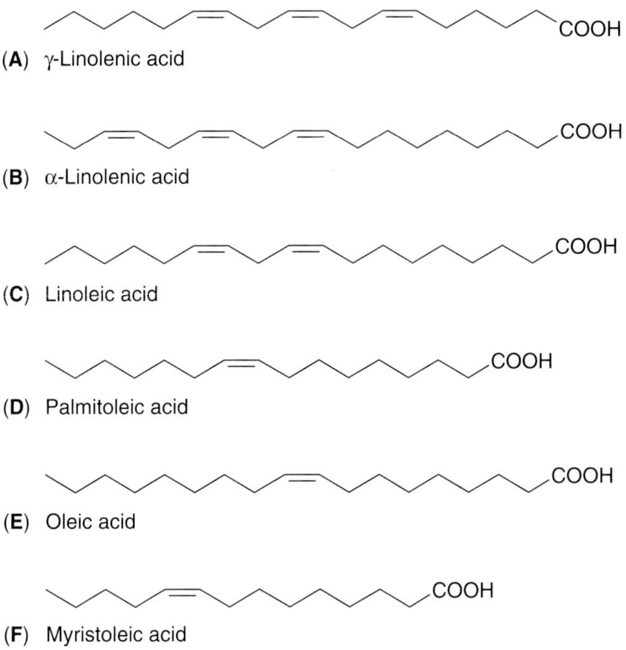

FIGURE 30 Fatty acids: (**A**) γ-linolenic acid, (**B**) α-linolenic acid, (**C**) linoleic acid, (**D**) palmitoleic acid, (**E**) oleic acid, and (**F**) myristoleic acid.

Specific type 1 inhibitors include the green tea catechin epigallocatechin-3-gallate (Fig. 31) ($IC_{50 \text{ type } 1} = 15 \, \mu M$) flavonoids such as baicalein (Fig. 32A) ($IC_{50 \text{ type } 1} = 29 \, \mu M$), quercetin (Fig. 32B) ($IC_{50 \text{ type } 1} = 23 \, \mu M$), fisetin (Fig. 32C) ($IC_{50 \text{ type } 1} = 57 \, \mu M$), and myricetin (Fig. 32D) ($IC_{50 \text{ type } 1} = 23 \, \mu M$), catechols such as nordihydroguaiaretic acid (Fig. 33) ($IC_{50 \text{ type } 1} = 19 \, \mu M$), as well as anthraquinoids such as alizarin (Fig. 34A) ($IC_{50 \text{ type } 1} = 23 \, \mu M$) and purpurin (Fig. 34B) ($IC_{50 \text{ type } 1} = 23 \, \mu M$) (47).

Azelaic acid (1,9-nonanedioic acid) (Fig. 35), occurring for example, in wheat, rye, and barley, was shown to be a competitive inhibitor of 5α-reductase. A complete inhibition was reached at a concentration of 3 mM. An additive

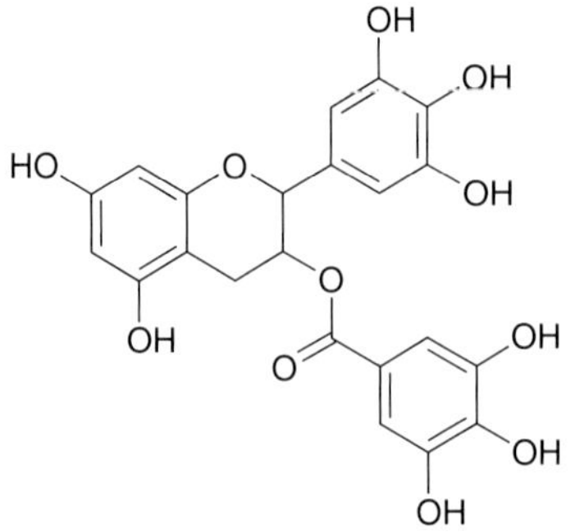

FIGURE 31 Epigallocatechin-3-gallate.

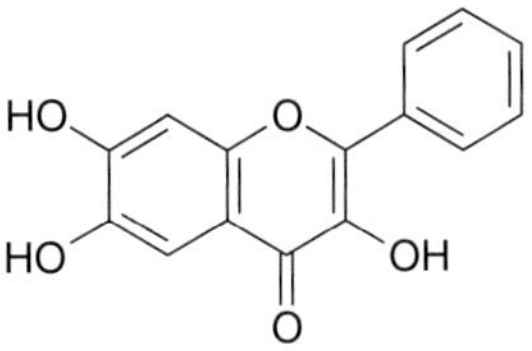

(**A**) Baicalein

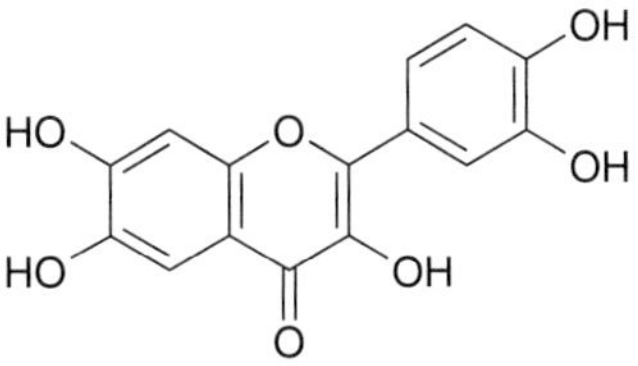

(**B**) Quercetin

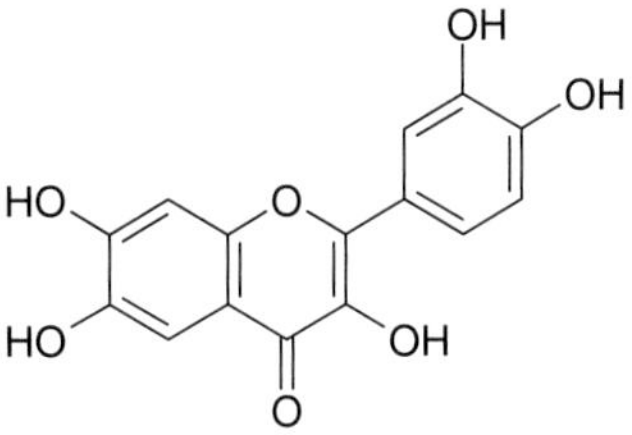

(**C**) Fisetin

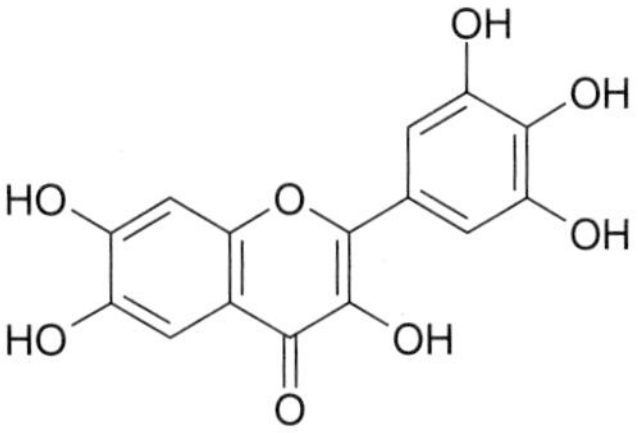

(**D**) Myricetin

FIGURE 32 Flavonoids: (**A**) baicalein, (**B**) quercetin, (**C**) fisetin, and (**D**) myricetin.

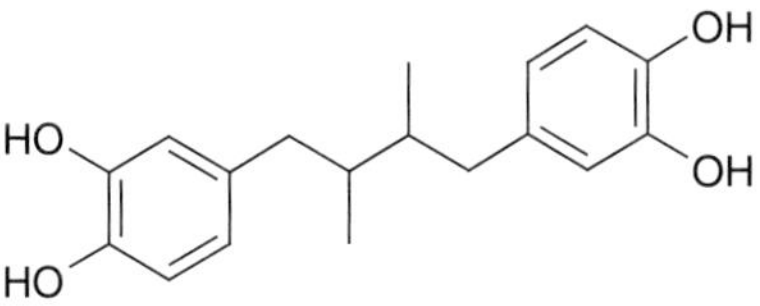

Nordihydroguaiaretic acid

FIGURE 33 Catechols: Nordihydroguaiaretic acid.

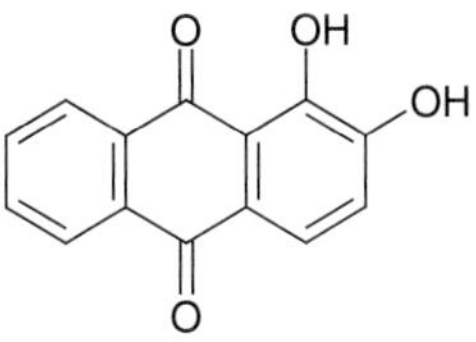

(A) Alizarin

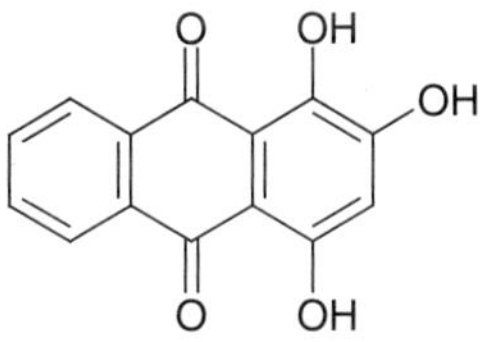

(B) Purpurin

FIGURE 34 Anthraquinoids: (**A**) alizarin and (**B**) purpurin.

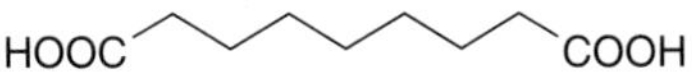

FIGURE 35 Azelaic acid.

inhibitory effect of zinc sulfate and azelaic acid on 5α-reductase activity was shown (49). Azelaic acid also possesses bacteriostatic activity to both aerobic and anaerobic bacteria including *Propionibacterium acnes*. Moreover, azelaic acid is an antikeratinizing agent, displaying antiproliferative cytostatic effects on keratinocytes, and modulating the early and terminal phases of epidermal differentiation. Therefore, several topical dermatological antiacne preparations containing a combination of a zinc salt and high concentrations of azelaic acid are available.

CONCLUSION

The most challenging and urgent work to achieve rigorous progress in the development of novel drugs, based on the inhibition of 5α-reductase, will be the purification of these enzymes, for which all efforts have failed so far because of their unstable nature during purification. Crystallization and X-ray diffraction structural analysis of the purified enzymes will be another important topic. Computer-supported molecular modeling, then, should provide directory data for developing more potent and selective inhibitors. On the other hand, the mechanism of action of enzymes and inhibitors needs to be further investigated. Steroidal inhibitors have already been extensively studied. However, developing of more efficient nonsteroidal compounds with simpler molecular structures and higher selectivity at lower costs is needed. This will also provide new information about enzyme and inhibitor interactions, and might lead to novel drugs that act differently from steroidal derivatives (6).

The prevalence of symptomatic benign prostatic hyperplasia is around 14% in men in their 40s, 24% in men in their 50s, and 43% in men beyond the age of 60. The number of patients undergoing operations for benign prostatic hyperplasia has decreased by approximately 60% in the United States over the past decade, due to the introduction of 5α-reductase inhibitors. Moreover, prostate cancer is the second leading cause of cancer death in males in the United States (20). Although acne is the most common skin disorder treated by dermatologists, it is, therefore, not surprising that the majority of the publications focus on the investigation of novel type 2 and dual acting 5α-reductase inhibitors. The contribution of DHT in the serum, which is partially derived from type 1 5α-reductase in the liver and the small amount of type 1 5α-reductase in the prostate, may play a role in maintaining prostatic enlargement. Thus, it is an effort to increase efficacy of treatment for benign prostatic hyperplasia that inhibits both types of 5α-reductase.

Beside the phytotherapeutic preparation Permixon®, to date Finasteride and Dutasteride are still the only synthetic 5α-reductase inhibitors, which are on the market as active ingredients in drugs. Anyhow, some inhibitors of type 1 isoenzyme have, meanwhile, been developed and studied in men with acne. To our knowledge, however, no successful outcomes have been published yet. The potential of drugs, such as Dutasteride that inhibits both the isoenzymes, for use in acne treatment remains to be determined.

Though systemically applied inhibitors of 5α-reductase could prove to be safe in women, they are currently not used because of potential fetal feminization and teratogenic risks (1). Currently published clinical results on acne treatment are rather disappointing (50,51). Therefore, effective topical applications may be a useful alternative. In humans, clinical responses to topical 5α-reductase inhibitors have been moderate, yet measurable. Actually, there exist no topical pharmaceuticals claiming exclusively 5α-reductase inhibition activity, although there are antiacne products on the market containing, for example, zinc acetate and azelaic acid, respectively. Most of the synthetic or phytochemical 5α-reductase inhibitors are still under in vitro investigation, animal studies, or clinical trials. Finally, it nevertheless remains to be pointed out that current research in acne therapy favors investigations of topical androgen receptor blockers over topical 5α-reductase inhibitors.

REFERENCES

1. Shaw JC. Hormonal therapies in acne. Expert Opin Pharmacother 2002; 3:865–874.
2. Thiboutot D, Jabara S, McAllister JM, et al. Human skin is a steroidogenic tissue: steroidogenic enzymes and cofactors are expressed in epidermis, normal sebocytes, and in immortalized sebocyte cell line (SEB-1). J Invest Dermatol 2003; 120:905–913.
3. Fritsch M, Orfanos CE, Zouboulis CC. Sebaceous are the key regulators of androgen homeostasis in human skin. J Invest Dermatol 2001; 116:793–800.
4. Zouboulis CC. Human skin: an independent peripheral endocrine organ. Horm Res 2000; 54:230–242.
5. Flores E, Bratoeff E, Cabeza M, et al. Steroid 5α-reductase inhibitors. Mini Rev Med Chem 2003; 3:225–237.
6. Li X, Chen C, Singh SM, et al. The enzyme and inhibitors of 4-ene-3-oxosteroid 5α-oxido-reductase. Steroids 1995; 60:430–441.
7. McConnel JD, Stoner E. 5α-reductase inhibitors. Adv Protein Chem 2001; 56:143–180.
8. Chen W, Zouboulis CC, Fritsch M, et al. Evidence of heterogeneity and quantitative differences of the type 1 5α-reductase expression in cultured human skin cells—evidence of its presence in melanocytes. J Invest Dermatol 1998; 110:84–89.
9. Chen W, Zouboulis CC, Orfanos CE. The 5α-reductase system and its inhibitors. Dermatology 1996; 193:177–184.
10. Cilotti A, Danza G, Serio M. Clinical application of 5α-reductase inhibitors. J Endocrinol Invest 2001; 24:199–203.
11. Randall VA. Role of 5α-reductase in health and disease. Baillière's Clin Endocrinol Metab 1994; 8:405–431.
12. Moore RJ, Wilson JD. Steroid 5α-reductase in cultured human fibroblasts. Biochemical and genetic evidence for two distinct enzyme activities. J Biol Chem 1976; 251:5895–5900.
13. Spera G, Lubrano C. 5α-reductases and their inhibitors. Int J Immunopathol Pharm 1996; 9:33–38.
14. Chen WC, Thiboutot D, Zouboulis CC. Cutaneous androgen metabolism: Basic research and clinical perspectives. J Invest Dermatol 2002; 119:992–1007.
15. Lopez-Solache I. Characterization and expression of 5α-reductase isoenzymes. Ph.D. dissertation, Laval University, Quebec, Canada, 1998.
16. Guarna A, Occhiato EG, Danza G, et al. 5α-Reductase inhibitors, chemical and clinical models. Steroids 1998; 63:355–361.
17. Thigpen AE, Cala KE, Russell DW. Characterization of Chinese hamster ovary cell lines expressing human steroid 5α-reductase isoenzymes. J Biol Chem 1993; 268:17404–17412.
18. Lopez-Solache I, Luu-The V, Seralini GE, et al. Heterogeneity of rat type 1 5α-reductase cDNA. Cloning, expression and regulation by pituitary implants and dihydrotestosterone. Biochem Biophys Acta 1996; 1305:139–144.
19. Levy MA, Brandt M, Sheedy KM, et al. Cloning, expression and functional characterization of type 1 and type 2 steroid 5α-reductases from Cynomolgus monkey: comparisons with human and rat isoenzymes. J Steroid Biochem Mol Biol 1995; 52:307–319.
20. Foley CL, Kirby RS. 5α-Reductase inhibitors: what's new ? Curr Opin Urol 2003; 13:31–37.
21. Thiboutot D, Bayne E, Thorne J, et al. Immunolocalization of 5α-reductase isozymes in acne lesions and normal skin. Arch Dermatol 2000; 136:1125–1129.
22. Kao JS, Garg A, Mao-Qiang M, et al. Testosterone perturbs epidermal permeability barrier homeostasis. J Invest Dermatol 2001; 116:443–451.

23.   Akamatsu H, Zouboulis CC, Orfanos CE. Control of human sebocyte proliferation in vitro by testosterone and 5α-dihydrotestosterone is dependent on the localization of the sebaceous glands. J Invest Dermatol 1992; 99:509–511.
24.   Thiboutot D, Knaggs H, Gilliland K, et al. Activity of 5α-reductase and 17β-hydroxysteroid dehydrogenase in the infrainfundibulum of subjects with and without Acne vulgaris. Dermatology 1998; 196:38–42.
25.   Nakayama O, Yagi M, Kioyto S, et al. Riboflavin, a testosterone 5α-reductase inhibitor. J Antibiot 1990; 43:1615–1616.
26.   Ahmed S. Molecular modelling of 5α-reductase inhibitors. Pharm Sci 1996; 2:251–253.
27.   Ahmed S, Denison S. Structure activity relationship study of known inhibitors of the enzyme 5α-reductase. Bioorg Med Chem Lett 1998; 8:409–414.
28.   Grisenti P, Magni A, Olgiati V, et al. Substrate interaction with 5α-reductase enzyme: Influence of the 17β-chain chirality in the mechanism of action of 4-azasteroid inhibitors. Steroids 2001; 66:803–810.
29.   Macchetti F, Guarna A. Novel inhibitors of 5α-reductase. Expert Opin Ther Patents 2002; 12:201–215.
30.   Amichai B, Grunwald MH, Sobel R. 5α-reductase inhibitors—a new hope in dermatology? Int J Dermatol 1997; 36:182–184.
31.   di Salle E, Guidici D, Radice A, et al. PNU 157706, a novel dual type 1 and 2 5α-reductase inhibitor. J Steroid Biochem Mol Biol 1998; 64:179–186.
32.   Ahmed S, Denison S. Mechanism based representation of the active site of 5α-reductase. Bioorg Med Chem Lett 1998; 8:2615–2620.
33.   Schwartz JI, Tanaka WK, Wang DZ, et al. MK-386, an inhibitor of 5α-reductase type 1, reduces dihydrotestosterone concentrations in serum and sebum without affecting dihydrotestosterone concentrations in semen. J Clin Endocrinol Metab 1997; 82:1373–1377.
34.   Chen C, Li X, Singh SM, et al. Activity of 17β-(N-alkyl/arylformamido) and 17β-[(N-alkyl/aryl) alkyl/arylamido]-4-methyl-4-aza-5α-androstan-3-ones as 5α-reductase inhibitors in the hamster flank organ and ear. J Invest Dermatol 1998; 111:273–278.
35.   Guarna A, Occhiato EG, Scarpi D, et al. Synthesis of benzo[c]quinolizin-3-ones: Selective nonsteroidal inhibitors of steroid 5α-reductase 1. Bioorg Med Chem Lett 1998; 8:2871–2876.
36.   Ishibashi K. 3-Oxo-4-aza-5α-androstane-17β-carboxamide derivatives with testosterone 5α-reductase inhibitory activity. Annu Report Sankyo Res Lab 2000; 52:1–14.
37.   Hirsch KS, Jones CD, Audia JE, et al. LY191704: A selective, nonsteroidal inhibitor of human steroid 5α-reductase type 1. Proc Natl Acad Sci USA 1993; 90:5277–5281.
38.   McNulty AM, Audia JE, Bemis KG, et al. Kinetic analysis of LY320236: competitive inhibitor of type 1 and non-competitive inhibitor of type 2 human steroid 5α-reductase. J Steroid Biochem Mol Biol 2000; 72:13–21.
39.   Baston E, Salem OIA, Hartmann RW. 6-Substituted 3,4-dihydro-naphtalene-2-carboxylic acids: synthesis and structure-activity studies in a novel class of 5-reductase inhibitors. J Enzyme Inhibition Med Chem 2002; 17:303–320.
40.   Baston E, Salem OIA, Hartmann RW. Cyclohex-1-ene carboxylic acids: synthesis and biological evaluation of novel inhibitors of human 5α-reductase. Arch Pharmacol Pharmacol Med Chem 2003; 1:31–38.
41.   Nakayama O, Hirosumi J, Chida N, et al. FR146687, a novel steroid 5α-reductase inhibitor: In vitro and in vivo effects on prostates. Prostate 1997; 31:241–249.
42.   Kojo H, Nakayama O, Hirosumi J, et al. Novel steroid 5α-reductase inhibitor FK143: Its dual inhibition against the two isoenzymes and its effect on transcription of the isoenzyme genes. Mol Pharmacol 1995; 48:401–406.
43.   Katashima M, Irino T, Shimojo F, et al. Pharmacokinetics and pharmacodynamics of FK143, a nonsteroidal inhibitor of steroid 5α-reductase, in healthy volunteers. Clin Pharmacol Ther 1998; 63:354–366.
44.   Sugimoto Y, Lopez-Solache I, Labrie F, et al. Cations inhibit specifically type 1 5α-reductase found in human skin. J Invest Dermatol 1995; 104:775–778.
45.   Iehle C, Delos S, Guirou O, et al. Human prostatic steroid 5α-reductase isoforms—a comparative study of selective inhibitors. J Steroid Biochem Mol Biol 1995; 54:273–279.

46. Picard-Lesboueyries E. Composition comprising 7-hydroxy DHEA and/or 7-keto DHEA and at least a 5α-reductase inhibitor. PCT Application WO 02/47644 A1.

47. Liao S, Hiipakka R. Method and compositions for regulation of 5α-reductase activity. US Patent Application Publication US 2003/0105030 A1.

48. Liang T, Liao S. Inhibition of steroid 5α-reductase by specific aliphatic unsaturated fatty acids. Biochem J 1992; 285:557–562.

49. Stamatiadis B, Bulteau-Portois MC, Mowszowicz I. Inhibition of 5α-reductase activity in human skin by zinc and azelaic acid. Br J Dermatol 1988; 119:627–632.

50. Leyden J, Bergfeld W, Drake L, et al. A systemic type I α-reductase inhibitor is ineffective in the treatment of acne vuljans. J Am Acad Dermatol 2004; 50:443–447.

51. Seiffert K, Seltmann H, Fritsch M, et al. Inhibition of 5 α-reductase activity in 5Z95 sebo-cytes and HaCaT keratinocytes in vitro. Norm Metab Res 2007; 35:141–148.

15 Sebum: Physical–Chemical Properties, Macromolecular Structure, and Effects of Ingredients

Linda D. Rhein
School of Natural Sciences, Fairleigh Dickinson University, Teaneck, New Jersey, U.S.A.

Joel L. Zatz and Monica R. Motwani
College of Pharmacy, Rutgers University, Piscataway, New Jersey, U.S.A.

INTRODUCTION

Sebum is a hallmark characteristic of oily skin, which typifies or is usually associated with acne-prone skin. The goal of this chapter is to present recent findings regarding the macromolecular structure of sebum and the influence of variations in composition of sebum on that macromolecular structure. It is further intended to discuss how these findings might relate to the pathogenesis of acne. In order to introduce a basis for this research, a brief review of the current knowledge of the composition of sebum is in order, although some repetition of information in other chapters on this subject is likely. After this review, the results of the thermal analysis of model sebum using differential scanning calorimetry (DSC) are presented along with an attempt to provide an explanation of the phase behavior, as it relates to sebum composition and to variations in the composition that might occur as part of a disease state such as acne. Further studies of the influence of vehicles on the phase behavior are presented, along with a discussion of how an imbalance in typical phase behavior may be relevant to the pathogenesis of acne.

Toward that end, our findings show that a model of sebum is a mixture of solid and liquid phases. We speculate that the liquid phase helps dissolve or "soften" the solid phase and that these two phases exist in a delicate balance. We further speculate that if this balance is altered, the consequences could be blockage of the sebaceous duct and of the infundibulum if the liquid part of sebum is too low and can no longer dissolve the solid part. This could result from action of *Propionibacterium acnes* bacteria on the sebum or from metabolic alterations in sebum composition in situ.

ORIGIN OF SEBUM

Sebum is the oily secretion of the sebaceous gland (Fig. 1). This "oil gland" is located juxtaposed to the hair follicle. The large ducts of the hair follicles are filled with this white pasty sebaceous material derived from the sebaceous gland. Sebaceous glands are generally found all over the body, except on the palms, soles, and dorsum of the feet (1). Most of the glands are associated with hair follicles and hence are termed pilosebaceous glands. In humans, they are concentrated on the scalp, forehead, and face, where there may be as many as 400 to 900 glands/cm^2 and up to 1600 glands/cm^2 on the nose (2). Sebaceous follicles are particularly

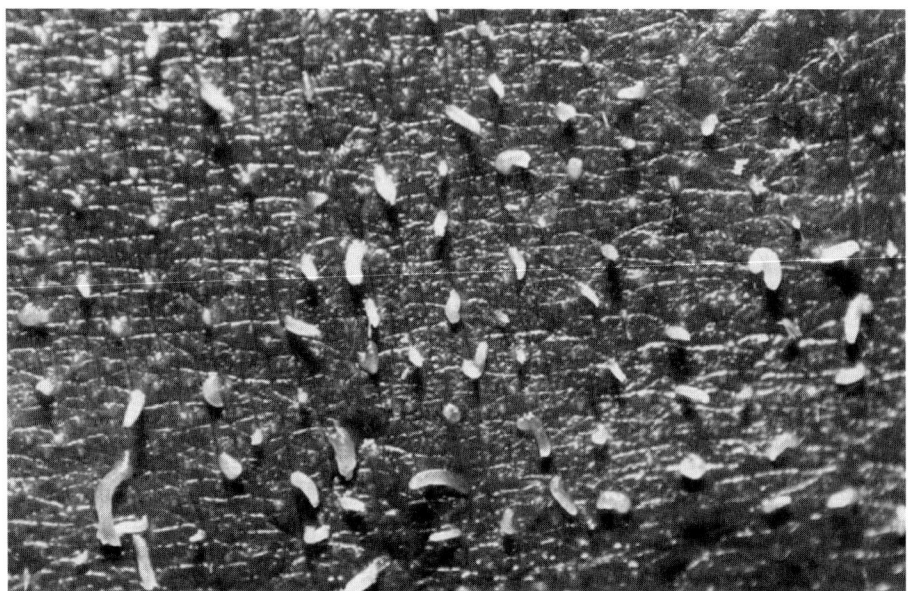

FIGURE 1   Sebum secretions from skin. *Source*: From Ref. 23.

abundant in the face, ear canal, v-shaped parts of the face, and chest, and on the sides of the upper arm. These skin areas are hence relatively greasy. The sebaceous gland, though present during childhood, is very small. At puberty, the gland becomes enlarged (3). This enlargement and increased activity of the sebaceous gland at puberty is primarily under androgen control (4).

SEBUM CHEMISTRY

The chemical composition and physical properties of sebum have been studied by several researchers and are discussed next.

Composition of Sebum

Knowledge of sebum lipid components helps us to consider how a penetrating molecule will react upon entering into the follicular canal and how this structure may theoretically be related to acnegenesis. The main lipids in human sebum are triglycerides, wax esters, and squalene with smaller proportions of cholesterol and cholesterol esters (4). Most importantly, free fatty acids (FFA) are often found in sebum and are formed from the triglycerides through the action of *P. acnes*. Bacterial lipases convert triglycerides to mono- and diglycerides as well as FFA in the sebum, many of which are unique to the sebaceous glands (5).

   The average composition of human skin surface lipid was given by Downing et al. (6) (Table 1) and of follicular casts by Nordstrom et al. (7). Note the variability in the amounts of triglycerides and FFA; this is attributed to the variable activity of the bacterial lipase, as discussed earlier. The activity of this enzyme seems to be an individual variable unique to each person's skin. The composition is compared with that of other animals in a summary table (Table 2). The wax and diol esters

TABLE 1 Average Composition of Human Skin Surface Lipid from the Forehead

Lipid class	Mean, weight (%)	Range, weight (%)
Triglycerides	41.0	19.5–49.4
Diglycerides	2.2	2.3–4.3
Fatty acids	16.4	7.9–39.0
Wax esters	25.0	22.6–29.5
Squalene	12.0	10.1–13.9
Cholesterol	1.4	1.2–2.3
Cholesterol esters	2.1	1.5–2.6

Source: From Ref. 6.

appear to be the predominant class of lipid in animals other than humans (8). Stewart et al. (9) have shown that wax esters are lipids that have their origin exclusively in the sebum that is derived from sebaceous gland's synthetic machinery via de nova synthesis. In fact, the same authors have proposed that the quantity of endogenous lipids synthesized de nova per cell relative to the sebocytes' original endowment of exogenously derived lipids is a major influence on the composition of secreted sebum.

The broad composition of the fatty acid components of various lipid classes found in sebum are given in Table 3 (10). Thirty percent to fourty three percent of the fatty acids are unsaturated. Around 85% are straight chains as opposed to branched and about 75% are even carbon chain lengths. The monounsaturated fatty acids of human sebum are characterized by the unusual placing of a double bond at position $\Delta6$; this differs from other animals where the $\Delta9$ monounsaturates are predominant (4). In fact, recent studies (11) have identified a $\Delta6$-desaturase found in differentiating the sebocytes from the suprabasal layer of the sebaceous gland; this enzyme forms the double bonds at the $\Delta6$ position. This suggests that the gland tightly regulates the formation of the $\Delta6$ fatty acids at the appropriate time during lipogenesis. These acids are found in greatest abundance in sebum from adults. Human sebum is unique in that it contains dienoic acids with double bonds at positions $\Delta5$ and $\Delta8$ and at positions $\Delta7$ and $\Delta10$. These constitute 2% to 3% of the total fatty acid content. The major form was identified as $18:2\Delta5, 8$ and, because of its presence in sebum, was named sebaleic acid (4). Branched chain acids are present, which are predominantly iso- and anteiso-isomers, but there are also smaller amounts of branched chain acids, in which the methyl branch occurs at other positions in the chain. Acids having two or three methyl branches may also be present. Up to half of the fatty acids of sebum are monounsaturated with double bonds in the unusual $\Delta6$ position. The monounsaturated fatty acids include iso- and anteiso-branched species, but no internally branched or multibranched species. The fatty alcohols of the wax esters contain chain branching

TABLE 2 Classes of Lipids in Weight Percent Present in the Sebum of Different Species

Lipid class	Human	Rat	Mouse	Hamster ear
Triglycerides	43	8	6	20
Squalene	12	—	—	—
Sterol and wax esters	26	44	15	68
Diol esters	—	—	66	—
Free sterols	1	6	13	2.9
Free fatty acids	16	1	1	5.5

Source: From Ref. 8.

TABLE 3 Fatty Acid Composition of Each Lipid Fraction Isolated from Sebum

Chain type (%)	Triglyceride	Cholesterol and hydrocarbon	Free fatty acid
Branched chains	15.0	13.6	12.4
Straight chains	84.9	86.4	87.5
Odd-carbon-number chains	22.5	26.2	21.8
Even-carbon-number chains	77.4	73.8	78.1
Saturated chains	70.9	56.2	69.7
Unsaturated chains	29.9	43.8	30.2

Source: From Ref. 10.

and unsaturation, similar to the fatty acids (12). The fatty acid composition of wax esters has been shown to vary with age in humans (4).

Several other authors have also examined the fatty acid and fatty alcohol components of the various lipid classes found in sebum. The major portion of the fatty acids in sebum are chain lengths of C16 carbons. However, after this, it depends on whether one is looking at saturated or unsaturated fatty acids (7,9,12,13). For example, for saturated fatty acids, the C14:0 exhibited the next higher fraction followed by C15:0, then C18:0. For unsaturated fatty acids, C16 and then C18 carbon chains predominate. The C16:1 chain is characterized by the large amounts of C16:1Δ6 fatty acids shown in follicular casts (7). The recent discovery of the Δ6 fatty acid desaturase in differentiating sebocytes was mentioned earlier. The straight chain fatty acids that are synthesized mainly by the sebaceous glands are C14:0, C14:1, C16:0, C16:1, and C18:2 Δ5,8, because these increased with increasing ratios of wax esters (of sebaceous origin) to cholesterol+cholesterol esters (both of exogenous origin) in sebum samples from different age subjects. Fatty acids that circulate in the blood, namely C18:0, C18:1, and C18:2 Δ9,12, tended to decrease with increasing ratios of wax esters to cholesterol + cholesterol esters, suggesting their exogenous origin in sebum. Stewart et al. (9) found that the fatty acids of triglycerides tended to follow the same compositions as the FFA except that they tended to have a higher level of saturated fatty acids. Although Nordstrom et al. (7) found that in follicular casts, the triglycerides lacked the C16:1Δ6 and there were significantly higher relative amounts of saturated fatty acids in these triglycerides.

Regarding the remaining lipid classes, Stewart et al. (9) reported that wax esters contained lower amounts of C18:0, C18:1, and linoleate than other lipid classes, suggesting that very few exogenous lipids get into the wax esters. Wax esters also contain more C14:1 and C16:1 and less C14:0 and C16:0 than other lipid classes. These findings suggest that there is some mechanism for differential distribution of fatty acids among the various lipid classes. Regarding the polyunsaturated fatty acids present in amounts less than 2% to 3%, linoleic acid (C18:2 Δ9,12) decreases and sebaleic acid (C18:2 Δ5,8) increases as the ratio of wax esters to cholesterol + cholesterol esters increases, leading again to the conclusion that linoleic acid is an exogenous lipid.

A feature of human sebum is its high squalene to the cholesterol ratio. The amount of cholesterol is very small compared to the amount of squalene. In fact, the sebaceous gland has an incomplete enzyme system and is unable to convert squalene to cholesterol (4). This suggests that the source of cholesterol in isolated sebum is of epidermal origin rather than sebaceous.

Copious amounts of phospholipids are required to support the cellular and subcellular membranes of the expanding sebaceous cells during their differentiation. In the final stages of differentiation, when the membranes are degraded, the phospholipids also disappear, and it is assumed that the fatty acids become esterified with whatever hydroxyl lipids that are available. These mechanisms explain why sebum does not contain phospholipids, despite the holocrine character of the sebaceous gland function (14).

Physical Properties of Sebum

The physical properties of sebum have been investigated a number of times. Braun-Falco et al. (15) claimed that a lipid obtained from the scalp using ether extraction is a liquid at body temperature. The fact that this lipid is obtained from the scalp, where usually no comedones are found, was ignored. Other workers (16–18) have also investigated the physical properties of sebum and its role in acnegenesis, without the concern that the sebum obtained was from the areas of the skin where acne does not normally occur. Hence, if any relationship does exist between the physical properties of sebum and acne, it would be erroneous to use these studies. Still other papers (19) used ether to extract it from the foreheads and this was then analyzed. Here again, only the surface lipid was analyzed and not the lipid from the inner acrofundibulum. Here, a major assumption was made that sebum is a liquid and hence flows out, and this was analyzed. It is reasonable to postulate that since sebum is a mixture of different substances, it will exist in more than one phase. Some phases may be liquids whereas others may be solids at body temperature.

Some of the physical properties have been enumerated. The physical properties of sebum are summarized in Table 4.

Freezing Temperature

Although Miescher and Schoenberg (20) isolated forehead sebum in normal volunteers and have assigned the freezing point of 33°C to 35°C to sebum, Butcher and Coonin (19) also isolated forehead sebum from normal volunteers and have ascribed a value of 15°C to 17°C. From these studies, it was not clear if sebum is a liquid or a solid at body temperature. Since sebum is a mixture of different

TABLE 4 Physical Properties of Sebum

Property	Forehead sebum (19)	Scalp sebum (16)
Specific gravity	0.91 g/cm^2	0.90 g/cm^2 for three normal samples
Surface tension	24.9 dynes/cm from 26.5°C–31°C	22.9 dynes/cm or six normal samples at 30°C
Viscosity	0.55 poise at 38°C	0.32 poise at 35°C and 0.82 poise at 25°C
	1.00 poise at 26.5°C Viscosity was discontinuous at 30°C due to separation of a precipitate in the sebum	
Melting point	Sample started to freeze at 30°C and then solidified at 15°–17°C	15–17°C

lipidic substances, it is assumed that it will not have a single freezing point, but rather a range of temperatures in which transitions from a liquid to a solid takes place. Butcher and Coonin (19) claim that the sebum sample started to freeze up to 30°C, but the whole sample solidified at 15°C to 17°C and stopped flowing.

Specific Gravity
The specific gravity of sebum given by Butcher and Coonin (19) from the forehead sebum of normal individuals was 0.911 ± 0.01 g/cm^3 for all samples. Burton (16) confirmed this for three normal subjects when scalp sebum was used.

Surface Tension
The surface tension (Table 4) at temperatures varying from 26.5°C to 31°C was found to be an average of 24.89 dynes/cm for forehead sebum of normal subjects. A very close value (22.9 ± 0.9–24.2 ± 1.1) was also obtained for scalp sebum of normal and acne patients.

Viscosity
The viscosity increased from 0.55 to 0.98 poise, as temperature decreased from 38°C to 28.5°C. The sebum separated into various components when the temperature was lowered from 29°C to 30°C and ceased to flow at 15°C to 17°C (19). Burton (16) reported a viscosity of 0.32 ± 0.03 poise at 35°C, 0.82 ± 0.22 poise at 25°C, and 1.71 ± 0.70 poise at 20°C. In addition, it was found that the viscosity of scalp sebum and forehead sebum was similar in normal individuals. Burton also reported that the mean viscosity of the sebum from 10 acne patients taking tetracycline was higher than with seven patients not taking tetracycline at 35°C.

IMPORTANCE OF SEBUM TO THE PATHOGENESIS OF ACNE

The role of sebum in acnegenesis is poorly understood. Acne vulgaris, a multifactorial disease of the skin, is found in areas rich in sebaceous follicles. It is characterized by seborrhea, disturbed keratinization in the follicles with comedones, and subsequent inflammatory papules, pustules and nodular abscesses, and scars (15). The pathology of acne is described in various other chapters in this book but a brief review here sets the stage for relevance of the studies of sebum described later in this chapter. There are three essential factors as a group that may cause acne.

1. There is an increase in androgen production in puberty, which induces enlargement of sebaceous follicles and increased sebum production (21).
2. Follicular hyperkeratinization leads to retention hyperkeratosis, that is, obstruction of the pilosebaceous duct by accumulation of an excessive amount of keratin as an important factor in the pathogenesis of acne (22).
3. *P. acnes* proliferate in the follicle, producing a variety of extracellular inflammatory products, which excite an inflammatory response (23).

The primary event in acne is faulty keratinization and the production of comedones. In the secondary stage, inflammation can occur in the comedones. Two pathways define the subsequent development of the lesions of acne. In the noninflammatory pathway, the microcomedo proceeds to mature into closed and open comedones through distention of the follicle wall and lumen. In the inflammatory pathway, the extracellular products of *P. acnes* incite inflammation. *P. acnes* colonization occurs relatively early in acne, and the production of extracellular products by this organism provides multiple potential mechanisms for the development of inflammation. Among the earliest findings, drugs that reduce fatty acids (FFA), such as tetracycline, are beneficial in inflammatory acne (24). It must be noted that skin surface-derived lipids produce an inflammatory papule or nodule when they are injected into the human skin (25). Furthermore, certain fractions of the sebaceous secretion, especially fatty acids and squalene, when applied to rabbits' ears promoted follicular hyperkeratosis and comedone formation (26–28).

In the absence of comedones, the large infundibulum channels are filled with the white pasty sebaceous material. It is the normal content of a sebaceous follicle, not of an acne lesion. Sometimes, the follicles are filled with a cocoon-type skeleton of corneocytes, having 20 to 40 cells surrounding the central fine hair, with a channel left free in the sebum of which *P. acnes* and staphylococci may be found (15). This is called a follicular filament or follicular cast. A comedo can arise from a follicular filament. It is believed that the lipid composition of the follicular casts may play a role in acne genesis. It was demonstrated by Nordstrom et al. (7) that about 29% of the net weight of follicular casts was lipid. In addition, the hydrolysis of the triglycerides in the follicular casts was much higher than on the skin surface.

The differences in the rate of sebum production in acne patients and normal controls have so far been the only consistent finding that links sebum secretion to acnegenesis (4,7). It has long been thought that acne is a result of an abnormality of sebum or sebaceous gland function. Yet, the current concept of follicular keratinization in the pathogenesis of the disease makes this relationship difficult to justify. However, four major reasons based on circumstantial but compelling evidence that link sebum to acne include:

1. Acne develops at puberty, when sebaceous glands become very active (29).
2. The rate of sebum secretion is generally higher in acne subjects than in normal individuals, though not all persons having high sebum secretion suffer from acne (30).
3. Some components of sebum are irritants and can be comedogenic in inflammatory acne.
4. Acne is improved by any modality that reduces sebaceous gland activity (31).

This indicates that sebum is probably an essential factor in the pathogenesis of acne, but not necessarily the only one.

It is possible that the changes in the horny layer could be the result of an alteration of the nature of the sebum, so that it causes keratinization of the duct and leads to comedone formation. The macromolecular structure of the sebum could change to a more crystalline state that forms a blockage and impedes its own flow through the sebaceous duct and infundibulum or alternatively cause irritation to the follicular epidermal lining. Gonzalez-Serva (32) and Abramovits and Gonzalez-Serva (33) have speculated that acne involves the build up of an intraductal calculus termed sebolith, which results from crystallization of sebum. They proposed that the sebolith punctures and erodes the follicular lining, leading to rupture and inflammation. The proliferation of bacteria could be the result of a change in sebum composition or structure, so that either it provides a richer, more bioavailable medium for bacterial growth or it no longer contains inhibitory factors. In such a manner, sebum can be involved. The authors believe that the characterization of the lipids of the sebaceous follicles and their physical behavior may provide more detailed information on the possible role of sebum in acne vulgaris.

Electron microscopy studies on comedones showed the presence of yeasts, bacteria, keratinized cells, sebum, and hairs. In these comedones, sebum was a ubiquitous component and appeared as an osmiophilic granular material, which varied in amount from scanty to abundant between the keratinized cells (34). Depressions between the microridges of the keratinized cells had the greatest propensity for sebum. Many yeast and bacteria occupied these sebum-rich areas and their surfaces were covered with fatty material.

The composition of the lipid components of comedones was also examined by Nicolaides et al. (13) and compared with the skin surface lipids. Chapter 3 by Dr. Wertz covers this in more detail, but findings relative to the purposes of this chapter are summarized here. The lipids in comedones contain all the same lipid classes as sebum, but some are in different proportions. Triglycerides represent only a small portion of the comedonal lipids (7%) and fatty acids represent 55% of the lipids. Wax esters are only 14% of the lipids compared with 24% in surface sebum. Free cholesterol is also much higher in comedonal lipids. Another notable difference is a larger amount of saturated fatty acids in comedonal lipids—about 70% of the comedonal FFA are saturated compared with only 65% of the surface sebum. The differences between comedonal and surface lipid reflect the contribution of epidermal lipids to the mix. Epidermal lipids do not contain any wax esters, and cholesterol is derived from epidermal lipid. Epidermal lipids also provide saturated fatty acids to the mix. The reduced amounts of triglycerides are due to nearly complete bacterial hydrolysis of this class to FFA.

Since sebum is a mixture of the different lipid components discussed earlier, it is important to understand how each component affects the macromolecular structure and the physical–chemical behavior of sebum, and how this is altered in diseases of the pilosebaceous unit, for example, acne. It is, therefore, useful to know how variations in the components, for example, concentration and ratio of different components, their carbon chain length, and the ratios of unsaturation to saturation, affect the macromolecular structure of sebum and how this relates to the composition of sebum in acne lesions in particular comedones. The ultimate goal is to determine how this composition can be altered in the skin of acne patients to correct the defects in the infundibulum and the sebaceous duct, and to facilitate penetration of anti-acne drugs into the pilosebaceous unit.

INVESTIGATIONS OF THE EFFECT OF VARIATIONS OF SEBUM COMPONENTS ON THE PHASE BEHAVIOR OF SEBUM

The presence of sebaceous secretions seen as a white pasty substance in the infundibulum, and the relationship between sebaceous activity and acnegenesis discussed earlier suggests that sebum macromolecular structure may play a role in the pathogenesis of acne. The physical properties of sebum, melting point, and viscosities in particular are important, as it would mediate the blockage of the sebaceous follicle. To evaluate this theory, we have examined the physical properties of the sebum components and their mixtures using DSC. The purpose was to examine parameters controlling the phase behavior of sebum (35). There are, however, physical limitations in collecting large amounts of sample from the skin surface and it is not easy to get "pure" sebum since it is contaminated with the varying amounts of epidermal lipids. Furthermore, sebum varies quantitatively from person to person and would contribute to the variability of the data. We (35) hence decided to carry out our experiments on a model sebum based on compositions given in the literature (Table 1). We have evaluated the effect of different ratios of lipid classes in a sebum model on phase behavior and on melting temperatures of these phases. In the models of sebum, the composition can be varied and the effect on the phase behavior can be determined by DSC. The aim of this research was to determine the effect of component characteristics on the phase behavior of the model sebum. In particular, we investigated the effects of the following on the melting behavior of the model sebum:

1. Carbon chain length of the triglycerides, fatty acids, and wax esters.
2. Ratio of unsaturated to saturated components in triglycerides, fatty acids, and wax esters.
3. Ratio of triglyceride to fatty acid content.
4. Effect of cosmetic additives.

Preparation of Lipid Samples and Differential Scanning Calorimetry Procedures

The ingredients for a particular model were weighed out and dissolved in a mixture of chloroform:methanol (3:1) (35). Small portions of the above model sebum were withdrawn and put on to a preweighed DSC pan. The solvent was evaporated and the weight of the pan was taken again. The difference gave us the weight of the lipid mixture and this weight was entered on the DSC run by computer. In the absence of chloroform–methanol cosolvent, the samples withdrawn were not uniform since there was a separation of the different phases. The DSC pan was then covered with an aluminum lid and run at a scan rate of 5°C/min from −50°C to 100°C using a Perkin–Elmer DSC-7. Each of the compositions was run in triplicates. For each individual component DSC runs were done in pure form, after dissolving in chloroform–methanol and evaporating the solvent. This was done to facilitate the identification of peaks. Polymorphic changes might occur when the individual components are dissolved in the cosolvent mixture, which is consequently evaporated. This step identifies if any such change has occurred.

The effect of the three different carbon chain lengths of sebum components, namely C14, C16, and C18, on phase behavior of sebum was examined. Major fatty acids of sebum fall in the carbon chain length of C14, C16, and C18, respectively, with negligible amounts of other carbon chain lengths (13). To investigate the phase transitions of sebum prepared with lipid classes with C14 carbon chains, the triglycerides, fatty acids, and wax esters in the sebum mixture were all of carbon chain length 14 (Table 5). Similarly, a sebum mixture for carbon chain length 16 and separately C18 was prepared. According to Table 1, sebum contains amounts of 41% triglycerides, 25% wax esters, and 16.4% FFA, and we used approximately that composition; the remainder was squalene.

The lipid classes are, however, a mixture of unsaturated and saturated components; therefore, these were varied also for our second objective. In Table 5, we have listed the ingredients used for the experiment. To study the effect of degree of saturation, the carbon chain length of all the components was kept constant and variation was done in the unsaturated and saturated portions. As an example, for the fatty acids, which made up 16.4% of the total, the ratio of unsaturated to saturated fatty acids was varied keeping the total to 16.4% of the sebum mixture.

TABLE 5 Lipids Used to Examine the Effect of Carbon Chain Length, Ratio of Unsaturated and Saturated Lipids, and the Ratio of Fatty Acid to Triglycerides in Sebum Model

Components of sebum model	Carbon chain length		
	14	16	18
Wax ester (unsaturated)	Oleyl oleate	Oleyl oleate	Oleyl oleate
Triglyceride (unsaturated)	Trimyristolein	Tripalmitolein	Triolein
Fatty acid (unsaturated)	Myristoleic acid	Palmitoleic acid	Oleic acid
Wax ester (saturated)	Myristyl myristate	Palmityl palmitate	Stearyl stearate
Triglyceride (saturated)	Trimyristin	Tripalmitin	Tristearin
Fatty acid (saturated)	Myristic acid	Palmitic acid	Stearic acid

Results of Phase Behavior of Model Sebum Mixtures
Model Sebum with C16 Carbon Chain Lipids and 1:1 Saturates to Unsaturates
Sebum was prepared with the C16 carbon chain species for each lipid class, also using a 1:1 mixture of saturated and unsaturated C16 fatty acid species for each lipid class. The carbon chain length of C16 is the major chain length in sebum lipid species in vivo. This sebum mixture contained

1. 41% triglyceride (ratio 1:1 tripalmitin/tripalmitolein),
2. 16.4% FFA (ratio 1:1 palmitic/palmitoleic),
3. 25% wax ester (ratio 1:1 oleyl oleate/palmityl palmitate), and
4. squalene, q.s.

A typical DSC thermogram of this model sebum has four distinct transitions that are assigned to different components in the sebum as shown in Figure 2A. The melting temperature referred to as Mp-1 through Mp-4 characterizes each of these transitions. Although Mp-1 and Mp-2 transitions occur below 0°C and represent the unsaturated portion, the other two transitions—Mp-3 and Mp-4—occur above 0°C and represent the saturated lipids. Thus, as the temperature is

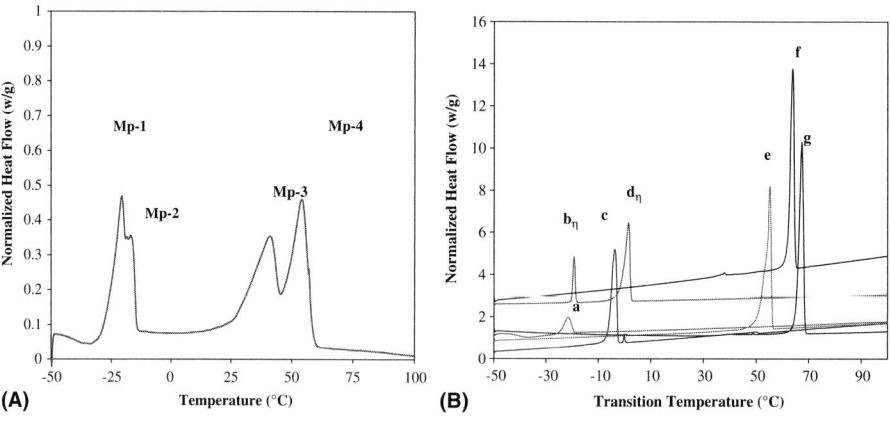

FIGURE 2 (**A**) Typical thermogram of a model sebum showing distinct melting transitions, Mp-1 to Mp-4. (**B**) Thermograms showing transition temperatures of individual components. Identifications are a. tripalmitolein m.p. = −21.184°C, b. α-palmitoleic acid m.p. = −18.7°C, c. oleyl oleate m.p. = −4.234°C, d. γ − palmitoleic acid = 2.1°C, e. palmityl palmitate = 55.166°C, f. palmitic acid = 63.866°C, and g. tripalmitin = 67.326°C.

increased from $-50°C$ to $0°C$, the unsaturated fractions of the lipid mixture melt (Fig. 2A). Standards were run and their transitions are shown in Figure 2B. The unsaturated triglycerides and unsaturated fatty acids overlap at approximately $-20°C$ in transition Mp-1 and the unsaturated wax esters (also with a small overlap with fatty acids), Mp-2 at approximately $-15°C$. As the temperature is further increased, the two saturated fractions of the model sebum melt (above $40°C$); one is designated as Mp-3 due to the saturated wax ester and then finally the last solid fraction of the model sebum melts at approximately $55°C$ and is designated as Mp-4—a transition represented by the overlap of saturated tripalmitin and palmitic acid. At $-50°C$, the sebum lipid mixture is still a solid, and by $100°C$, all components would have completely melted and the mixture is a liquid.

From the DSC profiles and melting endotherms, we can conclude that the model sebum both at room temperature and at the temperature of the skin ($32°C$ at the skin surface and closer to $40°C$ in the lower epidermis) is crystalline in nature. Generally, and as discussed by Motwani et al. (35), pure lipids or homogeneous systems yield single sharp peaks, whereas heterogeneous systems produce broad multiple peaks. If sebum was a homogeneous mixture, there would be one melting transition, but the presence of multiple melting transitions in the model sebum suggests that natural sebum has multiple phases. From the temperatures of these melting transitions, it appears that at skin temperature, some of the components of sebum are solids and some are liquids, which are not completely miscible with each other. The findings further suggest that the liquid phase probably helps solubilize the solid phase of the sebum. Therefore, it is likely that sebum exists in a macromolecular structure that is a delicate balance between the liquid and solid phases. This balance is determined in part by the ratio of saturated (solids) to unsaturated (liquids) species.

Effect of Varying the Ratio of Saturates to Unsaturates

The effect of degree of saturation on the phase transitions is shown in Figure 3A–C. The C16 lipid species were again used for these studies and each model sebum contained a different ratio of saturated to unsaturated fatty species. The transition temperatures are shown in relation to the percent of saturated components in each sample of model sebum in Figure 3. As the saturation increases (or unsaturation decreases), the intensity of the transitions for Mp-3 and Mp-4 (transitions for the saturated species) was greater and the intensities of Mp-1 and Mp-2 (transitions for the unsaturated species) was diminished, not surprising as their concentration was increasingly reduced. More interesting was that the temperatures where the phase transitions occurred decreased for the unsaturates and increased for the saturated species. The transition temperature for the unsaturated components (Mp-1 and Mp-2) decreases with a concurrent increase in the Mp-3 and Mp-4 for the saturates (Fig. 3B and C). This increase in transition temperature for the saturated compounds (Mp-3 and Mp-4) renders the sebum even more solid at the inner and outer temperature of skin.

As mentioned earlier, the presence of other substances decrease the melting point of the pure compounds. When there is more unsaturation than saturation, by the time the temperature is reached for the melting of the saturated compounds, some of the saturated portion dissolves in the already melted unsaturated portion and their melting point decreases. The more the unsaturation, the more the dissolving and hence higher decreases in the melting point. In these cases, the unsaturated portion acts as the solvent. When the percent of the saturated

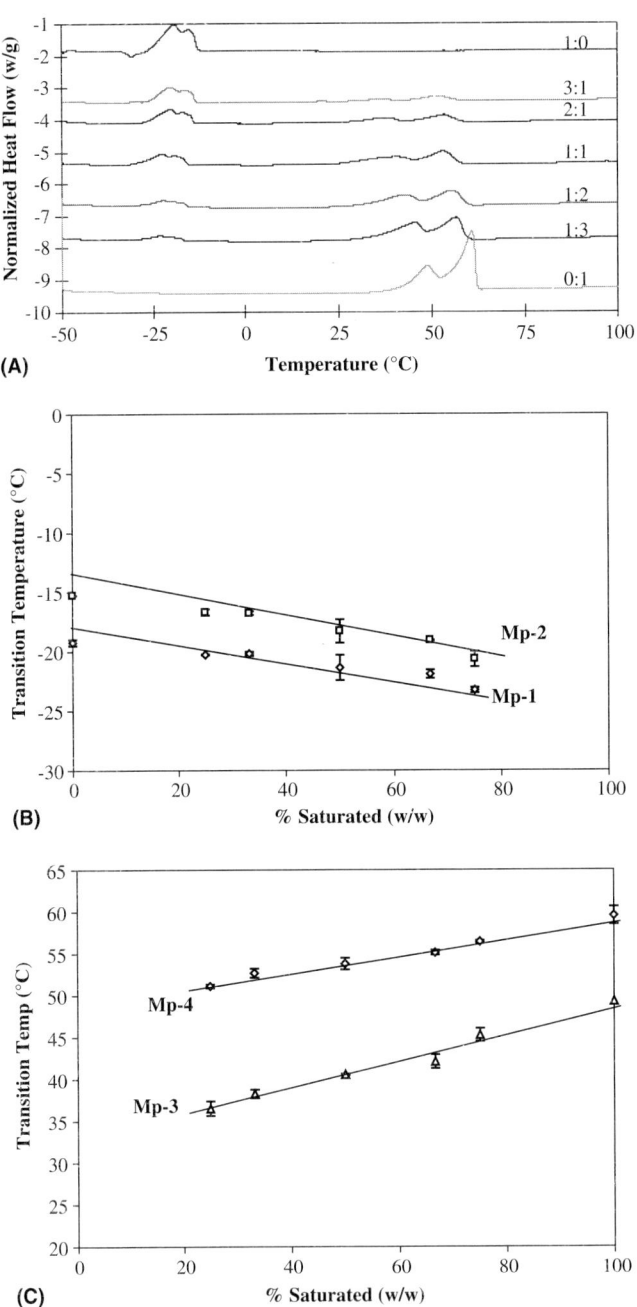

FIGURE 3 (**A**) Thermogram showing the effect of percent saturated in the model sebum for carbon chain length 16. Numbers on the side of thermograms indicate the ratio of unsaturation to saturation. (**B**) Effect of percent saturated on transition temperatures Mp-1 and Mp-2 for C-16 carbon chain. (**C**) Effect of percent saturated on transition temperatures Mp-3 and Mp-4 for C-16 carbon chain. *Note*: Error bars indicate the standard error of the mean of three replicates.

fraction is higher, it dissolves only partially in the diminished percent of the unsaturated portion. This is probably the reason that Mp-1 and Mp-2 are not affected as much as Mp-3 and Mp-4 with the increase in the percent saturated. The greater shift in transition temperature for Mp-3 than for Mp-4 means that the unsaturated portion is a "better" solvent for the wax esters (Mp-3) than the triglycerides and fatty acids (Mp-4). We are not sure as to why there is preferential dissolution of the wax ester fraction where the transition temperature shifted from 36°C to 50°C as compared with the combined fatty acid and triglyceride fraction (which exhibited the least change in transition temperature from 52°C to 60°C).

Effect of Varying the Carbon Chain Lengths
Similar results were also obtained for carbon chain length 14 and 18 compared with C16. From Figure 4A and B, it is obvious that as the carbon chain length increases, all the melting temperatures increase, which would be expected. Therefore, any change that results in an increase in average length of the carbon chains of

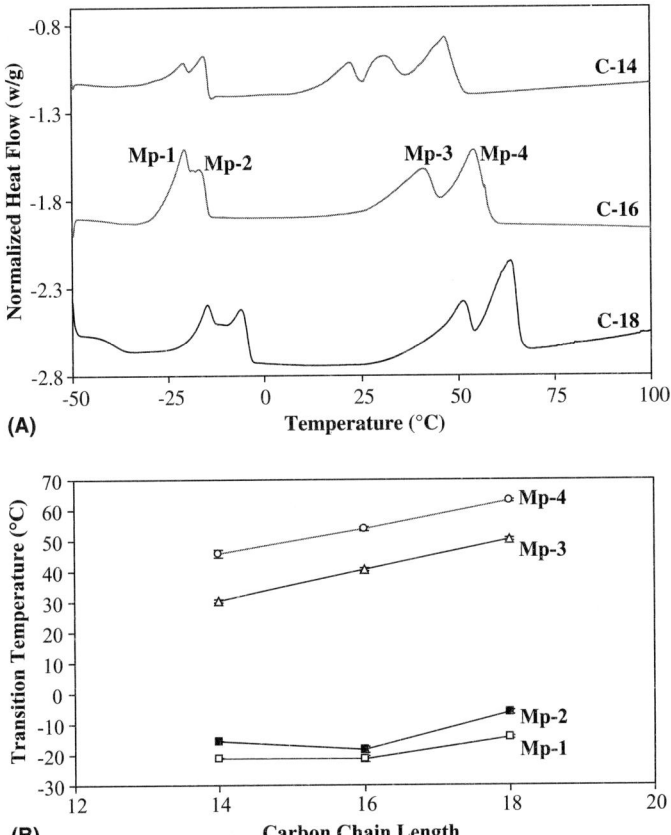

FIGURE 4 (**A**) Thermogram showing the effect of carbon chain length in the model sebum (ratio of unsaturation to saturation = 1:1). (**B**) Effect of carbon chain length on the transition temperature (ratio of unsaturation to saturation = 1:1). *Note*: Error bars indicate the standard error of the mean of three replicates.

sebum components could yield more of the solid phase at the physiological temperature of skin. The slopes of the unsaturated components are significantly smaller than the slopes of the saturated components, which means that the increase in carbon chain length affects the saturated portion more than the unsaturated portion. The shifts in the saturated portion are more relevant to in vivo skin temperatures.

Effect of Varying Ratios of Triglycerides to Free Fatty Acids

The last variable examined was varying the ratio of triglycerides to FFA. *P. acnes* hydrolyses triglycerides to fatty acids in the skin. It is hence necessary to examine the transition temperature of the model sebum when it contained different percentages of triglycerides and fatty acids. In these experiments, the ratio of unsaturated to saturated portion was maintained at 1:2 and the carbon chain length at 16. The wax ester fraction used in these experiments was palmityl myristate, and there was no unsaturated wax ester added. The reason why this wax ester was selected was because, according to Nordstrom et al. (7), this was the fraction that occurred most frequently. In Figure 5A–C, Mp-4 is ascribed to a mixture of palmitic acid (m.p. = 63°C) and tripalmitin (m.p. = 68°C). The three figures show the effect of decreasing the relative amount of triglycerides and increasing fatty acids. MP-4 decreases from 59°C to 48°C, as the percentage of triglyceride decreases. The shift in Mp-3 was very small as the percent of triglycerides decreased (fatty acid increases), which was not unexpected. The decrease in the Mp-4 transition temperature when fatty acids increases still leaves it much higher than that of the skin (32°C to 40°C), and it is probably not going to have a significant impact on physiological conditions of the skin because it remains in the solid state.

Effect of Ingredients on the Phase Behavior of Sebum

An additional question is what types of ingredients can aid the solubilization of sebum. Such ingredients could be incorporated into acne treatment products that would solubilize sebum to help "soften" the blocked infundibulum. This could potentiate delivery of drugs into the follicle to treat the other components of acne, for example, exfoliating drugs and antimicrobials. The goal was to identify different vehicles that affect the thermal behavior of sebum monitored by DSC.

For this purpose, the model sebum mixture was prepared based on a composition discussed in the previous section (35,36). The test vehicle was added in a concentration of 15% of the weight of sebum. Small portions of the above mixture were put on a preweighed DSC pan. These were run from −50°C to 100°C at 5°C/min. In the model sebum, four distinct transitions were observed. Mp-1 and Mp-2 (which occurred below 0°C) and Mp-3 and Mp-4 (which occurred above 30°C), ingredients that affected Mp-3 and Mp-4 were considered for further analysis. The reason again is that on addition of different substances to the model sebum, the changes that occur near the body temperature are physiologically more important; therefore, we have concentrated on the effect of vehicle on the two transitions Mp-3 and Mp-4—the transitions for the solid phases of sebum. If an interaction occurs between a component of the model sebum and the ingredient, generally there is a decrease in the transition temperatures along with a decrease in the heat associated with the same. A decrease in transition temperature or the heats of transition (area under the curve for the transition) indicates dissolution of the sebum component in the vehicle below its usual melting temperature. This can be considered

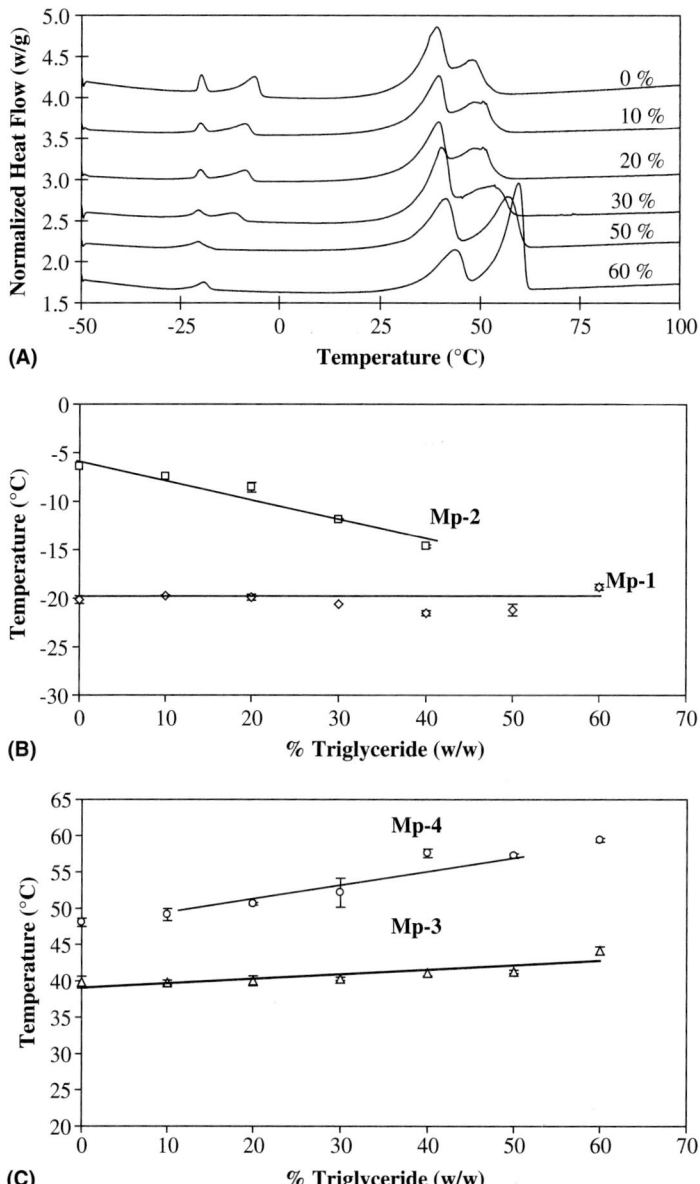

(A)

(B)

(C)

FIGURE 5 (**A**) Representative thermogram showing the effect of percent triglyceride in the model sebum. Numbers on the side of thermograms indicate the percent of triglycerides. (**B**) Effect of percent triglycerides on the transition temperatures Mp-1 and Mp-2 for C-16 (ratio of unsaturation to saturation = 1:2). (**C**) Effect of percent triglycerides on the transition temperatures Mp-3 and Mp-4 for C-16 (ratio of unsaturation to saturation = 1:2). *Note*: Error bars indicate the standard error of the mean of three replicates.

as a measure of miscibility of the vehicle with the sebum component associated with that transition. Heats of transition were too variable to assess reliably.

The effect of vehicles on Mp-3 and Mp-4 transitions of model sebum (control) is plotted in Figure 6A and B, respectively. Several vehicles reduced the transition temperatures; however, there was only slight correlation between vehicles that affect both, transitions for saturated wax esters and fatty acids/triglyceride. This would be logical since Mp-3 is the transition for the wax ester, whereas Mp-4 is a combination peak for the wax fatty acid and triglyceride. If a vehicle interacts with one component of the model sebum, it is not necessary that it will also interact with the other component.

Numerous vehicles have been examined and are reported elsewhere (36); a few are discussed here for demonstration purposes. In general, we can see from Figure 6A that the hydrophobic materials [e.g., isopropyl myristate (IPM), oleic

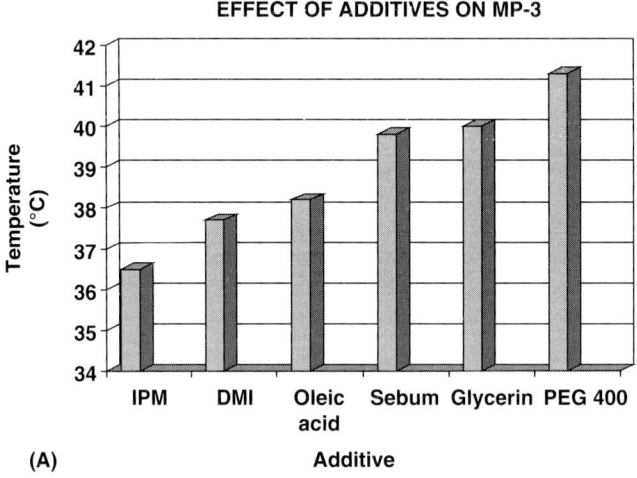

(A)

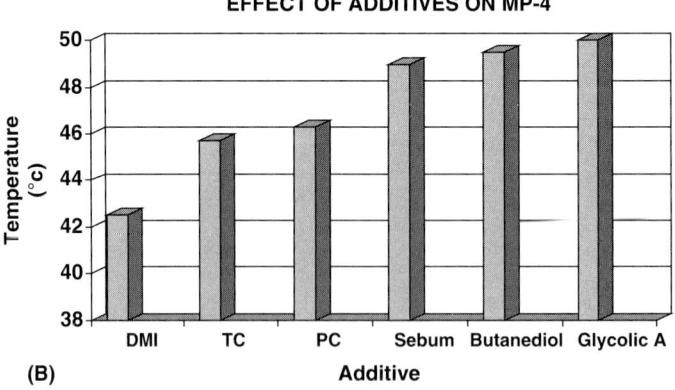

(B)

FIGURE 6 (**A**) Effect of cosmetic additives on Mp-3 for model sebum. (**B**) Effect of cosmetic additives on Mp-4 for model sebum. *Note*: The model sebum without any additives is included as the control (additive present at 15% w/w). *Abbreviations*: DMI, dimethyl isosorbide; IPM, isopropyl myristate; OA, oleic acid; PC, phosphatidyl choline; TC, transcutol.

acid (OA)] are more effective in lowering Mp-3, whereas the polar materials (glycerine and PEG-400) actually raise Mp-3 above sebum. This can be in part because sebum is made up of a mixture of nonpolar lipids and the hydrophobic vehicles are easily miscible. Similarly, another set of vehicles, which are miscible with the triglyceride and fatty acid fraction of sebum (represented by a reduction in the Mp-4 transition), are seen in Figure 6B [dimethyl isosorbide (DMI), transcutol, and phosphatidyl choline]. Other more polar vehicles are not miscible, such as butanediol and glycolic acid. On examining the data (Fig. 6) closely, it is seen that some of the vehicles show miscibility with sebum are also good skin permeation enhancers like IPM (37), oleic acid (38), transcutol (39), and DMI (40), whereas some such as glycolic acid (41) are known to not be skin permeation enhancers. Similarly, glycerin is a humectant and does not act as a permeation enhancer. In our DSC studies too, glycerin did not show much effect on Mp-3 and Mp-4, which means it is not miscible with the model sebum (36). It is interesting to note that the permeation enhancers also interact with sebum and are miscible with some of its components, as shown by our experiments. Isopropyl myristate is known to be a permeation enhancer and increases follicular delivery (42), and its presence led to a considerable decrease in the Mp-3 peak. It is possible that the increase in permeability is due to the increased miscibility with sebum and hence higher follicular delivery. Many other vehicles tested (36) in our studies have not been tested earlier for follicular delivery. This method may help us to identify other potential vehicles for follicular drug delivery.

Summary of Findings

We conclude that under the experimental conditions, the unsaturated lipids help dissolve the saturated lipids. As the proportion of the saturated, solid components (associated with the Mp-3 and Mp-4 peak) increase, it is more unlikely that the liquid components will be able to dissolve the solid under physiological conditions of the skin. Hence, if *P. acnes* action preferentially increases the relative percent of longer chains and more saturated constituents, producing more solids, these will not be dissolved by the skins' natural liquid oils. These solids may plug the pilosebaceous ducts and the infundibulum.

Nicolaides et al. (13) reported that comedonal material is relatively more saturated whereas sebum collected from the skin surface is more unsaturated. Additionally, it is well-published that there is a deficiency in polyunsaturated fatty acids, such as linoleic and sebaleic acids, in sebum from acne patients (14); this would result in relatively more of the saturated components. The findings suggest that conversion of triglycerides to FFA by the *P. acnes* may not have the largest physiological consequences as far as the physical properties of sebum are concerned, providing that the concentration of the saturated forms relative to the unsaturated species does not change. However, if relatively more of the longer chain, saturated fatty acid species are produced by the bacterial hydrolysis within the infundibulum, the balance between the liquid and solid phases will be altered.

Actual sebum may lie somewhere in between all the model sebum that we have investigated, and a portion of it may be solid at physiological temperatures of 32°C to 40°C. Further, the presence of the solid portion depends in a large part on the presence of the unsaturated or liquid portion of the sebum. The fact that sebum may exist in different phases has also been suggested by Burton (16).

Butcher and Coonin (19) also showed that although some components of forehead sebum started to solidify at 30°C, it completely solidified at 15°C to 17°C. These studies are in agreement with the present studies that sebum does not exist as one phase but rather as a mixture of a solid and a liquid at skin temperature. DSC of scalp sebum has been done by Bore et al. (18). Their results also confirm the presence of multiple phases in sebum. Their samples were also mixtures of solids and liquids at body temperature. They showed that as the percentage of unsaturated portion increased, the viscosity of the sample decreased. We showed that as the unsaturated portion increases, the saturated portion's melting temperature decreased, which in turn may contribute to the decreased viscosity.

Vehicles were also identified, that can "soften" the solid components of sebum. Some of these are known penetration enhancers such as IPM, OA, and transcutol. These vehicles are miscible with the solid components (Mp-3 and Mp-4). The effect of these ingredients on delivery of polar and nonpolar anti-acne treatment drugs would be interesting and is the subject of future investigations.

The most important finding from this research is that the mixture of sebum lipids exists in multiple phases—liquids and solids—and that the average carbon chain length and degree of saturation controls the relative amounts of these phases. Whether the presence of an excessive amount of the solid phase of sebum in the follicle plays a role in the pathogenesis of acne still remains to be investigated. The presence of excessive amounts of the solid phase would render it difficult for the liquid phase to dissolve the solid phase and could plausibly lead to altered sebum flow and blockage of the pilosebaceous duct, as is known to occur in acne patients. Gonzalez and Kroumpouzos reported the presence of polarizable crystals in comedonal sebum (32), supporting this view.

CONCLUSIONS

In this chapter, the composition of sebum has been described and the relevance of alterations in sebum composition to the pathogenesis of acne discussed. Excessive sebum production is generally associated with acne. Comedonal sebum appears to be enriched in saturated fatty acids compared with skin surface lipids. Sebum appears to be a mixture of solid and liquid phases, as evidenced by the appearance of the four transitions in the thermal analysis. The liquid phase of sebum comprising unsaturated lipid species facilitates dissolution of the solid phase of sebum comprising saturated species. If this balance is suboptimal, it could lead to blockage of the pilosebaceous duct. These two appear to be in a delicate balance. In acne, it seems that this balance is disrupted probably due to the metabolic activity of *P. acnes*, producing relatively more of the saturated solid components found in the comedones; these would presumably cause the blockages in the pilosebaceous unit. This thermal analysis method can be used to identify cosmetic ingredients that facilitate dissolution of sebum, thereby reducing the blockage and influencing the penetration of certain types of acne medications to the pilosebaceous unit.

During the preparation of this chapter, others have proposed new strategies to solubilize sebum components. The use of triblock surfactants and hydrophilic and hydrophobic linker molecules efficiently form single phase microemulsions during emulsification. This new approach allows suppression of undesirable lamellar phases that usually dominate the aqueous behavior of surfactant-triglyceride mixtures (43,44).

REFERENCES

1. Strauss JS, Pochi PE. Histology, photochemistry and electron microscopy of sebaceous glands in man. In: Gans O, Steigleder GK, eds. Hanbuch der Haut-und Geschlechtskrankheiten; Normale und Pathologische Anatomie der haut I. Berlin: Springer-Verlag, 1968:184–223.
2. Pagnoni A, Kligman AM, Gammal S, Stoudemayer T. Determination of density of follicles on various regions of the face by cyanoacrylate biopsy: correlation with sebum output. Br J Dermatol 1994; 131:862–865.
3. Strauss JS, Downing DT, Ebling FJ. In: Goldsmith LA, ed. Biochemistry and Physiology of Skin. Vol. 1, Oxford University Press, 1983:569–595.
4. Thody AJ, Shuster S. Control and function of sebaceous glands. Physiol Rev 1989; 69(2):383–416.
5. Nicolaides N, Ansari MNA. The dienoic fatty acids of human surface lipid. Lipids 1969; 4:79–81.
6. Downing DT, Strauss JS, Pochi PE. Variability of the chemical composition of human skin surface lipids. J Invest Dermatol 1969; 53:322–327.
7. Nordstrom KM, Labows JN, McGinley KJ, Leyden JJ. Characterization of wax esters, triglycerides, and free fatty acids of follicular casts. J Invest Dermatol 1986; 86(6):700–705.
8. Lauer AC, Ramachandran C, Lieb LM, Niemiec S, Weiner ND. Targeted delivery to the pilosebaceous unit via liposomes. Adv Drug Deliv Rev 1996; 18:311–324.
9. Stewart ME, Steele WA, Downing DT. Changes in relative amounts of endogenous and exogenous fatty acids in sebaceous lipids during early adolescence. J Invest Dermatol 1989; 92:371–378.
10. Kosugi H, Ueta N. The fatty acid composition of sebum. Jpn J Exp Med 1977; 47:335.
11. Gordon GL, Hsuan JS, Stenn K, Prouty SM. The identification of delta-6 desaturase of human sebaceous glands: expression and enzyme activity. J Invest Dermatol 2003; 120(5):707–714, erratum in J Invest Dermatol 2003; 121(3):434.
12. Nicolaides N. The monoene and other wax alcohols of human skin surface lipid and their relation to the fatty acids of this lipid. Lipids 1969; 2:266–275.
13. Nicolaides N, Ansari MN, Fu HC, Lindsay DG. Lipid composition of comedones compared with that of human skin surface in acne patients. J Invest Dermatol 1970; 54(6):487–495.
14. Downing DT, Stewart ME, Wertz PW, Strauss JS. Essential fatty acids and acne. J Am Acad Dermatol 1986; 14:221–225.
15. Braun-Falco O, Plewig G, Wolff HH, Winkelmann RK. Diseases of sebaceous follicles. In: Braun-Falco O, Plewig G, Wolff HH, Winkelmann RK, eds. Dermatology. Berlin: Springer-Verlag, 1991:716–743.
16. Burton JL. The physical properties of sebum in acne vulgaris. Clin Sci 1970; 39:757–767.
17. Bore P, Goetz N, Caron JC. Differential thermal analysis of human sebum as a new approach to rheological behavior. Int J Cosmet Sci 1980; 2:177–191.
18. Bore P, Goetz N. A physical method for qualitative examination of human sebum. J Soc Cos Chem 1977; 28:317–328.
19. Butcher EO, Coonin A. The physical properties of human sebum. J Invest Dermatol 1949; 12:249–254.
20. Miescher G, Schoenberg A. Unterchungen uber die funktion der talgdrusen. Bulletin der Schweizerischen Akademie der Medizinischen Wissenschaften 1944; 1:101–107.
21. Ebling JF. Effects of steroids on the skin. Biochem Soc Trans 1976; 4:597–602.
22. Cunliffe WJ, Perera WDH, Tan SG, Williams M, Williams S. Pilosebaceous duct physiology. Br J Dermatol 1976; 94:431–434.
23. Plewig G, Kligman AM. Acne and Rosacea. Berlin: Springer-Verlag, 1975, p. 59.
24. Freinkel RK, Strauss JS, Yip SY. Effect of tetracycline on the composition of sebum in acne vulgaris. N Engl J Med 1965; 273(16):850–854.
25. Strauss JS, Pochi PE. Intracutaneous injection of sebum and comedones. Arch Dermatol 1965; 92:443–456.
26. Kligman AM, Katz AG. Pathogenesis of acne vulgaris I. Comedogenic properties of human sebum in external ear canal of the rabbit. Arch Dermatol 1968; 98(1):53–57.

27. Kligman AM. Pathogenesis of acne vulgaris II Histopathology of comedones induced in the rabbit ear by human sebum. Arch Dermatol 1968; 98:58–66.
28. Kanaar P. Follicular-keratogenic properties of fatty acids in the external ear canal of the rabbit. Dermatologica 1971; 142:14–22.
29. Jacobsen E, Billings JK, Frantz RA, Kinney CK, Stewart ME, Downing DT. Age related changes in sebaceous wax ester secretion rates in men and women. J Invest Dermatol 1985; 85(5):483–485.
30. Strauss JS, Pochi PE, Downing DT. Acne: perspectives. J Invest Dermatol 1974; 62(3):321–325.
31. Cotterill JA, Cunliffe WJ, Williamson B. Sebum excretion rate and biochemistry in patients with acne vulgaris treated by oral fenfluramine. Br J Dermatol 1971; 85:127–129.
32. Gonzalez-Serva A, Kroumpouzos G. Demonstration of polarizable crystals in fresh comedonal extracts. Acta Derm Venereol 2004; 84(6):418–421.
33. Abramovits W, Gonzalez-Serva A. Sebum, cosmetics and skin care. Dermatol Aspects Cosmet 2000; 18:617–620.
34. Wilborn WH, Montes LF, Lyons RE, Battista GW. Ultrastructural basis for the assay of topical acne treatments. transmission and scanning electron microscopy of untreated comedones. J Cutan Pathol 1978; 5:165–183.
35. Motwani M, Rhein L, Zatz J. Differential scanning calorimetry studies of sebum models. J Cosmet Sci 2001; 52:211–224.
36. Motwani M, Rhein L, Zatz J. Influence of vehicles on the phase transitions of model sebum. J Cosmet Sci 2002; 53:35–42.
37. Gorukanti SR, Li L, Kim KH. Transdermal delivery of antiparkinsonian agent, benztropine.I. Effect of vehicles on skin permeation. Int J Pharm 1999; 192:159–172.
38. Tanojo H, Boelsma E, Junginger HE, Ponec M, Bodde HE. In vivo human skin permeability enhancement by oleic acid: a laser Doppler velocimetry study. J Control Release 1999; 58:97–104.
39. Mura P, Faucci MT, Bramanti G, Corti P. Evaluation of transcutol as a clonazepam transdermal permeation enhancer from hydrophilic gel formulations. Eur J Pharm Sci 2000; 9:365–372.
40. Squillante E, Needham T, Maniar A, Kislalioglu S, Hossein Z. Codiffusion of propylene glycol and dimethyl isosorbide in hairless mouse skin. Eur J Pharm Biopharm 1998; 46:265–271.
41. Hood HL, Kraeling ME, Robl MG, Bronaugh RL. The effects of an alpha hydroxy acid (glycolic acid) on hairless guinea pig skin permeability. Food Chem Toxicol 1999; 37(11):1105–1111.
42. Kogan A, Garti H. Microemulsions and transdermal delivery vehicles. Adv Colloid Interface Sci 2006; 123–126:369–385.
43. Komesvarakul N, Sanders MD, Szekeves E, et al. Microemulsions of triglyceride-based oils: the effect of co-oil and salinity on phase diagram. J Cosmet Sci 2006; 57(4):309–325.
44. Huang L, Lips A, Co CC. Microemulsions of triglyceride sebum and the role of interfacial structure on bicontinuous behavior. Langmuir 2004; 20(9):3559–3563.

16 Targeted Delivery of Actives from Topical Treatment Products to the Pilosebaceous Unit

Linda D. Rhein
School of Natural Sciences, Fairleigh Dickinson University, Teaneck, New Jersey, U.S.A.

Joel L. Zatz and Monica R. Motwani
College of Pharmacy, Rutgers University, Piscataway, New Jersey, U.S.A.

INTRODUCTION

Delivery of topical acne medications has focused on two challenges during the past decade. First, delivering the drug to the pilosebaceous unit (PSU) is required for treating diseases such as acne that have their origin in that unit. The other challenge is delivering medications such as exfoliating agents via controlled release systems that keep the irritation caused by these drugs in abeyance. Follicular delivery involves depositing drugs in the hair follicle, hair shaft, sebaceous glands, and all components of the PSU. It is hypothesized that vehicles, which are miscible with sebum, may help the active ingredient concentrate preferentially in the PSU. Such a preferential accumulation can be advantageous for increasing the transport of the drugs through the skin, as well as for targeting the drug to achieve therapeutic efficacy in the PSU itself. Knowledge of sebum lipid components helps us to consider how a penetrating vehicle will react upon entrance into the follicular canal. Additionally, these systems must release drugs into the follicle slowly over time, as well as target their delivery into the epidermis in the follicle via partitioning from slow release agents and mild vehicles so that the system is non-irritating. The major goals of this chapter are:

1. To review methods/models used to study penetration of and actions of ingredients within the PSU,
2. To review the fundamental research on technologies that target drugs to the PSU,
3. To review investigations of different vehicle effects on the thermal behavior of model sebum and their role in targeting delivery of acne medications to the PSU, and
4. To discuss recent advances in new drug delivery technologies in marketed or newly developed topical acne treatments.

The overall goal of this chapter is to summarize the state-of-the-art knowledge of targeting follicular delivery identifying strategies that could potentially provide effective topical anti-acne products.

SEBACEOUS GLANDS AND THE PILOSEBACEOUS UNIT

Sebaceous glands are generally found all over the body, except on the palms, soles, and dorsum of the feet. Most of the glands are associated with hair follicles and hence are termed pilosebaceous glands. In humans, they are concentrated on the scalp, forehead, and face, where there may be as much as 320 glands/cm^2 on the lateral regions of the face to as much as 1600 glands/cm^2 on the alae nasi (1). Sebaceous follicles are particularly abundant in the face, ear canal, v-shaped parts of the face and chest, and on the sides of the upper arm. These skin areas are hence relatively greasy. They are also the regions where acne lesions seem to accumulate. There are a number of dermatological disorders involving the pilosebaceous structures, including acne, seborrhea, androgenic alopecia areata, and some skin cancers (2). Because the sebaceous gland is the primary source of the skin surface lipids covering large portions of the anatomy, understanding the anatomy and the properties of this skin appendage and its secretions becomes important to understanding the pathogenesis of acne, the subject of this book.

Sebaceous glands are multiacnar glands associated with hair follicles. They usually consist of a single lobule (acinus) or collection of lobules that open into a system of ducts, which in the case of pilosebaceous glands open into the piliary gland (Fig. 1).

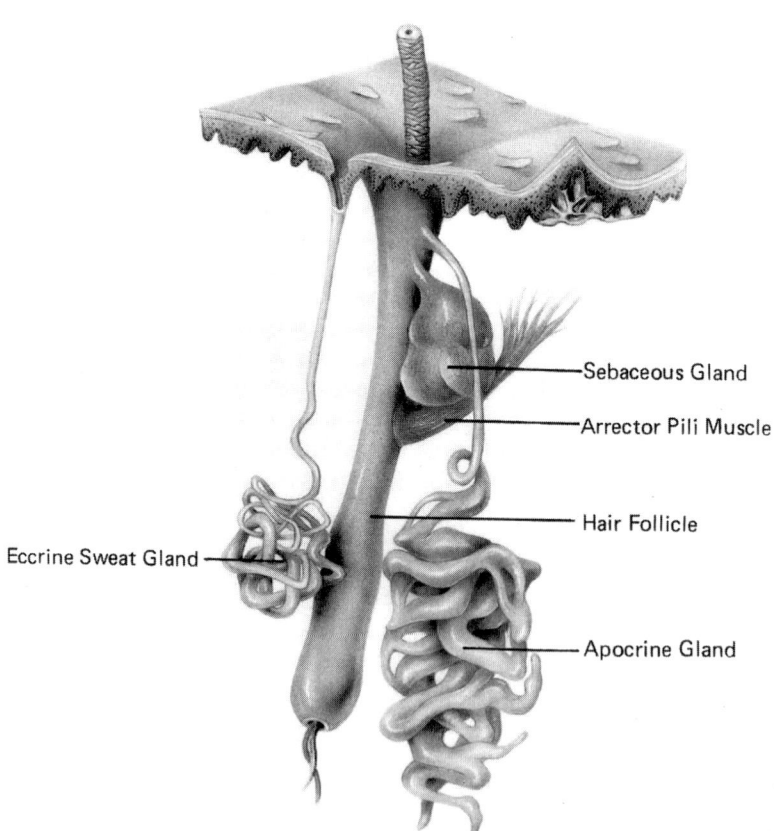

FIGURE 1 (*See color insert.*) Schematic representation of the pilosebaceous unit and associated skin appendages. *Source*: From Ref. 70.

A sebaceous follicle consists of four parts (3):

1. The infundibulum, which is coated with keratinized epithelium
2. The large sebaceous gland acini (or lobes)
3. The small vellus hair structure
4. The sebaceous duct, via which the sebaceous gland lobes (sebaceous gland acini) open into the infundibulum.

The large, cauliflower–like, lobed acini produce the sebum, and its chemical composition and physical properties are also described in other chapters and by Thody and Shuster (4). The secretory duct, the infundibulum is a long duct lined by keratinocytes. After differentiating, the keratinocytes produce corneocytes, which are ejected outward; that is, into the lumen. The infundibulum consists of a distal part adjoining the epidermis, the acroinfundibulum. The infrainfundibulum is the lower part of the infundibulum and shows a keratinization differing from that of the epidermis. The corneocytes produced here are brittle and small. Human follicles can range in diameter from 10 to 70 μm (5).

There are two different types of sebaceous cells: the lipid-producing cells of the acinus and the stratified squamous epithelium of the duct, which is continuous with the wall of the piliary canal and the surface epidermis (4). Sebaceous glands are composed of undifferentiated, differentiated, and mature cells. The sebaceous glands are holocrine (self-destruct), and their secretion, sebum, is formed when the fully mature, lipid-rich cells die and disintegrate. This results because there is a large reserve of fully synthesized sebum contained in the follicular reservoir; that is, in the upper portions of the hair follicle and the orifice to the sebaceous gland. This source of sebum is not depleted, even by repeated solvent extractions. Thus, after careful cleansing of the skin, sebum contained in the follicular reservoir initially appears to flow out on to the skin surface at a constant rate over a several hour period, until the amount of sebum normally present on the skin surface is reached. After the normal level of sebum is reached, no further increase in the sebum concentration is observed (6). Once on the surface of the skin, the sebum has already been chemically modified by microorganisms in the PSU and becomes mixed with the lipids of epidermal origin (4). Hence, the term sebum is more precisely reserved to describe the lipid content of the sebaceous glands, and the term skin surface lipid is used to describe the lipid mixture on the skin surface. However, the composition of the sebum from the surface may not be the part that, is involved in acne.

ACNE

While subsequent chapters cover the pathogenesis of acne in great detail, a brief overview will be provided here to set the stage for the discussion of delivery drug. Acne vulgaris, a multifactorial disease of the skin, is found in areas rich in sebaceous follicles. It is characterized by seborrhea, disturbed keratinization in the follicles with comedones, and subsequent inflammatory papules, pustules, and nodular abscesses and scars (3,7). In the absence of comedones, the large infundibulum channels are filled with white pasty material. It is the normal content of a sebaceous follicle, not of an acne lesion. Sometimes, the follicles are filled with a cocoon-type skeleton of corneocytes, with 20 to 40 cells surrounding the central fine hair, with a channel left free in which sebum, *Propionibacterium acnes*, and staphylococci may be found (3). This is called a follicular filament or follicular cast. A comedo can arise from a follicular filament. It is believed that the lipid composition of the follicular casts may play a role in acnegenesis and in targeting therapies (6,7).

The primary event in acne is faulty keratinization and the production of microcomedones. The initial noninflammatory lesions of acne result from alterations in the follicular epithelium, as demonstrated both physiologically and by light and electron microscopic level (7). The proliferation and retention-type hyperkeratosis develops in the infundibulum, which expands like a balloon. Two pathways define the subsequent development of the lesions of acne. In the noninflammatory pathway, the microcomedo proceeds to mature into closed and open comedones through distention of the follicle wall and lumen. Accumulation of corneocytes continues with the conversion of the follicle epithelium to the comedo epithelium. Open comedones arise from closed ones by continuous growth, sometimes directly from microcomedones without the intermediate stage. This plug consists of a very densely packed set of several hundred closely adhering corneocytes, together with sebum and *P. acnes*. Exfoliating drugs, such as salicylic acid (SA) and retinoic acid (RA), are often used to treat these types of lesions. In the inflammatory pathway, the extracellular products of *P. acnes* incite inflammation. *P. acnes* colonization occurs relatively early in acne, and the production of extracellular products by this organism provides multiple potential mechanisms for the development of inflammation. Among the earliest findings was that drugs that reduce free fatty acids (FFA), such as tetracycline, are beneficial in inflammatory acne (8). It must be noted that skin surface-derived lipids produce an inflammatory papule or nodule (9) and/or follicular hyperkeratosis and comedones when they are injected into human skin or rabbit ears (10–12).

PRINCIPLES OF THERAPY AND TYPES OF DRUGS DELIVERED IN TOPICAL ACNE TREATMENTS

Four principles have been used to treat acne on an individualized basis, depending upon the clinical presentation (13).

1. Correcting the defect in keratinization, for example, SA, RA
2. Decreasing sebaceous gland activity, for example, antiandrogens
3. Reducing the population of *P. acnes*, for example, antibiotics, benzoyl peroxide
4. Producing an anti-inflammatory response, for example, benzoyl peroxide

In mild acne that consists mainly of comedones, it is important to correct the defect in keratinization using exfoliating agents. In inflammatory acne, it is important to reduce the population of *P. acnes* in the follicle and the generation of extracellular products of the organism and reduce the inflammatory effects. In more severe, inflammatory acne that has proven to be resistant to therapy, it is important to consider adding a drug that decreases sebaceous gland activity. Since the comedo is the initial noticeable lesion even in inflammatory acne, it is important to correct the defect in keratinization in all cases of acne (13).

FOLLICULAR ROUTE

The follicular route is important for drug penetration as well as localized action to treat acne. Targeted delivery of active compounds to the PSU or its components can help treat a follicular disease, which for the purposes of this chapter is acne. Drug delivery through the follicular route has recently generated a growing interest. Appendages account for only 0.1% to 1% of the surface area of skin and only 0.01% to 0.1% of the skin volume. Thus, because of this, these appendages were not considered important routes for drug delivery (14). The maximum flux is low because of this—$0.5-1 \times 10^{-6}$ cm/hr. In contrast, the flux across stratum corneum (SC) is higher, 10^{-3} cm/hr, due to the large surface area, but there is a lag time because of the slow diffusivity across the intercellular lipid. This is when the PSU becomes important (14). In order to influence the flux of compounds across skin significantly, the diffusion coefficient would have to be more than three orders of magnitude higher than across the intercellular lipid domains or the corneocytes of the SC. It is because of this that the shunt pathways that represent areas of discontinuities/areas of invagination in the SC will become important for the delivery of molecules that exhibit a slow rate of percutaneous penetration and they will be particularly important during the early stages immediately after topical application. Figure 2 is a hypothetical representation of this phenomenon showing greater penetration of the drug into the appendagial shunt at early time points. The nature of the drug and the vehicle, however, can greatly influence these differences. Increasingly, the PSU is gaining acknowledgment as a complex, dynamic structure that may contribute significantly to passive transport of compounds to the skin. There are several objectives of follicular delivery:

1. Reducing or bypassing the transepidermal route,
2. Increasing drug concentration in the PSU,
3. Increasing the therapeutic index of the drug,
4. Decreasing toxicity of the drug, and
5. Reducing the high dose of the applied drug and reducing the frequency of administration.

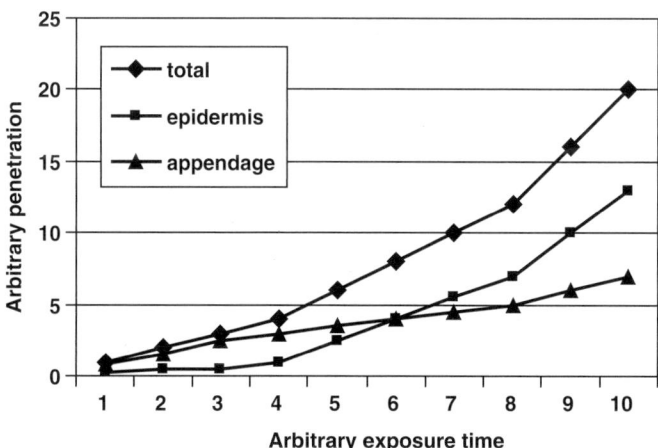

FIGURE 2 Hypothetical comparison of penetration of a topical medication into the skin. Note that the appendagial shunt pathway is the favored pathway during early time points while the epidermis becomes important during the later time points (14). The extent of this difference depends on the nature of the drug and vehicle.

BARRIERS AGAINST DRUG DELIVERY TO THE FOLLICLES

Several sites are present within the follicle that represent potentially significant targets for drug delivery, but these may be limited by the structural aspects of the hair follicle and its chemical environment (14,15). Getting the drug to these sites is also limited by the chemical nature of the drug, for example, hydrophobic or hydrophilic. Aspects of the hair follicle structure that may impede drug delivery are the following.

1. The glass membrane surrounding the entire follicle and the keratinous layers of the inner and outer sheaths may physically restrict the passage of chemical agents deep within the follicle.
2. Sebum flow into the hair follicle may represent a physical barrier to drug delivery from some formulations. The effect of sebum composition on delivery of compounds into the follicles is not known. It is, however, likely that in the sebum-filled follicle, efficient drug delivery, and pharmacological activity would depend on the interaction of drug and sebum and the physicochemical properties of the vehicle.
3. Optimum particle size requirements may also be required to traverse the hair follicle. It was found (16) that delivery of polystyrene beads into the hair follicle was size-dependent. Beads between 5 and 7 μm in diameter were optimally deposited deep within the follicle, whereas smaller or larger beads were more likely to be localized in the SC and skin surface.

ROLE OF SEBUM IN THE FOLLICULAR ROUTE

Sebaceous glands connected to the hair follicle by ducts release sebum into the upper third of the follicular canal, creating an environment enriched in neutral, nonpolar lipids. Among mammals, sebum composition varies considerably. It has been reported that the sebum-enriched environment of the hair follicle that invaginates the epidermis into the dermis could provide significant lipoidal pathway for the transport of large lipophilic molecules. Chapter 15 shows a comparison of sebum composition among different species commonly used in percutaneous absorption studies (Table 2 in that chapter). Wide variations in sebum composition among species should be considered before extrapolating data from animal to human studies. However, knowledge of sebum lipid components and their physical chemical interactions helps us to consider how a penetrating vehicle will react upon entrance into the follicular canal.

The use of vehicles that are compatible with sebum to selectively transport drug via the transfollicular pathway is certainly not a new concept (17). The basis for understanding a vehicle's effect on the delivery into the sebum-rich areas, such as the hair follicle, appears to be fully explained by conventional solubility properties. The Hildebrand coefficients for model sebum compositions demonstrate that sebum is overall a nonpolar, oily material, with a Hildebrand coefficient of approximately 7.5 to 8.0 $cal^{1/2}/cm^{3/2}$. Some authors believe (6) that many polar vehicles used in topicals, vehicles such as water, propylene glycol (PG), and ethanol would be too polar to be readily soluble in sebum. Hence, to deliver relatively polar drugs, if the vehicle is not specifically designed to solubilize sebum, there would be little chance to effectively deliver the drug to the deeper portions of the hair follicle. Hydrophilic or marginally hydrophobic drugs would not be

TABLE 1 Deposition of Drugs into the Pilosebaceous Unit

Relative compatibility of drug with sebum[a]	Relative compatibility of vehicle with sebum[b]	Amount in sebaceous glands
Incompatible	Incompatible	0
Incompatible	Compatible	+
Compatible	Incompatible	+
Compatible	Compatible	+++

[a]Compatibility in terms of partitioning and solubility/miscibility of drug with components of sebum.
[b]Compatibility in terms of miscibility of vehicle with components of sebum.

expected to be highly compatible with the sebum. For hydrophobic drugs, the transport of the drug is predominantly follicular and is brought about by cotransport of the drug dissolved in the oil phase into and across the PSUs (17). The efficiency of such a follicular enhancement in drug transport would depend on the solubility of the drug in the vehicle and the compatibility of the vehicle, with the sebum-rich lipid environment within the follicles. The deposition of a drug into sebaceous glands follows the rank order suggested in Table 1 (17). Thus, sebum therefore may represent a significant physical barrier to drug delivery from some formulations.

It has been reported that the highest pilosebaceous penetration occurred with vehicles that were mixtures of various solvents, interface active agents, coupling agents, and solubilizers (18). Studies identified isopropyl myristate, glyceryl dilaurate (GDL), and polyoxyethylene-10-stearyl ether (POE-10) as being effective at delivering drugs into the pilosebaceous duct because of their compatibility with sebum. Studies have suggested that the follicular delivery may be dependent on the physicochemical properties of the drug and/or vehicle (19,20). The lipoidal environment of the follicular canal may favor certain drugs and manipulating formulation factors, and thereby may enhance delivery of vehicles and drugs by the follicular delivery route. Solvents, which interact with sebum, thus were opening the passageway for drug deposition within the follicle.

Since sebum is a mixture of different components, it is important to characterize it. It is useful to know how variations in the components, their carbon chain length, and the ratios of unsaturation to saturation affect the physical but thermal behavior of sebum. This will provide direction on how to manipulate these properties with topical delivery systems. The thermal behavior of sebum in response to these variables has been reviewed in Chapter 15. Vehicles that alter this behavior have also been reviewed in that chapter and in Motwani et al. (20). These are discussed later in this chapter in relation to drug delivery.

MODELS USED TO STUDY FOLLICLES

A major limitation in elucidating the follicular pathway is the current lack of an adequate pharmacokinetic model that can clearly distinguish transfollicular from transepidermal percutaneous absorption. Animal models and human models can be used to study follicular delivery. The experiments can be in vivo or in vitro. These models can further be divided into models for studies of diseases and models to investigate follicular delivery. To date, the following models (Table 2) have been used and details on each model are given after the table, along with studies using these models in the next section.

TABLE 2 Animal and Human Models for Follicular Delivery

Model	Comment
Rabbit ear model	Used to assess comedogenicity of cosmetic chemicals
Rhino mouse model	Has large comedonal cysts; used to assess effectiveness of exfoliatitng agents
Macaque monkey model	Frontal scalp baldness; used to assess delivery of antiandrogens and their effect on hair growth
Hamster ear model	Has large sebaceous glands; similar to humans; used to assess drug delivery by isolation of glands
Rat model	Similar to humans; heat treat to remove epidermis containing sebaceous glands
Guinea pig model	Hairy epidermis on back and nonhairy epidermis behind the ears used to compare follicular and nonfollicular delivery
Human model	Best for studying anti-acne drug efficacy; cyanoacrylate glue or skin biopsy used to study follicular delivery by isolating follicular casts

Rabbit Ear Model

Kligman and Kwong (21) proposed this model for studying the comedogenic potential of substances commonly found in cosmetic formulations. This model is very well-suited for assessing comedogenic compounds that are encountered in the etiopathogenesis of acne vulgaris, acne cosmetica, chloracne, cutting oil acne, pitch acne, pomade acne, and tar acne (22). The procedure involves applying a comedolytic substance using a glass rod over the undersurface during a two-week period. After the animal is sacrificed, skin is sampled up to the level of the cartilage and is immersed in 60°C water for two minutes, after which the epidermis is peeled off, with the follicular extensions still attached. The comedones can be observed under the microscope. For quantitative studies, the number of comedones can be counted and compared to comedones induced by other comedogenic substances.

Rhino Mouse Model

This model was used extensively by Kligman and Kligman (23). The skin of the rhino mouse, which is an allelic of the hairless mouse, contains deep dermal cysts and a huge number of utriculi filled with keratinous debris that resembles comedones. The horny cells do not contain *P. acnes*, but like in human acne, the sebaceous glands shrink as the pseudocomedones enlarge. They concluded that the rhino mouse is a suitable model for assessing chemicals that effect epithelial differentiation (retinoids) or that promote loss of cohesion between horny cells (descaling agents). In the procedure, formulations are applied to the dorsal trunk of the mouse for a specified period and then the skin sections are histologically examined. The procedure involves application of the test substances to the entire dorsal trunk for a specified time.

Macaque Monkey Model

This model has been used to study drugs affecting hair growth. This species exhibits baldness due to hormonal and genetic factors, which is similar to androgenic alopecia (19). The stumptailed macaque monkey model exhibits a species-specific frontal scalp baldness that coincides with puberty at a rate of nearly 100% in both sexes.

Uno and Kurata (24) investigated the effects of topically applied minoxidil and diazoxide on hair growth in bald macaque monkeys and they studied the activity of 5-α reductase inhibitors in nonbald monkeys. Hair and follicular growth were evaluated by obtaining phototrichograms (gross photographs and images of frontal scalps) after closely clipping the hairs and folliculograms (4 mm punch biopsies embedded in paraffin, serially sectioned and stained). The rate of DNA synthesis in the follicular cells was also determined. The phototrichograms revealed a conversion of short vellus hair to long terminal hairs, and the folliculograms showed enlarged follicles. The DNA synthesis studies indicated an increased rate of follicular cell proliferation. This model therefore appears to have promise for further work related to human androgenic alopecia.

Hamster Ear Model

Matias and Orentreich (25) examined this model by planimetry of peeled off skin instead of routine vertical histological sections. This model has been proposed as a model system for human sebaceous glands because of the similarities in morphology and in turnover time (26). In this case, each sebaceous gland unit consists of an infundibular canal, several large lobulated acini with 6 to 20 layers of sebocytes, and one centrally located piliary unit. Male hamsters are large, and the size of their sebaceous glands is similar to that of humans. Microscopic observation of the sebaceous glands from biopsies detects pilosebaceous drug deposition.

Rat Model

This model has been used extensively by Illel et al. (27). The isolation procedure produces both follicle-free and follicular skin. The hairless rat model is chosen because the sebaceous glands density and size are closely related to those of human forehead skin. The process involves inducing anesthesia to the animals, after which the animals are treated by immersion of the back in 60°C water for one minute. The epidermis is removed from this treated area. The subsequent healing is monitored histologically and transepidermal water loss measurements (TEWLs) are done. After 9 to 10 weeks, the epidermis and horny layer regrow as a continuous layer, without the pilosebaceous structures, and the TEWL returns to normal, thereby indicating normal barrier properties. In this model, the SC looks normal, but the epidermis looks hyperplastic. The permeation is done in vitro to see the differences between follicle and follicle-free skin. However, aside from the pain and suffering inflicted on the animal and the time involved in developing the follicle-skin, there is the question of structural composition and permeability behavior of the newly regrown tissue compared with the normal epidermis of hairless rat skin and whether the comparison between the two tissue types is valid. A hairless rat has also been used without the treatment mentioned earlier, with autoradiography to give a visual impression of the follicular route (28).

Guinea Pig

Wahlberg (29) used hairy and nonhairy skin of guinea pigs to demonstrate the delivery into the follicles. For the hairy skin, the back of the guinea pig was used, whereas for the nonhairy skin, the area behind the ears of guinea pigs, which is completely devoid of hair follicles and of sebaceous and sweat glands, was used.

However, the physiological differences between the two areas make it difficult to justify its use. Also, in some cases, different strains of guinea pigs (hairy and hairless) (30) have been used to investigate the importance of follicles. However, direct comparison due to differences in species is difficult.

Human Model

The human skin contains acne-prone areas with numerous huge sebaceous follicles—an ideal site for acne vulgaris and other such follicular diseases. The human model can be used for both investigating follicular diseases as well as follicular delivery. The human skin is generally investigated by the noninvasive cyanoacrylate technique or the skin biopsy technique, the details of which are given in the next section.

METHODS TO INVESTIGATE DEPOSITION INTO THE FOLLICLES

The skin is a multilayered organ, complex in structure and function, composed of outer epidermis and inner dermis. There are various potential pathways for permeation through the SC, including the transepidermal (or "bulk") and the transappendageal (or "shunt") routes. The transepidermal route across the continuous SC and the epidermis comprises two routes of entry: the intercellular spaces, consisting of bilayers of lipids, and the intracellular or transcellular route through the keratin of the dead cornified cells (corneocytes). The transappendageal route comprises transport via both the sweat glands, hair follicles with their associated sebaceous glands. Capillaries closely surround both the follicles and the sweat glands, and rapid absorption of permeating molecules is assumed once the molecules have passed through the follicular walls. An important aspect to consider for transdermal delivery is the mechanism of penetration, that is, the fractional contribution of the bulk strata versus the appendageal pathway to the total absorption. Some of the techniques, both qualitative and quantitative, are summarized next.

Skin Biopsy Techniques
Noninvasive Cyanoacrylate Technique
Marks and Dawber (31) expanded the ancient technique to remove horny cell layers by presenting a very potent glue—cyanoacrylate—and termed it skin surface biopsy. This technique was used for excavation of follicular contents, analogous to the painful squeezing of sebaceous filaments. It involves placing a drop of adhesive on a clean region of the skin and then gently pressing a slightly moist glass slide on top of the area. After 30 to 40 seconds, the slide is removed along with the superficial horny layer of SC and follicular casts. Lavker et al. (32) have investigated the earlier events of comedo formation in relation to the bacterial contents using this technique. Mills and Kligman (33) used this model to assay comedolytic substances. Microcomedones were induced on the back of adult males by a two-week occlusive exposure to 10% crude coal tar. The test agents were then applied for two weeks and the reduction in the density of microcomedones is determined by the noninvasive cyanoacrylate technique. This method was used to screen anti-acne formulations. Mills et al. (34) analyzed SA levels in sebaceous follicles after topically applying it in a 2% hydroalcoholic vehicle or gel base.

Azelaic acid (20%) (AzA) cream was used on human volunteers for the treatment of acne (35). Surface AzA was removed by washing with acetone and then collected the follicular casts using follicular biopsy method and analyzed by HPLC method. Initial samples were taken in five minutes and thereafter over a period of five hours, five times with no fixed intervals.

Invasive Technique
Often, a full thickness biopsy containing several sebaceous follicles is needed. Biopsies are inevitable if sebaceous glands are to be investigated. It has been used for human tissues where the tissue is used within 24 hours of excision (36). After the permeation experiments in vitro, the SC is removed by stripping and then the biopsies are taken from the formulation-treated skin. The biopsies are immersed in $CaCl_2$ for a few hours and then the epidermis and dermis is separated. Under microscopic observation, the epidermis with the attached PSU is removed from the dermis. These sebaceous glands are cut off from the under side of the epidermis and then analyzed by a suitable analytical technique.

Mechanical Separation of the Follicles
This has been documented recently by Lieb (37). The procedure involved using the Syrian hamster ear as a model. The scheme involved mounting the ears, ventral side up on the diffusion cells, which maintained the temperature at 32°C. An aliquot of the test preparation was then applied to the skin surface. At predetermined time intervals, the skin specimens were separated by gentle peeling or scraping into three layers: epidermis, ventral dermis, and dorsal dermis. The sebaceous glands in the ventral dermis were removed by gentle dragging of a dull scalpel across the bottom surface of the layer. The pilosebaceous material appeared as a milky material. The scraping process was considered complete when the skin areas previously containing glands appear empty under the microscope. The scraped sebaceous glands and skin layers were assayed separately by scintillation counting.

Follicle-Free Models
This has been explained earlier in the rat model. Illel and Schafer (38) reported the first systematic, quantitative in vivo studies of follicular delivery using this method. By employing the Franz diffusion cell method, it is possible to compare penetration of drug across both follicle-free and normal skin (30).

Skin Autoradiography by Computerized Image Analysis
In this technique, the spatial distribution of a radiolabeled substance within a biological specimen is detected by exposure of the specimen to radiation-sensitive film. The main drawback of qualitative autoradiography is that it merely enables visualization but not quantification of the penetrant in the skin. Furthermore, the signals appearing on the images generally represent the tissue-bound residues rather than the freely diffusable substance. The technique, therefore, only provides an indication of drug transport through the integument.

Some workers have used quantitative autoradiography (39). With this method, it is possible to visualize and measure by means of a software program the concentrations in the hair follicle, glands, and various skin layers without resorting to mechanical horizontal sectioning. The general procedure involves freezing the test skin sample at $-130°C$, and then vertically sectioning them by cryostat in order to yield 6-μm thick slices. These sections are then fixated on glass slides, placed in film cassettes, and covered by tritium-sensitive autoradiography film. Following a four- to seven-week exposure period, the autoradiograms are developed. An imaging system consisting of a video camera, high-resolution light microscope, IBM-compatible computer, and appropriate software transforms the optical density readings of the experimental autoradiograms into drug concentrations values and projects the resultant digitized images on a TV screen, where they are displayed in pseudocolor mode. This provides a more visually meaningful picture of drug localization. In addition to autoradiography, the original skin sections are stained with hematoxylin and eosin dye. In the final step, the instrumentation is used to superimpose the autoradiography image with the histological image. The computerized system is then used to quantify drug deposition densities into drug concentration. These values require reference to calibration graph data, which are derived from a separate set of experiments. In these calibration experiments, good reproducibility was shown between the optical density readings of standard sections containing the same drug concentration (40).

Confocal Laser Microscopy

This method depends upon the analysis of re-emitted light, with the measuring depth dependent upon the beam wavelength. However, in fluorescence spectroscopy, the remitted light is detected after passing a second monochromator, that is, only a specific emission wavelength is detected. The procedure involves application of a self-fluorescent marker in a formulation on the skin. After a predetermined time, the diffusion cells are dismantled and the area of the skin exposed to treatment is punched out. The peeling and scraping technique previously described is used to mechanically isolate the sebaceous glands. The scraped glands are then suspended in a buffer and sonicated in order to release the fluorescent marker. This solution could then be assayed for the marker with a fluorescent microscope. This technique has been used quantitatively by Weiner et al. (18).

Horizontal Sectioning of Strata

This technique involves the application of the test compound (typically radiolabeled) to a specific area of skin. After a defined exposure time, the excess drug is removed. The horny layer is stripped off by the consecutive application of an adhesive tape. The underlying tissue can then be excised, and the epidermis and dermis are sectioned parallel to the skin surface with a freezing microtome. The quantity of drug in each horny layer strip or tissue slice can be determined by using a suitable analytical technique. From the derived data, it is possible to generate a profile representing drug concentration versus depth for the investigated tissue. A disadvantage of this technique is the fact that unless sufficient data is available from the literature about the thickness of each skin layer at the required regional site, preliminary experiments are needed to assess this. Another major limitation of this technique is that it does not yield any data about penetrant concentrations in the PSUs. It usually has to be used in conjunction with other techniques described earlier (41).

REVIEW OF INVESTIGATIONS OF DELIVERY VIA
THE FOLLICULAR PATHWAY
Mathematical Considerations

Scheuplein in 1967 (42) did the mathematical modeling for follicular delivery of small molecular weight electrolytes and nonelectrolytes. He used reported values of thickness, diffusion constant, area of each layer of the skin. According to him, during the initial part of the experiment, the shunt pathway (follicular and sweat glands) is dominant and that introduces the lag period. At steady state, the transepidermal route is dominant. The point at which the shunt pathway becomes equal to the bulk pathway is around 300 seconds, as per these calculations. According to the paper, the concentration levels in the neighborhood of the ducts and the follicles may be very much higher than in the bulk of the epidermis in the early stages of diffusion, before steady-state diffusion is achieved for small molecules (ordinarily within the first one hour after application of an aqueous solution). The reason for this behavior arises from the limited area of the skin surface occupied by these appendages, their relatively large diffusion constants, and the nonlinear character of diffusion prior to steady state. Usually, measurements of skin permeability done in vitro are invariably measurements of steady state because it is quite difficult to detect concentrations within the first few minutes. However, this calculation was only for small hydrophilic molecules and has been shown to fail many times because it does not take into consideration the nature of the vehicle.

This theory was then extended in another report (43), where it was found that more polar steroid molecules in aqueous solutions had a longer lag time than the nonpolar ones. The reason given for this was that the diffusion constant of polar molecules is smaller and they tend to prefer the follicular route as compared with the epidermal route, and hence the long lag times and small fluxes (Fig. 2).

In still another paper (44), aqueous ibuprofen solution penetration was monitored through hydrated human skin. The parameters of the experiment obtained were fitted into the equation as given by the authors, accounting for the shunt and bulk pathway. It was found that the shunt accounted for almost 25% of the total permeation at steady state. Also, in the presence of shunt pathway, the lag time was eight minutes, which would have otherwise been 92 minutes in the absence of the appendages.

Studies Done to Investigate Physicochemical Properties
of Drug and Follicular Deposition

The importance of the appendages was shown by Kao et al. (45) in mouse skin. Three different strains of mice were used: the normal-haired mice, the nonhaired mice, and the intermediate fuzzy-haired mice. The actives, benzopyrene and testosterone, in acetone under nonoccluded conditions were then applied to the excised dorsal skin organ culture of the mice and the permeation monitored hourly by scintillation counting for 16 hours. Some of the preparations were also investigated by fluorescence microscopy. It was concluded that the hair follicles could contribute significantly to skin permeation, although there were differences in the different strains of the mice. Testosterone permeated to a higher degree than benzopyrene. It was found that for testosterone, permeation was rapid, peak absorption was observed, and peak absorption was higher and faster than in fuzzy-haired or hairless skin. Hence, it was concluded that testosterone that is absorbed extensively, the transappendageal route, played an important role in the beginning of the experiment, but later the percutaneous absorption was important. For benzopyrene, that was less well-absorbed and peak absorption was not seen during the course of the experiment, indicating that the transappendageal route is the dominant route. It is not explained how the permeation took place for 16 hours after acetone had evaporated.

Skin permeation of two steroids, hydrocortisone ($\log P = 1.61$) and testosterone ($\log P = 3.32$), in 95% ethanol in water was evaluated in vivo on normal and artificially damaged hairless mouse skin in which sebaceous glands disappeared during healing (41). The test compounds were applied for 0.5, 2, and 6 hours. The results indicated that the permeation into the dermis and epidermis was more through the normal skin than appendage-free skin. It was postulated that sebaceous glands probably contributed to the penetration of hydrocortisone and testosterone. Testosterone, which is a more lipophilic molecule, was found at a higher concentration than hydrocortisone in the SC. It was also observed that in the case of normal skin, the epidermal and dermal amounts of these drugs increased with application time, but this increase was smaller in the case of scar skin. It was hypothesized that the sebaceous glands acted as reservoir for the steroids. In these experiments, it was not mentioned whether they were carried out under occluded conditions and if the vehicle evaporated before the end of the experiment.

In another study done by Hueber et al. (41), percutaneous absorption of steroids on human skin was examined in vitro. Percutaneous absorption studies on four steroids—progesterone ($\log P = 3.87$), testosterone ($\log P = 3.32$), estradiol ($\log P = 2.49$), and hydrocortisone ($\log P = 1.61$)—were done using freshly excised normal and scar (obtained from abdominal and mammary plasties) human skin. The steroids were dissolved in 95% ethanol in water and applied. The experiments were carried out for eight hours for progesterone and testosterone and up to 24 hours for estradiol and hydrocortisone. It was found that permeation of the steroids was significantly greater in normal skin as compared to scar skin. The fluxes obtained for progesterone and testosterone were significantly higher in normal skin than in scar skin. The fluxes of estradiol and hydrocortisone became significant after four hours. From the percentage absorbed {[(Normal skin – scar skin)/normal skin] ∗ 100}, it was also concluded from the study that transfollicular absorption was higher for progesterone and testosterone, the more lipophilic steroids, than for estradiol and hydrocortisone. It was not mentioned if the experiment was carried out under occluded or nonoccluded conditions.

Viprostol is a synthetic PGE_2, is a vasodilator, and its deposition was monitored in the skin, following application in different animals (mouse, rat, guinea pig, rabbit, and monkey) using scintillation counting and autoradiography (46). The active was incorporated in petrolatum base. Autoradiography was done only for mice and monkeys. In mice, the radioactivity was visible in SC and the hair shafts by 30 minutes. In two hours, radioactivity was also visible throughout the viable epidermis and only the hair shaft had considerable radioactivity. Skin taken after 12 hours indicated the presence of radioactivity well down in the follicle and, after 72 hours, radioactivity was visible only in the hair shaft and hair follicle. The monkey skin also showed a similar pattern, but the time was longer. By scintillation counting, it was concluded that the drug was present in the skin for a relatively long period, following removal of the drug from the application site. The authors indicated that there was formation of a significant drug depot in the skin and that viprostol penetrated through the follicular route.

Rutherford and Black (47) used autoradiography to study the localization of germicides in guinea pig skin. The deposition of two germicides, zinc pyride-2-thione 1 N oxide [zinc pyrithione (PTO)] and zirconium pyride-2-thione 1 N oxide (zirconium PTO), from shampoos in guinea pig skin was investigated. Application on the skin was rubbed for 10 minutes, after which the animals were killed and the skin excised. Both germicides were observed in the SC, hair follicles, and sebaceous glands. However, while zirconium PTO was detected in the upper epidermis, zinc PTO was not. It was concluded that zinc PTO's solubility in sebum may allow it to become localized in the hair follicle, zirconium PTO is not soluble in sebum, and this causes it to penetrate the dermis. This suggested that the physicochemical properties of the drug influence delivery into the PSU.

Studies Done to Investigate Vehicle Effects on Follicular Deposition
Vehicles Containing Organic Solvents
MacKee et al. (48) were among the first to investigate the nature of vehicle influencing the deposition of iron, bismuth, sulfonamide compounds, and dyes in both guinea pigs and human skin. The penetration was monitored for 5, 30, and 60 minutes. The vehicles investigated were (*i*) ointment bases, which included lanolin, (*ii*) organic solvents, which included PG, (*iii*) aqueous solutions, (*iv*) mixtures of water, surface active agents, and solubilizers, (*v*) mixtures of organic solvents, surface active agents, solubilizers, and coupling agents, (*vi*) mixtures of organic solvents, surface active agents, and solubilizers, (*vii*) mixtures of organic solvents, water, surface active agents, and solubilizers, and (*viii*) mixtures of organic solvents, surface active agents, and water. None of the studies were above one hour. Histological examination of the skin biopsies was done to investigate the distribution of the "active." There was little or no penetration seen by the ointment bases, or by PG, better penetration with the aqueous solutions with the surface-active agent and best penetration with the combination vehicles. The authors first suggested the follicular route as being important for delivery of actives. In this particular study, the time in which it was carried out was very short, and it is possible that due to the viscosity of the oleaginous bases, the effect was not visible until one hour.

Rutherford and Black (47) used autoradiography to study the localization of germicides in guinea pig skin. A trichlorocarbanilide (TCC) compound in soap vehicle resulted in predominantly transepidermal penetration through the skin, whereas follicular deposition occurred with a nonsoap detergent. Application on the skin was rubbed for 10 minutes, after which the animals were killed and the skin excised. They concluded that the vehicle influenced the penetration route.

Montagna (49) studied penetration and local effect of vitamin A on the skin of the guinea pig. The effect of vehicles, linoleic acid, oleic acid, alcohol, and chloroform and a paste made of petrolatum, zinc oxide, and talcum on penetration of the 0.5% vitamin A active was investigated. Specimens of skin were in contact with these agents for 10 minutes, one hour, and two hours and, in some cases, four and eight hours, after which skin biopsies were taken. The penetration was tracked by the fluorescence of vitamin A. It was found that the penetration of the active (dissolved in alcohol and chloroform) into the PSU was seen very quickly (in 10 minutes). In oleic acid, the penetration to the sebaceous ducts took almost two hours. With linoleic acid, it was almost four to eight hours before fluorescence could be detected in the sebaceous ducts. With the paste, it was even slower. The author concluded that the speed of vitamin A depended on the vehicle used. It is possible that viscosity effects played a role in delivery to the PSU.

Estradiol distribution and penetration was penetration of studies in rat skin after topical application, by high-resolution autoradiography (50). Estradiol in different concentrations was applied in vehicles dimethyl sulfoxide (DMSO), ethylene glycol, and sesame oil in vivo. It was observed that the rate of estradiol localization in the sebaceous glands was dependent on the vehicle and dose. At the end of two hours, the rate of deposition of the drug into the sebaceous glands was more with DMSO as compared to ethylene glycol. The concentration of estradiol is found to be the highest in the sebaceous glands at the end of two hours, after which it starts to decrease. It was observed that radioactivity was retained in the sebaceous glands for 24 hours or longer in low but significant amounts in all vehicles, suggesting that a drug depot effect may occur within the PSU.

The importance of the appendageal pathway was also observed in the percutaneous absorption of 5% pyridostigmine bromide (hydrophilic) through various vehicles, which was evaluated using normal and appendage-free scar rat skin in vitro during 72 hours (51). It was found that the drug absorbed was higher from nerol 8% in ethanol, followed by azone 5% in ethanol–PG (90:10), followed by DMSO 10% in ethanol. PG 10% in ethanol inhibited pyridostigmine absorption as compared to the control, which was an ethanolic solution. In all cases, the absorption through the appendage-free skin was lower than the absorption through control skin. The percentage of appendageal pathway was calculated by the formula (1-Scar skin flux/normal skin flux) ∗ 100. It was found that in the first four hours, the appendageal absorption was most for the DMSO solution, followed by the proplylene glycol in ethanol, followed by ethanol, then azone solution, and then the nerol solution. At the end of 72 hours, proplylene glycol in ethanol had the highest percentage of appendageal transport, followed by DMSO, and the others were not that significant. The authors suggested that the enhancers (Nerol, azone) affected the structure of the epidermis, whereas the other solvents (DMSO, ethanol, and PG) were incorporated in the sebum and dragged the drug into the sebaceous ducts. These experiments were done under occlusion. It was concluded that ethanol, DMSO, and PG in ethanol favored the transfollicular pathway, but the other vehicles did not. Since ethanol is primarily a lipid solvent, it can solubilize sebum and allow the migration of the active in the sebaceous glands, explaining why it is primarily transfollicular. It was concluded that by using the right vehicle it was possible to favor the transfollicular pathway and target the drug.

Radiography was used quantitatively by Fabin et al. (39). Two drugs, tetrahydrocannabinol (THC) and oleic acid, were evaluated for delivery into hairless rat skin appendages with different vehicles in vivo. These vehicles included polyethylene glycol 400 (PEG 400), transcutol, and PG:ethanol (7:3). It was found that after two hours, THC had the highest penetration from transcutol and the lowest from PEG 400. After two hours, distribution of THC and oleic acid from transcutol was not very different. At 24 hours, the transcutol system had delivered the maximum THC in the different skin layers and PEG 400 delivered the lowest. At 24 hours more, THC had been delivered in the different layers of the skin compared two hours. It appears that there is a time-dependent effect in the distribution and localization of the drug in the follicle. In the same experiments, when oleic acid was added as a vehicle to the PG:ethanol system, the penetration of THC after two hours was much higher with compared to when oleic acid was not added. It was concluded that the presence of oleic acid in the delivery system applied to the skin could increase penetration to all the strata of the skin, including the appendages.

The percutaneous absorption of RA was monitored in haired and hairless guinea pigs with the expectation that drug penetration would be lower in hairless guinea pigs because they have fewer hair follicles (30). RA was formulated in a 0.025% in an ethanolic gel formulation together with and without polyolprepolymer (PP-2) at 10%. In vitro permeation was monitored on haired and hairless guinea pigs for 24 hours. It was observed from penetration profile that hairless guinea pig skin was more permeable to RA than haired skin despite the lower follicular density. This was attributed to the different strains having different thickness of the SC and different structure rather than greater follicular density. It was suggested that a depot of RA was formed in the hair follicle of the hair guinea pig due to the PP-2. The addition of PP-2 to the formulation decreased the penetration of the drug. It is possible that by addition of a polymer, the viscosity of the formulation increased and hence there was decrease in the penetration.

In summary, from these studies it can be concluded that vehicles that interact with sebum seem to be delivering the drug into the PSU. If sufficient time is given for the experiment to run, then the more viscous materials may help in delivering the drug. Viscosity of the vehicle may play a role in the delivery.

Vehicles Made of Liposomes

Liposomes have become popular in the delivery of drugs to the PSU. In a study done by Li et al. (52), liposomes made of phosphatidylcholine (PC)-containing calcein dye were investigated for delivery to the PSU using mouse skin histocultures by confocal microscopy. It was found that liposomes-entrapped dye became associated with the hair follicles in contrast to free dye without liposomes in 20 minutes. In a similar study (53) done by the same authors, liposome, made of PC, mediated targeted delivery of melanin and into the hair follicles of histocultured mouse skin in 12 hours was reported. This was monitored by fluorescence microscopy. Similarly, DNA encapsulated liposomes were shown to target the hair follicle of histocultured mouse skin in 44 hours, as shown by autoradiography (54). For all these studies, the entrapped drug was separated from the free drug using gel filtration. It could be concluded that it takes longer for larger molecules to be targeted to the PSU.

Liposomes have been used by Lieb et al. (18) for delivery into the PSU of the hamster ear in vitro. Carboxyfluorescein (CF) encapsulated in multilamellar vesicles was prepared. The multilamellar vesicles were made of PC:Cholesterol (CH):Phosphatidylserine (PS) in the ratio of 1:0.5:0.1, respectively. Other vehicles containing the same concentration of CF were also used, which included HEPES buffer (pH = 7.4), 5% PG in HEPES, 10% ethanol in HEPES, and 0.05% sodium lauryl sulfate in HEPES. In vitro diffusion studies for 24 hours, quantitative fluorescence microscopy, and scraping technique was done to investigate the deposition into the follicles. It was found that the most intense fluorescence was observed with the liposomal formulations, whereas the other formulations were not much different from each other.

Liposomes made of PC:CH and PS at a mole ratio of 1.0:0.5:0.1 were made containing 0.5% cimetidine (55) and were evaluated for deposition into the PSU of hamster ears. Nonionic liposomes made of GDL:CH:POE-10 at a weight ratio of 57:15:28 containing cimetidine were also evaluated in vitro and in vivo. These formulations were compared with (*i*) aqueous solution of pH = 8.3, (*ii*) 50%

alcohol solution of pH = 7.4, (*iii*) aqueous solution of pH = 5.5, (*iv*) phospholipid liposome pH = 5.5, (*v*) phospholipid liposome pH = 8.3, (*vi*) nonionic liposome of pH = 5.5, and (*vii*) nonionic liposome of pH = 5.5. At pH = 8.3, the drug is predominately unionized. In vitro deposition studies were done on excised hamster ears when the formulation was applied for 24 hours, after which the cells were dismantled and the distribution of the drug in the various strata of the skin was determined. In the in vitro studies, the aqueous solution showed significant deposition into the sebum-rich PSU of the hamster ear. In the in vivo studies done similarly, after 12 hours, maximum deposition in the PSU was observed by the phospholipid liposome at pH = 5.5 as compared to the 50% alcohol solution at pH = 7.4 and the nonionic liposome at pH = 5.5. Therefore, when bioassay was done and a decrease in size of the sebaceous glands was monitored, it was found that only the hydroalcoholic solution and the nonionic liposomes suppressed the growth of the glands. From these studies it was found that there were discrepancies in the in vivo and the in vitro data, and caution needs to be exercised about the activity of the drug in specific tissue.

Influence of nonionic liposomal composition on topical delivery of alpha interferon (α-IFN) into PSUs was done using the hamster ear model (56). The deposition of hydrophilic protein, α-IFN into the PSU and other strata of the hamster ear 12 hours after topical in vivo application from three nonionic formulations, a phospholipid formulation, and an aqueous control was determined. The deposition of cyclosporin (CsA), a hydrophobic peptide into the PSUs and other strata of the ear using the same liposomal formulations and a hydroalcoholic control, was also done. The nonionic liposome (Non-1) was made with GDL, POE-10, and CH, Non-2 was made with GDS (glyceryl distearate) and POE-10 and CH, and Non-3 was made with POE-10 and CH. The liposomal formulation was made from PC:CH and PS at a mole ratio of 1.0:0.5:0.1. The analysis was done the scintillation counting. The deposition α-IFN of into the PSUs was in the order: Non-1 >> PC > Non-2 > Non-3 = Aq. The deposition of CsA into the PSUs was in the order: Non-1 >> Hydroalcoholic solution > PC > Non-2 = Non-3. It was concluded that in spite of differences in the hydrophobicities of the peptide drugs, Non-1 liposome significantly enhanced the deposition into the PSUs. Hence, the vehicle carrying the drug made a major impact on the deposition irrespective of whether it was hydrophilic or hydrophobic. CsA was, however, deposited to a greater extent than α-IFN. It was explained that since GDL melted at 30°C, it was able to cause some fluidization of the liposomal bilayer and partial release of its contents like POE-10 at body temperature, whereas GDS melted at 54°C and hence did not cause this fluidization.

Expression plasmid DNA for the human interleukin-1 receptor antagonist (IL-1ra) protein was formulated with nonionic:cationic (NC) liposome and PC:cationic (PC) liposomes and applied to auricular skin of hamsters (57). Confocal microscopy identified delivery of the plasmid DNA proximal to the perifollicular cells. In the second part of the study, the skin was treated for three days with the NC liposomes and had statistically significant levels of transgenic IL-1ra present for five days post-treatment. The results indicated that the NC liposomes could deliver expression plasmid DNA to perifollicular cells and mediate transient transfection in vivo. The control formulations were made with empty niosomes, that is, no DNA, and were done with infinite dosing. The control used should have been empty niosomes with the plasmid DNA outside it and would have indicated if drug or niosome had the property of reaching the follicle.

The sebaceous gland deposition of isotretinoin after topical application on human facial skin in vitro was measured 16 hours after application by taking skin biopsies and separation of the skin compartments (58). Ethanolic gel was the control and was compared with a liposomal formulation, Natipide II (made of PC) formulation, and a mixed micelle formulation. All the experiments were performed with skin from the periauricular skin of women undergoing plastic surgery. Autoradiography and fluorescence microscopy elucidated the penetration pathway of the active. The results showed that neither the liposomes nor the mixed micellar system revealed an improved sebaceous gland deposition of isotretenoin as compared with the ethanolic gel.

The significance of the sebaceous gland pathway in the cutaneous permeation of an antiandrogen, RU58841 in liposomes, was studied with normal and scar skin in hairless rat (59). RU 58841 was made into a liposomal formulation containing lipoid E 100-35 and α-tocopherol in a phosphate buffer of pH = 7, whereas the control solution was made of ethanol PG:water (40:10:50 w/w). The in vitro cutaneous permeation studies were carried out for 24 hours. The cumulative percentage of RU 58841 absorbed was three-fold higher through normal skin after 24 hours, whereas that of the liposomes was four-fold higher through normal skin as compared to scar skin. However, the permeation of the ethanolic solution was much higher through normal skin as compared to the liposomal formulation through the skin. In in vivo studies carried out for 24 hours, it was found that the epidermis and dermis of normal skin contained more amounts of the active than the scar tissue. An autoradiography showed that with the ethanolic solution, the drug was mainly localized in the SC/epidermis and with the liposomes it was localized in the sebaceous glands. The overall permeation was, however, higher through the normal skin for the ethanolic solutions as compared to the liposomal solutions. When the correction for targeting was applied, liposomes targeted better than the ethanolic solution.

Mechanism of Action of Liposomes
Weiner et al. (60) have hypothesized the use of liposomes in the following way. For hydrophobic drugs, a major fraction of the added drug would be encapsulated or intercalated within the bilayers of the liposomes. The transfer of drug from the lipid bilayers into the skin could occur as long as the bilayers were in liquid crystalline state. If the liquid crystalline phase is altered to the gel state, transport of the drug would cease or be negligibly low. Dehydration of liposomal suspensions has been shown to reduce transitions from the liquid crystalline phase to the gel state. If, however, dehydration was complete and the bilayers were transformed from the liquid crystalline state to a gel state, then the transfer of the drug would cease. If dehydration to an equilibrium stage occurs, wherein a constant amount of water is always retained, then the transport of the drug is steady and continuous. A second consequence of dehydration involves the formation of a strong adhesive patch of the liposomal bilayers on the skin. The formation of such patches maximizes the intimacy of contact between the drug-laden bilayers and the skin.

For hydrophilic drugs, too, a similar mode of action is explained. Liposomal systems that undergo total dehydration, drug transport ceases, as the drug is no longer in a dissolved state. For liposomal systems that retain a constant amount of water within the bilayers following dehydration to an equilibrium, drug transport would continue over extended periods. A major consequence of dehydration for hydrophilic drugs involves the enhancement or enrichment of drug concentration in the aqueous phase of the bilayers, leading to an enhancement in flux of drug into and across skin. When a follicular pathway is present, upon dehydration, the liposomal bilayers can partition and can pack into the follicular ducts containing the lipids. The filling of the follicular openings with the liposomal bilayers not only results in entrapped drugs being carried into the follicles, but also allows partitioning of free drugs into the bilayer matrix within the follicles.

Vehicles Made of Lipid Melts

In these studies, the melted form of the lipid components, which were used to make the niosomes (namely, GDL:CH:POE-10), were evaluated as a vehicle for the transport of CsA and other agents into and through hairless mouse skin (58,60,61). The experiments were carried out under nonoccluded conditions. At predetermined times of two, four, eight and 24 hours, the diffusion setup was dismantled and the drug in various strata of the skin determined using stripping and digesting of the skin using scintillation counting. The profiles of the extent and uptake of CsA from the lipid melt formulations are similar to those of the liposomal formulations of the same compositions. In these same experiments, the ratio of GDL to POE-10 was varied. In all these formulation, CH was kept at a constant concentration of 15% and GDL to POE-10 ratios examined were 0:85, 15:70, 45:40, and 57:28. It was found that the 45:40 lipid melt was more effective in delivery of the active into and through the mouse skin. The authors explained that that particular combination of lipid melt had the lowest melting point ($\sim$23°C) and that was responsible for the better uptake. Nevertheless, the remaining melts (except 0% GDL) were also liquids at body temperature and the melting point does not seem to explain the point enough. The microautoradiographs and light microscope images also confirm these results. It was thus concluded that the similarity of the kinetic profiles for CsA transport into and across living skin strata of hairless mice from the liposomal and lipid melt formulations along with the microautoradiographic evidence for localization within the PSUs implied that transport of CsA into the highly hydrophilic viable skin strata occurs mainly via the follicular route.

Similar studies were also done on the delivery of hydrocortisone (hydrophobic) and mannitol (hydrophilic) through the same lipid-based formulations in and through hairless mouse skin in vitro (62). The results after 24 hours indicated that the extent of hydrocortisone uptake rose with increasing the GDL to POE-10 ratio, whereas for mannitol, the uptake was the opposite decreasing with increase in this ratio in liposomes. Lipid melt formulations for mannitol were not made because it is a hydrophilic drug and niosomes of the above compositions along with water were made. From the autoradiographic studies, it was reported that the nonionic lipid-based formulations were predominantly transfollicular. It was also suggested that a hydrophilic molecule like mannitol could not partition into the lipid environment of the sebum-filled follicles or into and across the SC and was transported mainly via the transepidermal route. This suggested that the two macromolecules were transported through the skin via two different pathways. It was thus was possible to tailor formulations for specific and targeted delivery across a certain route.

Studies Done on Microbeads: Size Effects on Follicular Deposition

Fluorescent polystyrene (16) microbeads of different sizes were made in aqueous medium and Miglyol® (hydrophobic vehicle) as suspensions and were applied on live female hairless rat's back and freshly excised human skin. Suspensions were applied with massaging for five minutes. The experiment was carried on for 15 minutes, after which skin biopsy was done and observed under a fluorescent microscope. It was found that the best follicular penetration was observed with the most lipophilic vehicle Miglyol®. The 9- to 10-μm beads concentrated at the opening of the follicles, but did not penetrate; however, the 7-μm beads were frequently observed deep down in the follicular canal, but rarely penetrated the SC. The smallest beads <3 μm penetrated the follicles well, but were also observed in the superficial layers of the SC.

In the same paper, poly β-alanine beads labeled with dansyl chloride were formulated in an aqueous gel, hydroalcoholic gel, and silicone oil. The suspensions were applied to the rat's back and human skin. Here too, the best results were observed with the most lipophilic vehicle (silicone oil). The 5 μm showed selectivity for the follicular canal.

The site-specific delivery of adalapene to the hair follicles was attempted both in vivo and in vitro (63). The drug was loaded in 50:50 poly (DL-lactic–coglycolic acid). Different sizes (1, 5, and 20 μm) of the microspheres were evaluated in vitro by investigating cutaneous penetration of the microspheres through human skin and the female hairless rat skin. The permeation was allowed to proceed for 35 and 300 minutes, after which the cells were dismantled and the skin samples were frozen and then evaluated by fluorescence microscopy. It was found that the 1-μm microspheres were randomly distributed into the SC and hair follicles. The 20-μm microparticles did not penetrate the skin and remained on the surface where the 5 μm were found in the hair follicles. In addition, a time-dependent effect was seen in this evaluation where greater penetration was observed after 300 minutes than after 35 minutes.

RECENT ADVANCES IN THE DELIVERY OF TOPICAL ANTI-ACNE MEDICATIONS

This section reviews the most recent research advances in technology being marketed or being developed to deliver acne treatment medications to the target lesions. Two types of technologies are discussed. One is a recent technological approach based on lipid melts and particulates that target drugs to the PSU. Second is controlled release technology that delivers the drug into the PSU more slowly over time, and thereby provides milder topical treatment systems. These are based on the fundamental research findings reviewed in the last section and have been applied specifically to the delivery of antiacne drugs to the target site.

Advances in Use of Lipid Melts to Deliver Anti-acne Drugs to the Pilosebaceous Unit

The present authors, Rhein et al. (64), have investigated further the use of lipid melts to deliver SA to the PSU. It is hypothesized that vehicles that are miscible with sebum or a part of it will be effective in preferentially delivering drugs to the sebaceous glands. In a previous chapter, we have characterized model sebum based on its thermal behavior (Chapter 15) and identified four melting transitions by differential scanning calorimetry corresponding to four different species: Mp-1 and Mp-2 are transitions at $-15°C$ and $-20°C$ for the unsaturated triglycerides/fatty acids (overlapped) and the wax esters and Mp-3 and Mp-4 at $+40°C$ and $+55°C$ are for saturated triglycerides/fatty acids (overlapped) and wax esters, respectively. We refer to that chapter for detailing this information. In that chapter, we have also identified vehicles that are miscible with sebum because they lower the melting point of the solid components (saturated triglycerides/fatty acids and wax esters, Mp-3 and Mp-4), and thereby enhance their dissolution by the liquid components in sebum. In this chapter, we have investigated the follicular delivery of SA using some of those vehicles; the hamster ear model discussed earlier was used to quantify delivery of SA.

The strategy of using lipid melts to deliver drugs to the PSU can be achieved in two different ways. For hydrophobic drugs, lipid melts (combination of vehicle and sebum) can "soften" if not liquefy the solid components of sebum and the drug will essentially be solubilized in the sebum along with the vehicle; the drug is thus cotransported into the sebum along with the vehicle. For hydrophilic drugs, the vehicle serves a different function which is to facilitate partitioning of the drug from the vehicle into the sebum. We have therefore characterized two types of vehicles for effectiveness at delivering drugs, in particular SA into the PSU. These are fatty vehicles and polar vehicles, and are shown in Table 3 along with the percentage of delivery of SA from the vehicle into the sebaceous follicle and also the solubility of SA in the vehicle.

Comparing the solubility of SA in the vehicle and the delivery into the sebaceous glands, it was found that for fatty vehicles as the solubility of SA increased in the vehicles, more drug was delivered into the sebaceous glands (Table 3). For the polar vehicles, however, the trend was the opposite, that is, as solubility increased, delivery to the sebaceous gland went down (Table 3). This led to the conclusion that the mechanism of the drug delivery into the follicle was different for the two types of vehicles. It appears that the fatty vehicles are miscible with sebum and hence the increase in solubility leads to higher follicular delivery, as SA is cotransported with the vehicle into the sebum. In the case of the polar vehicles, the decrease in follicular delivery with increase in solubility leads us to believe that it is a partitioning effect, that is, the more soluble in the polar vehicle the less likely SA is to partition into the sebum.

TABLE 3 Solubility of Salicylic Acid in Fatty and Polar Vehicles and Extent of Delivery to Hamster Sebaceous Glands

Vehicle	Applied SA dose in sebaceous gland (% of applied dose)	Solubility of SA in vehicle (mg/mL)
Fatty vehicles		
IPM	28	47
Glycerid acid, MSO	24	43
OA	17	41
L	14	40
Polar vehicles		
G	17	15
MP	9.7	210
PG	10	280
B	10	300
DMI	6.8	380
Diethylene glycol monoethyl ether (T)	8	465

Abbreviations: B, butanediol; DMI, dimethyl isosorbide; G, glycerin; IPM, isopropyl myristate; L, labrafil M 2125CS; MP, MP diol; MSO, maleated soyabean oil; OA, oleic acid; PG, propylene glycol; SA, salicylic acid; T, transcutol.
Source: From Ref. 64.

We then correlated the SA delivery with the results of DSC studies. The DSC of a model sebum showed four major transitions: Mp-1, Mp-2, Mp-3, and Mp-4. Of the four melting transitions in sebum described earlier, Mp-3 and Mp-4, transitions for the solid part of sebum occurred between 40°C and 55°C; these are the most meaningful transitions of the saturated and, therefore, solid species (saturated-fatty acid, triglycerides, and wax esters) that exist at the physiological temperature of skin. This solid part offers the challenge for drug delivery and dissolution of solid sebum in the follicle. The effect of the vehicles on Mp-3 and Mp-4 has been tabulated in Table 4. The delta values in the table are the difference between the transition of the model sebum and the model sebum plus vehicle. It was found that as the percent of drug delivered into the sebaceous glands increased as ΔMp-3 increased for fatty vehicles (Fig. 3). ΔMp-3 is the difference in the Mp-3 transition temperature of model sebum and the Mp-3 transition temperature of the model sebum treated with fatty vehicle. It is a measure of the effect of the vehicle on the Mp-3 fraction of model sebum and a higher number indicates higher miscibility of the vehicle with that fraction of sebum. This means that the higher the miscibility of the fatty vehicle with the Mp-3 fraction of sebum, the higher is the follicular deposition of SA using the vehicle.

Similarly for the polar vehicles as the effect on Mp-4 increases, the percent of drug delivered in the sebaceous glands decreases (Fig. 4). ΔMp-4 is referred to as the difference in the Mp-4 transition temperature of model sebum and the Mp-4 transition temperature of the model sebum and polar vehicle. ΔMp-4 is a measure of the effect of the vehicle on the Mp-4 fraction of model sebum and a higher number indicates higher miscibility of the vehicle with that fraction of sebum. These results can be explained by the fact that sebum is made up of nonpolar components. If a vehicle does not interact with sebum (as is observed from its noneffect on Mp-4), it would mean that it is polar in nature and there would be a pronounced partitioning effect. The more soluble the drug is in the polar vehicle the less likely it is to penetrate into the sebaceous gland. Glycerine is a good

TABLE 4 Effect of Polar and Nonpolar Vehicles on the Transition Temperatures of Model Sebum

Vehicle	Mp-4 (°C)	Mp-3 (°C)	ΔMp-3[a] (°C)	ΔMp-4[a] (°C)
Model sebum (control)	48.83 (0.22)	39.74 (0.43)	—	—
Fatty vehicles				
MSO	45.29 (0.73)	37.42 (0.42)	2.32	3.54
IPM	45.88 (0.31)	36.51 (0.62)	3.23	2.95
OA	46.22 (0.27)	38.12 (0.55)	1.62	2.61
L	46.36 (0.27)	38.37 (0.07)	1.37	2.47
Polar vehicles				
G	49.11 (0.29)	39.81 (0.17)	−0.07	−0.28
B	47.02 (0.022)	40.41 (0.18)	−0.67	1.81
MP	46.61(0.45)	39.46 (0.43)	0.28	2.22
PG	Not observed	38.92 (0.18)	0.82	—
DMI	41.97 (0.45)	37.67 (0.27)	2.07	6.86
T	43.86 (0.22)	38.97 (0.12)	0.77	4.97

[a]Delta values are the differences between the transition of the model sebum and the model sebum containing the vehicle.

Abbreviations: B, butanediol; DMI, dimethyl isosorbide; G, glycerin; IPM, isopropyl myristate; L, labrafil M 2125CS; MP, MP diol; MSO, maleated soyabean oil; OA, oleic acid; PG, propylene glycol; T, transcutol.

Source: From Ref. 64.

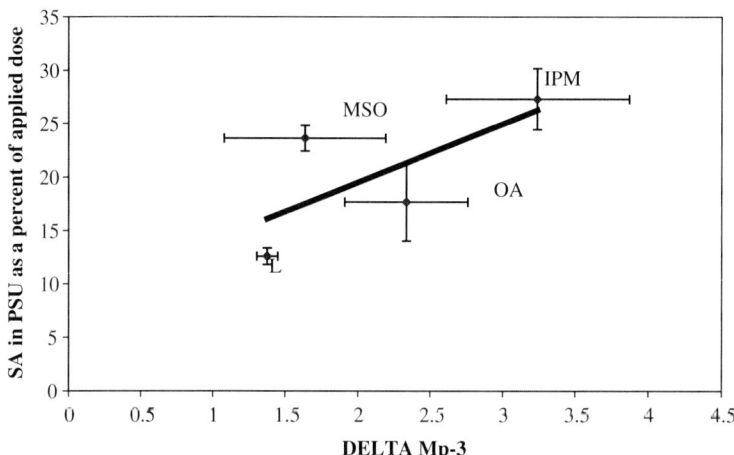

FIGURE 3 Correlation of the percent of salicylic acid in sebaceous glands to ΔMp-3 for fatty vehicles. *Note*: ΔMp-3 is designated Delta Mp-3. *x*-axis error bars indicate the standard error of the mean of three experiments and *y*-axis error bars indicate the standard error of the mean of six experiments. *Abbreviations*: IPM, isopropyl myristate; MSO, maleated soybean oil; OA, oleic acid. *Source*: From Ref. 64.

example; SA is delivered to sebaceous gland better compared to the other polar vehicles yet glycerine does not miscible with Mp-3 or Mp-4. SA therefore partitions better into the gland from glycerine. We would, however, anticipate that a more hydrophilic drug will present great difficulty partitioning from glycerine to the

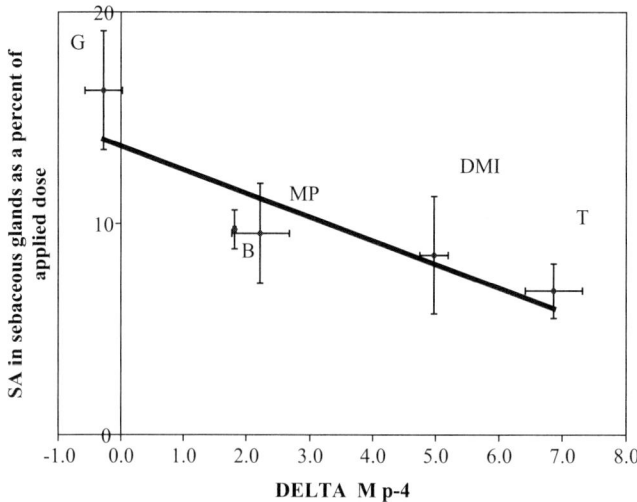

FIGURE 4 Correlation of the percent of salicylic acid in sebaceous glands to ΔMp-4 for fatty vehicles. *Note*: ΔMp-4 is designated Delta Mp-4. *x*-axis error bars indicate the standard error of the mean of three experiments and *y*-axis error bars indicate the standard error of the mean of six experiments. *Abbreviations*: B, butanediol; DMI, dimethyl isosorbide; G, glycerin; MP, MP diol; SA, salicylic acid; T, transcutol. *Source*: From Ref. 64.

gland. These results further strengthen our theory of the miscibility of the fatty vehicles and the partitioning of the polar vehicles. Future research will investigate challenges of delivery of other drugs of varying hydrophilicity.

Delivery of Adapalene to the Pilosebaceous Unit
Using Polymeric Microspheres

A classic execution of a targeted delivery system for the anti-acne medication, adapalene, was done by Galderma Researchers (63,65–68). Adapalene is the chemically stable form of naphthoic acid. It binds in skin to the RA receptor subtypes RAR gamma in the epidermis and RAR beta in the dermal fibroblasts activating differentiation specific genes and is a fast-acting anti-acne treatment. Researchers there have investigated the use of particulate microspheres to deliver this anti-acne medications to the PSU. The drug is entrapped inside the microspheres. Shroot et al. (65) and Allec et al. (66) have discovered that delivery of the microspheres to the PSU depends on the size of the sphere. The composition of the microspheres is 50:50 poly(DL-lactic–coglycolic acid) and they are impregnated with adapalene using the solvent evaporation technique. Depending on the stir rate and emulsification technique, spheres of different diameter can be formulated, 1, 5, and 20 μm with corresponding doses of adapalene of 0.01%, 0.05%, and 0.1%.

The hairless mouse model along with full thickness human skin described earlier was used to assess site of penetration of the microspheres (63). The spheres were applied topically and the location of the spheres was determined using fluorescence microscopy and scanning electron microscopy. What was discovered was that spheres of 5 μm primarily were localized within the PSU and penetration depth was time-dependent. On the other hand, larger spheres, >10 μm, remained on the skin surface and smaller spheres, <3 μm, penetrated both the PSU and the epidermis.

One could naively argue that smaller spheres would more effectively treat acne because they penetrate both the PSU and the epidermal surface since PSUs occupy only 0.1% of the epidermal surface. However, acne is a disease of the PSU and further studies showed that formulations of microspheres that target penetration to the PSU provide similar efficacy without irritation, a known side effect of other anti-acne medications such as tretinoin (68). This suggests that penetration through the epidermis rather than the PSU tends to deliver drugs into and through the living tissue and into the systemic circulation more readily, thus causing irritation. These results also suggest that the target site for optimal treatment of the disease is the PSU where acne develops. However, more research is needed to confirm these findings.

Controlled Release Systems

Various controlled release formulations are now on the market that are designed to deliver the acne medication into the skin more slowly to avoid an initial burst during the first few hours. Such an initial burst of drug and/or enhancers can lead to irritation that is frequently observed with acne medications and is the subject of numerous consumer complaints in the marketplace. However it is not known whether these technologies preferentially deliver the medicament to the PSU. Bertek and GlaxoSmithKline employ a polyurethane polymer technology— PP-2 that alters the activity of the free drug in the respective formulations. Bertek markets such a technology with RA and GlaxoSmithKline markets a similar technology with SA. Rhein et al. (69) published studies showing the benefit of the controlled release PP-2 in controlling delivery of SA with regard to irritation reduction; however, they failed to demonstrate the benefit of this technology to the resolution of acne. Additionally, while studies were done to show targeted delivery to the cutaneous epidermis, no penetration experiments were done on the PSU versus epidermis.

CONCLUSIONS AND FUTURE DIRECTIONS

Numerous methods have been reviewed that enable the researcher to study targeted delivery of acne medications and enhancers to the PSU. The current status of drug delivery to the PSU for the potential treatment of acne has been summarized in this chapter. Techniques to deliver anti-acne drugs have been summarized, along with methods to assess transfollicular delivery. What is eminently clear is that the biochemistry and physiology of the PSU is not well-understood fundamentally and the pathogenesis of acne as it progresses within the PSU is also not well-understood. It appears to be a chance occurrence that a delivery vehicle is formulated that targets delivery of anti-acne medications to the PSU with some fundamental learning emerging form it. The knowledge is thus very much in the rudimentary stages, given that the structure of sebum then manipulating the phase behavior by the appropriate chemical enhancers such as liposomes and fluidizing agents is feasible. It seems that by knowing the chemical structure of the active, that is, hydrophobic or hydrophilic in nature among other things, topical delivery vehicles can be developed that potentiate penetration into the PSU.

Future strategies will likely embrace new delivery devices to target the PSUs (71). Some of these are microneedle-based delivery systems, microfluid devices, sonophoresis, iontophoresis, and even magnetic modulation. The future of such techniques should yield interesting developments in the treatment of acne via the PSU. The continuing issue is the unavailability of an appropriate in vitro model. Directions of future developments have been review by Meiden et al. (72). A new in vitro skin sandwich model that mimics transfollicular penetration is discussed. Confocal laser scanning microscopy is the most focused direction as a noninvasive methodology for deriving high resolution images of the PSU the principal advantages is its capacity for in vivo application, good time-resolution and the ability to visualize at multiple depths parallel to the sample surface without the need for mechanical sectioning (73). The combination use with confocal Raman spectroscopy is another promising tool for analyzing follicular drug delivery. New developments in innovative liposomes and microspheres continue to be on the forefront (74,75). The porcine ear is emerging as an in vitro model that may better mimic human skin (76). Latest techniques being studied for follicular delivery is to remove the sebum plug and then apply treatment which greatly potentiates delivery to the PSU (74). The key decision of the researcher is whether they are targeting the PSU or is the intent transfollicular penetration. This will dictate the strategy to a large extent and the delivery systems required. The more formidable question is what is the appropriate pharmacology that identifies more effective actives targeting the appropriate site within the PSU? The delivery aspects will be tailored to that active depending on its chemical nature and the target site. Perhaps some of these questions are also answered in other chapters in this book.

REFERENCES

1. Pagnoni A, Kligman AM, Gammal S, Stoudemayer T. Determination of density of follicles on various regions of the face by cyanoacrylate biopsy: correlation with sebum output. Br J Dermatol 1994; 131:862–865.
2. Gupchup GV, Zatz JL. Targeted delivery to pilosebaceous structure. Cosmet Toileteres 1997; 112:79–87.
3. Braun-Falco O, Plewig G, Wolff HH, Winkelmann RK. Diseases of sebaceous follicles. In: Braun-Falco O, Plewig G, Wolff HH, Winkelmann RK, eds. Dermatology. Berlin: Springer-Verlag, 1991:716–743.
4. Thody AJ, Shuster S. Control and function of sebaceous glands. Physiol Rev 1989; 69(2):383–416.
5. Odland GF. Structure of the skin. In: Goldsmith LA, ed. Biochemistry and Physiology of the Skin. Oxford: Oxford University Press, 1985:3–63.
6. Osborne DW, Hatzenbuhler DA. Influence of skin surface lipids on topical formulations. In: Osborne DW, Amann AH, eds. Topical Drug Delivery Formulations. New York: Marcel Dekker, Inc., 1990:69–86.
7. Gollnick H. Current concepts in the pathogenesis of acne. Drugs 2003; 63(15):1579–1596.
8. Freinkel RK, Strauss JS, Yip SY. Effect of tetracycline on the composition of sebum in acne vulgaris. N Engl J Med 1965; 273(16):850–854.
9. Strauss JS, Pochi PE. Intracutaneous injection of sebum and comedones. Arch Dermatol 1965; 92:443–456.
10. Kligman AM, Katz AG. Pathogenesis of acne vulgaris I. comedogenic properties of human sebum in external ear canal of the rabbit. Archiv Dermatol 1968; 98(1):53–57.
11. Kligman AM. Pathogenesis of acne vulgaris II histopathology of comedones induced in the rabbit ear by human Sebum. Archiv Dermatol 1968; 98:58–66.
12. Kanaar K. Follicular-keratogenic properties of fatty acids in the external ear canal of the rabbit. Dermatologica 1971; 142:14–22.
13. Strauss JS. Sebaceous gland, acne and related disorders-an epilogue. Dermatology 1998; 196:182–184.
14. Schaefer H, Redelmeie TE. Biological factors influencing percutaneous absorption. Principles of Percutaneous Absorption. New York: Karager, 1996:189–212.
15. Lauer AC, Ramachandran C, Lieb LM, Niemiec S, Weiner ND. Targeted delivery to the pilosebaceous unit via liposomes. Adv Drug Deliv Rev 1996; 18:311–324.
16. Schaefer H, Watts F, Brod J, Illel B. Follicular penetration. In: Scott RC, Guy RH, Hadgraft J eds. Prediction of Percutaneous Penetration: Methods, Measurements and Modeling. London: IBC Technical Services, 1990:163–173.
17. Shyamla JC. Follicular delivery of erythromycin from nonionic liposomes and emulsion. Doctoral Dissertation, 1997.
18. Lieb L, Ramachandran C, Egbaria E, Weiner N. Topical delivery enhancement with multilamellar liposomes into pilosebaceous units: I In vitro evaluation using flouresent techniques with the hamster ear model. J Invest Dermatol 1992; 99(3):108–113.
19. Lauer AC, Lieb LM, Ramachandran C, Flynn GL, Weiner ND. Transfollicular drug delivery. Pharm Res 1995; 12(2):179–186.
20. Motwani M, Rhein L, Zatz J. Influence of vehicles on the phase transitions of model sebum. J Cosmet Sci 2002; 53:35–42.
21. Kligman LH, Kwong T. An improved rabbit ear model for assessing comedogenic substances. Br J Dermatol 1979; 100:699–702.
22. Plewig G. Models to study follicular diseases. In: Plewig G, ed. Skin Models to Study Function of the Disease of the Skin. Berlin: Springer Verlag, 1986:13–23.
23. Kligman LH, Kligman AM. The effect on rhino mouse skin of agents which influence keratinization and exfoliation. J Invest Dermatol 1979; 73:354–358.
24. Uno K, Kurata K. Chemical agents and peptides affect hair growth. J Invest Dermatol 1993; 101(1):143S–147S.
25. Matias JR, Orentreich N. The hamster ear sebaceous glands I examination of regional variation by stripped skin planimetry. J Invest Dermatol 1983; 81:43–46.
26. Plewig G, Luderschmidt C. Hamster ear model for sebaceous glands. J Invest Dermatol 1977; 68:171–176.

27. Illel B, Schaefer H, Wepierre J, Doucet O. Follicles play an important role in percutaneous absorption. J Pharm Sci 1991; 80(5):424–427.
28. Waranuch N, Ramachandran C, Weiner ND. Controlled topical delivery of cyclosporin A from nonionic liposomal formulations: mechanistic aspects. J Liposome Res 1998; 8(2):225–238.
29. Wahlberg JE. Transepidermal or transfollicular absorption? Acta Derm Venereol 1968; 48:336–344.
30. Hisoire G, Bucks D. An unexpected finding in percutaneous absorption observed between hairy and hairless guinea pig skin. J Pharm Sci 1997; 86(3):398–400.
31. Marks R, Dawber RPR. Skin surface biopsy: an improved technique for the examination of the horny layer. Br J Dermatol 1971; 84:117–123.
32. Lavker RM, Leyden JJ, MCGinley KJ. The relationship between bacteria and the abnormal follicular keratinization in acne vulgaris. J Invest Dermatol 1981; 77:253–255.
33. Mills OH, Kligman AM. Is sulfur helpful or harmful in acne vulgaris? Br J Dermatol 1972; 86:620–627.
34. Mills OH, Berger RS, Cardin CW, Erekuff GG, Smiles KA. Analysis of salicylic acid levels in the sebaceous follicles. Poster Presented at the Annual Meeting of the Society of Investigative Dermatology, 1995.
35. Bojar RA, Cutcliffe AG, Graupe K, Cunliffe WJ, Holland KT. Follicular concentrations of azelaic acid after a single topical application. Br J Dermatol 1993; 129:399–402.
36. Tschan T, Steffen H, Supersaxo A. Sebaceous gland deposition of isotretinoin after topical application: an *in vitro* study using human facial skin. Skin Pharmacol 1997; 10:135–143.
37. Lieb LM. Formulation factors affecting follicular (pilosebaceous route) drug delivery as evaluated with hamster ear model. College of Pharmacy, University of Michigan, Doctoral Dissertation, 1994.
38. Illel B, Schaefer H. Transfollicular percutaneous absorption: skin model for quantitative studies. Acta Derm Venereol (Stockh) 1988; 68:427–430.
39. Touitou E, Fabin B. Localization of lipophilic molecules penetrating rat skin *in vivo* by quantitative autoradiography. Int J Pharm 1991; 74:59–65.
40. Touitou E, Meidan VM, Horwitz E. Methods for quantitative determination of drug localized in the skin. J Control Release 1998; 567–572.
41. Hueber F, Wepierre J, Schaefer H. Role of transepidermal and transfollicular routes in percutaneous absorption of hydrocortisone and testosterone: *in vivo* study in the hairless rat. Skin Pharmacol 1992; 5:99–107.
42. Scheuplin RJ. Mechanism of percuatneous Absorption II. Transient diffusion and the relative importance of various routes of skin penetration. J Invest Dermatol 1967; 48(1):79–88.
43. Scheuplin RJ, Blank IH, Brauner GI, MacFarlane DJ. Percutaneous absorption of steroids. J Invest Dermatol 1969; 52(1):63–70.
44. Keister JC, Kasting KB. The use of transient diffusion to investigate transport pathways through the skin. J Control Release 1986; 4:111–117.
45. Kao J, Hall J, Helman G. *In vitro* percutaneous absorption in mouse skin: influence of skin appendages. Toxicol Appl Pharmacol 1988; 94:93–103.
46. Nicolau G, Baughman RA, Tonelli A, McWilliams W, Schiltz J, Yacobi A. Deposition of viprostol in the skin following topical administration to laboratory animals. Xenobiotica 1987; 17(9):1113–1120.
47. Rutherford T, Black JG. The use of autoradiography to study the localization of germicides in skin. Br J Dermatol 1954; 81(suppl 4):75–87.
48. MacKee MG, Sulzberger MB, Herrmann F, Baer RL. Histological studies on percutaneous penetration with special reference to the effect of vehicles. J Invest Dermatol 1945; 6:43–61.
49. Montagna W. Penetration and local effect of vitamin A on the skin of the guinea pig. Proc Soc Exp Biol Med 1969; 86:668–672.
50. Bidmon HJ, Pitts JD, Solomon HF, Bondi JV, Stumpf WE. Estradiol distribution and penetration in rat skin after topical application, studied by high resolution autoradiography. Histochemistry 1990; 95:43–54.

51. Bamba FL, Wepierre J. Role of appendageal pathway in the percutaneous absorption of pyridostigmine bromide in various vehicles. Eur J Drug Metab Pharmacokinet 1993; 18(4):349–353.
52. Li L, Margolis LB, Lishko VK, Hoffman RM. Product-delivering liposomes specifically target hair follicles in histocultured intact skin. In Vitro Cell Dev Biol 1992; 28A:679–681.
53. Li L, Lishko VK, Hoffman RM. Liposomes can specifically target entrapped melanin to hair follicles in histocultured skin. In Vitro Cell Dev Biol 1993; 29A:192–194.
54. Li L, Lishko VK, Hoffman RM. Liposome targeting of high molecular weight DNA to the hair follicles of histocultured skin:a model for gene therapy of the hair growth process. In Vitro Cell Dev Biol 1993; 29A:258–260.
55. Lieb LM, Flynn GL, Weiner ND. Follicular (pilosebaceous unit) deposition and pharma-cological behavior of cimetidine as a function of formulation. Pharm Res 1994; 11(10):1414–1423.
56. Niemiec S, Ramachandran C, Weiner ND. Influence of nonionic liposomal composition on topical delivery of peptide drugs into pilosebaceous units: an *in vivo* study using the hamster ear model. Pharm Res 1995; 12(8):1184–1188.
57. Niemiec S, Latta JM, Ramachandran C, Weiner ND. Perifollicular transgenic expression of human interleukin-1 receptor antagonist protein following topical application of novel liposome-plasmid DNA formulations *in vivo*. J Pharm Sci 1997; 86(6):701–708.
58. Tschan T, Steffen H, Supersaxo A. Sebaceous gland deposition of isotretinoin after topical application: an *in vitro* study using human facial skin. Skin Pharmacol 1997; 10:135–143.
59. Bernard E, Dubois J-L, Wepierre J. Importance of sebaceous glands in cutaneous penetration of an antiandrogen: target effect of liposomes. J Pharm Sci 1997; 86(5): 573–578.
60. Weiner ND, Ramachandran C, Lieb LM, Egbaria K. Deposition of liposomally associated substances in the skin strata and the pilosebaceous structures. J Pharm Sci 1994; 83(9):1196–1199.
61. Weiner ND. Targeted delivery of macromolecules via liposomes. Int J Pharm 1998; 162:29–38.
62. Waranuch N, Ramachandran C, Weiner ND. Controlled topical delivery of hydrocorti-sone and mannitol via select pathway. J Liposome Res 1999; 9(1):139–153.
63. Rolland A, Wagner N, Chatelus A, Shroot B, Schaefer H. Site specific drug delivery to the pilosebaceous structures using polymeric microspheres. Pharm Res 1993; 10(12):1738–1744.
64. Rhein L, Motwani M, Zatz J. Deposition of salicylic acid into hamster sebaceous glands. J Cosmet Sci 2004; 55(6):519–531.
65. Shroot B, Michel S, Allec J, Chatelus A, Wagner N. A new concept off drug delivery for acne. Dermatology 1998; 196:165–170.
66. Allec J, Chatelus A, Wagner N. Skin distribution and pharmaceutical aspects of adapa-lene. J Am Acad Dermatol 1997; 36S:119–125.
67. Rolland A, Wagner N, Chatelus A, Shroot B, Schaefer H. Site specific drug delivery to pilosebaceous structures using polymeric microspheres. Pharm Res 1993; 10:1738–1744.
68. Waugh J, Scott IJ. Adapalene: a review of its use in the treatment of acne vulgaris. Drugs 2004; 64:1465–1478.
69. Rhein L, Chaudhuri B, Jivani N. Targeted delivery of salicylic acid to from acne treat-ment products into and through the skin: role of solution and ingredient properties and relationships to irritation. J Cosmet Sci 2004; 55:65–80.
70. Montagna W, Kligman A, Carlisle K. Atlas of Normal Human Skin, Plate 107. New York, NY: Springer-Verlag, 1992:226.
71. Willie JJ. Skind delivery systems: transdermals, dermatologicals, and cosmetic actives. In: Willie J, ed. Blackwell Publishing Limited, 2006.
72. Meidan VM, Michael C, Bonner MC, Michniak BB. Transfollicular drug delivery—is it a reality. Intl J Pharmaceutics 2005; 306(1–2):1–14.
73. R. Alvarez-Román RA, Naik A, Kalia YN, Fessi H, Guy RH. Visualization of skin penetration using confocal laser scanning microscopy. Eur J Pharmaceutics and Bio-pharmaceutics 2004; 58(2):301–316.

74. Toll R, Jacobi U, Richter H, Lademann J, Schaefer H, Blume-Peytavi U. Penetration profile of microspheres in follicular targeting of terminal hair follicles. J Invest Dermatol 2004; 123(1):168–176.
75. Jung S, Otberg N, Thiede G, et al. Innovative liposomes as a transfollicular drug delivery system: penetration into porcine hair follicles. J Invest Dermatol 2006; 128(8):1728–1732.
76. Jacobi U, Kaiser M, Toll R, et al. Porcine ear skin: an in vitro model for human skin. Skin Res Technol 2007; 13(1):19–24.

Topical Therapy and Formulation Principles

Steve Boothroyd
Department of Research and Development, Reckitt Benckiser PLC, Hull, U.K.

INTRODUCTION

Other chapters have discussed the biology and medical consequences of acne, and with it the types of actives required to be delivered to resolve them. This chapter focuses on the actives and the delivery vehicle used, and considers the myriad types of formulation available.

This is not intended to be a truly comprehensive and in-depth study, since space does not permit it. Rather, it is designed to inform and, hopefully, excite interest and provide a starting platform for further investigation and experimentation. Some guideline formulations will be given, but there are other sources that offer these in greater number. Suppliers of raw materials are always valuable sources of starting formulary, some of which may already have undergone some performance testing. As with all published formulae, the principle of caveat emptor applies, and the formulator should always confirm that the product performs to the required standards.

The sections within this chapter are intended to form the basis of the information that needs to be generated in developing the product. Although this may not seem relevant in this context, the risks associated with the formulation are such that a wide range of proof should be established. Some of this is prescribed in legislation, and the requirements this imposes on formulations will be discussed.

Formulations are much more than a simple mix of chemicals with long and often incomprehensible names. The formulation is the long-term success story of a product in that:

- It carries the active and ultimately determines whether or not the active delivers the desired benefits.
- It can influence a user's desire to continue using the product to obtain the full benefit of the active.
- For commercial products, persuading consumers to make an initial purchase requires good marketing; getting them to purchase it a second time (and hopefully more) requires a good formulation.

It is important to note that the majority of topical acne treatment products are commercial in nature, purchased directly from a store shelf or pharmacy counter. Consumer promotion and advertising are an integral part of this market place, and the formulator of such products must be aware of and take into account the demands of these consumers.

Before a product can be considered fit for release to the consumer, consideration must be given to the following points:

- Does the product meet the brief set by the marketing team and will it satisfy the end consumer's needs?

- Does it conform to the product description, advertising, and any claims that may be made?
- Is it economically viable?
- Does it infringe others' intellectual property rights?
- Is it safe for its intended purpose?
- Is it stable and will it remain fit for the purpose for a reasonable length of time?
- Can it be manufactured reproducibly and in reasonable quantities to satisfy consumer demand?

Failure to satisfy these principles increases the risk of issues arising in the market place and, with it, potential harm to the user and commercial damage to the producer. As with many things, preparation is the key and a clear strategy of how these points will be addressed should be in place before the formulation is considered. Careful planning, sound scientific skills, and a robust process will ensure the ultimate end point—a successful product.

In treating acne, we are attempting to:

- Clear existing lesions and prevent the formation of new ones.
- Relieve the discomfort from the biophysical process of acne formation and therapy.
- Reduce inflammation.
- Minimize the negative psychological effects.

The physical/chemical activities that the product will be attempting to deal with are:

- Reducing excess oil.
- Controlling the bacteria associated with acne.
- Reducing the effects of hyperkeratinization.
- Unclogging pores.

The extent of the condition will dictate the type of active required:

- Moderate-to-severe drug products, some requiring a physician's prescription.
- Mild-to-moderate mixture of drug products that do not require a physician's prescription and more cosmetic products from a range of producers, for example, Clearasil® (Reckitt Benckiser Inc., New Jersey, U.S.A.), Clean & Clear® (Johnson & Johnson Corporation, New Jersey, U.S.A.), and Neutrogena® (Neutrogena Corporation, California, U.S.A.).

The formulator must consider the technical characteristics of maintaining and delivering the drug active alongside the need for an elegant product that the user will enjoy using. Although this may sound incongruous, a product that is enjoyable to use is more likely to be used as required and, therefore, deliver the full benefit of the active.

Formulating the product, that is, putting a mixture of ingredients together, is only the first stage and in doing so the formulator must always bear in mind the basic principles outlined earlier. In order to do that, a clear understanding of what is required allows a robust strategy to be developed, reducing time wasted on unnecessary formulation.

FORMULATION STRATEGY

A clear brief or desired end point is essential for an effective strategy. Once obtained, there are three routes the formulator can take:

- Modify an existing product with a known history.
- Use or modify a formulation obtained from the literature.
- Devise an entirely new formulation.

The route taken will clearly be dictated by a number of factors, but will include such things as the degree of risk the formulator is able to take and the timescales in which the product has to be delivered. The first route is clearly the lowest risk, as there will be information on many of the key factors required for a successful development. The second route provides for somewhat higher risk in that the product may not have undergone a complete evaluation.

The final route clearly has the highest risk but offers the greatest flexibility for incorporation of actives, and allows for significant innovation. A clear view of the intended application and all claims that will be made about the product are essential. The starting point will be the active, or actives, and the formulation should be built with the view to maximizing performance, safety, and stability. It is important to remember that this must include end-user compliance; petrolatum may be the best carrier for a topical active, but it would not be the most likely base to ensure continued use. The complexity of factors in producing novel formulations is shown in Figure 1 (1).

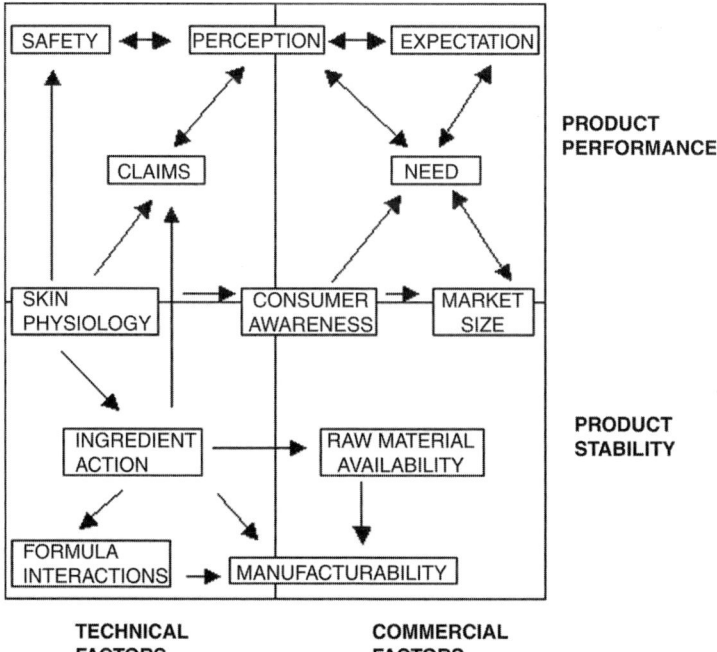

FIGURE 1   There are clearly inter-related events that must be taken into account when formulating new products. They are not mutually exclusive and it is important to consider all possibilities during the whole process of development. *Source*: From Ref. 1.

Acne treatments fall within three major regulatory areas:

- Licensed prescription or licensed over-the-counter (OTC) medicines.
- Monographed OTC medicines.
- Cosmetics.

Regulations exist in all countries concerning most, if not all, of these three areas. Although somewhat easier in the European Union (EU), where there is harmonization of regulations, formulators should confirm that the ingredients used and products produced comply with local regulations, especially where they are likely to be sold in different countries. While the International Conference on Harmonization of Technical Requirements for Registration of Pharmaceuticals for Human Use (ICH) has attempted to introduce a degree of harmonization in certain areas, it should be remembered that products considered drugs in one country are cosmetics in another.

Even with increasing harmonization, formulators should be aware of the local regulatory status of their product as this may affect:

- The type of claims that can be made.
- The status of certain ingredients such as sunscreens, colors, preservatives, and herbal extracts in terms of ability to use and level.
- The statutory warnings that require displaying for the product, actives, and excipients.
- The quality standards of the actives and excipients used in the formulation.
- The type and extent of the testing required to bring the product to market.

Regulations constantly change and formulators require up-to-date knowledge on the legal requirements and the implications that these may have on the formulation of topical acne products.

In the next section, the range of technologies available for use will be discussed.

PRODUCT TYPES

There are six major technology areas that formulators may wish to utilize, as shown in Table 1.

Emulsions

An emulsion is a dispersion of two immiscible liquids in the form of droplets. The majority of emulsions fall into one of two types, as shown in Figure 2.

The following general characteristics of emulsions are displayed in Table 2. Emulsions are thermodynamically unstable, which means they are always attempting to return to their natural, single-phase states. This is overcome through the addition of energy in two forms:

- Mechanical energy through the use of high shear mixers.
- Chemical energy through the use of emulsifiers.

In practice, both forms of energy would be used to deliver a longer-term stable product.

TABLE 1 Available Product Technologies for Topical Therapy

Technology area	Pros	Cons
Emulsion systems	Multiphase allows for incompatible materials Range of textures Wide range of claims possible Relatively low cost Good format for treatment	Variability in manufacture High temperature stability can be difficult to achieve
Detergent (surfactant) systems	Removes sebum effectively Easy to manufacture Can incorporate hard-to-dissolve ingredients	Wash off; risks low level of active remaining on skin after use
Solutions	Easy to manufacture Wide range of solvents available	Can be difficult to apply
Gels	Easy to use Easy to manufacture Range of textures possible	Limited range of solvents can be gelled
Ointments	Highly emollient reducing risk of wash off of active	Can be quite greasy Difficult to incorporate water soluble actives
Soap	Removes sebum effectively Easy to use	High pH reducing range of actives that may be incorporated Reduced skin tolerance Wash off only risks low level of active remaining on skin after use

Note: The range of products available for use is wide, and careful consideration should be given to the best type to achieve maximum active delivery and good patient compliance.

Emulsifiers are materials that have an affinity for both the oil and water phases, and as such, sit at the interface of the two phases. There are a number of types, as shown in Table 3.

Anionic emulsifiers have increasingly become replaced by nonionic systems, as they offer the formulator much greater flexibility in terms of range, end product characteristics, mildness, and compatibility with actives. Cationic emulsifiers are only rarely used.

With the myriad of emulsifiers that are available for the formulator, the choice is not an easy one. Considerations such as compatibility with actives and excipients and finished product stability are clear priorities, but significant thought should be given to ease of use (both in terms of laboratory and large scale), safety profile, supply chain and, of course, price.

For systems in which the formulator has decided to use nonionic emulsifiers, help is available in deciding the type of emulsifier. Known as the Hydrophilic–Lipophilic Balance (HLB) system, it gives the formulator an indication (within a

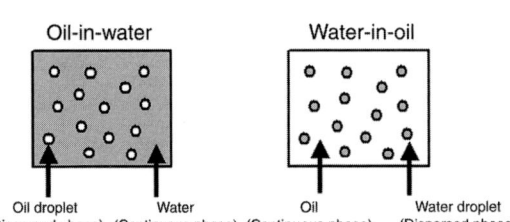

FIGURE 2 Within the two most common types of emulsion the oil-in-water shown (*left*) is the preferred choice for many formulations.

TABLE 2 Comparison Between Two Most Common Emulsion Types Seen in Topical Therapy

Characteristic	Oil-in-water	Water-in-oil
Predominant phase	Water	Oil
Typical oil content	5–20%	50–90%
Conducts electricity	Yes	No
Preservation required	In most cases	Not always

Note: Water in oil systems tend to have a heavier, greasier feel that may not be suitable for skin types who often suffer from acne. The higher level of water in oil-in-water systems is used to produce emulsions that are light and elegant.

given molecule) of the balance between affinity for oil and water. HLB uses a simple numbering system to indicate the relative balance. In the system, 1 represents highly lipophilic (oil-loving) and 20 represents highly hydrophilic (water-loving). Figure 3 illustrates how this is achieved in practice.

The HLB number is determined experimentally by producing emulsions with oils of known HLB, or by theoretical calculation based on the chemistry of the molecule. A blend of high and low HLB emulsifiers will generally be more effective than a single emulsifier that yields an equivalent HLB, as illustrated in Figure 4.

The types of oils used in the formulation will determine the required HLB number. Formulators need to consider the type of emulsion they are intending to make as this can affect the choice of emulsifier system required. For example, to emulsify Paraffinium Liquidium (2):

Required HLB for oil in water: 10–12

Required HLB for water in oil: 4–5

The choice of oils will be determined by the desired texture of the finished product. Such blends are determined by trial and error until optimum product performance is achieved. Other ingredients that might form part of the emulsion system include humectants, water phase thickeners, such as carbomer and xanthan gum, preservatives, and fragrance.

Surfactant Systems

An important part of acne treatment is ensuring that the affected area is kept clean. This product category is clearly important in achieving this objective. Although the emulsifiers, described in the previous section, are surfactant in nature, their concentration is significantly lower than that found in many washing products such as shampoos and shower gels.

TABLE 3 Basic Emulsifier Categories

Emulsifier type	Charge	Example
Anionic	Negative	Sodium stearate
Cationic	Positive	Palmitamidopropyl trimonium chloride
Nonionic	Neutral	Polysorbate 20

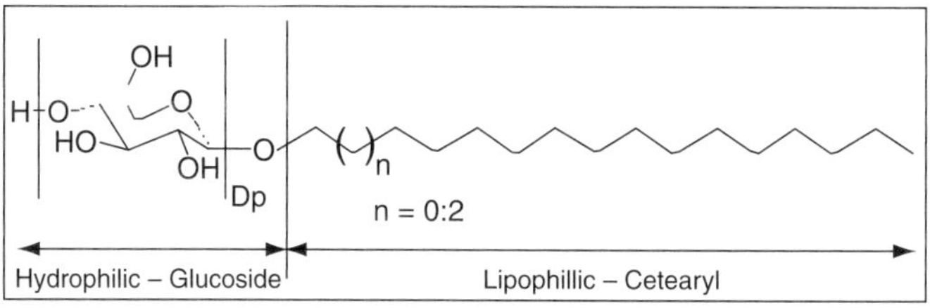

H$-$O--- OH
HO O
OH O$\left(\right)_n$
Dp
$n = 0:2$

Hydrophilic – Glucoside | Lipophillic – Cetearyl

FIGURE 3 Nonionic emulsifier, Cetearyl Glucoside [Tego® Care CG90 (Goldschmidt GmbH, Essen, Germany)], illustrating the balance between hydrophilic and lipophilic entities. The Hydrophilic–Lipophilic Balance of this molecule is 11 ± 1 and by manipulating the number of units on either side, changes the balance and with it the likelihood of being able to produce different emulsion types. *Source*: Diagram courtesy Degussa Goldschmidt Personal Care.

The classification given in Table 3 remains applicable here, although Table 4 indicates the relative merits of these materials for this application.

The primary purpose of surfactant products in acne applications is the removal of surface oils. While it is possible to add active ingredients to such systems, formulators must remember that they are wash-off products and the degree of deposition of active can vary.

Formulating surfactant products is not simply a matter of maximizing the level of surfactant. Even in oily skin, excessive defatting remains a problem, and the balance between cleanliness and drying/irritation should be taken into account. Due to their nature, surfactants tend to form the micellular structure shown in Figure 5.

This is an important property as it helps to explain the mechanism by which the products remove oil and prevent re-deposition. The surfactant reduces the surface tension of the oil on the skin, allowing dispersion of the unwanted oil in the surfactant system. The lipophilic core of the micelle is where the oil is held.

Formulators must also be aware of the reverse happening with a detrimental effect on product performance. Such situations may occur where actives have significant affinity for the surfactant micelle, and the active ingredient becomes effectively trapped and is removed on rinsing. This is most likely to occur with lipophilic actives, or in anionic systems with small cationic materials due to charge coupling.

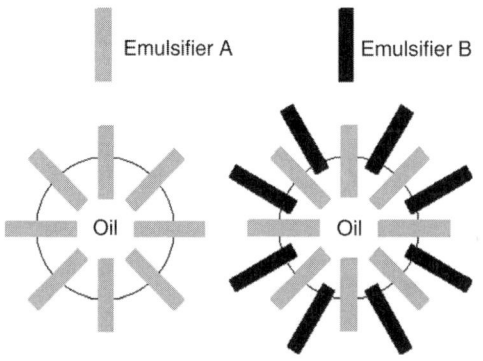

FIGURE 4 A greater degree of emulsifier packing in an oil droplet is possible when using a mix of emulsifiers. In this example, emulsifier A is more lipophilic (lower hydrophilic–lipophilic balance) than emulsifier B.

TABLE 4 Basic Surfactant Categories

Surfactant type	Charge	Properties
Anionic	Negative	High levels of flash foam
		Offer wide variety of foam quality
		Excellent primary surfactant
		Wide range of types available
		Choice of counter ion important in terms of irritancy potential
Amphoteric	Overall neutral due to positive and negative charges present within one molecule	Substantive to skin
		Good secondary surfactant
Cationic	Positive	Substantive to the skin offering conditioning but increased risk of irritation
		Do not produce high levels of foam
		Not widely used
Nonionic	Neutral	Often used as secondary surfactants to stabilise foam
		Often used as primary surfactant in milder products
		Generally produce low levels of flash foam

Note the additional types available in surfactants to be used in this application compared to emulsifiers. Amphoterics, although possessing an overall neutral charge, have very different properties compared to the nonionics.

There is a range of anionic surfactants that the formulator may consider. The most popular is based on alkyl ether sulfates, such as sodium or ammonium lauryl ether sulfate. The extent of ethylene oxide addition determines the overall properties of the surfactant. Two or three units are the most common format combining good surfactancy; ammonium salts produce richer creamy foam than the more open but equally copious sodium version. For the equivalent degree of ethoxylation, magnesium salts show more mildness than their sodium counterpart and increasing the number of ethoxylated units also increases mildness (3). Alkyl ether sulfates provide the backbone to many wash products, given their ease of handling, wide range of stability, and cost.

Other commonly used primary surfactants include those from groups such as sarcosinates and sulfosuccinates. These ingredients offer greater mildness (3) and conditioning than alkyl ether sulfates, but their cost-performance ratio has not led to their

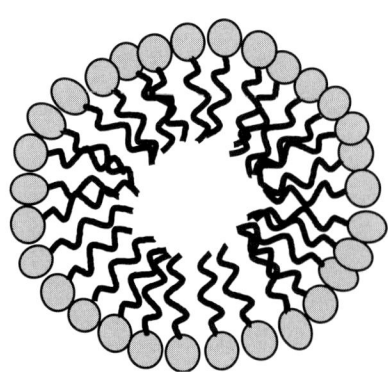

FIGURE 5 In micelles, the hydrophobic tails point into the center, creating a void into which oil and particulate matter can be captured and retained.

TABLE 5 Other Components that May be Found In a Surfactant Product

Component	Function
Viscosity modifier/thickening agents	Changes product rheology, e.g., salts (type depends on the counter ion of the surfactant) Carbomer, PEG 6000 distearate
Pearlizing agents	Improves visual appearance of products, e.g., glycol distearate
Cationic polymer	Improved skin/hair feel, e.g., polyquaterniums, proteins
Moisturizers/refatting agents	Reduce skin dryness, e.g., glycerin, PEG 7 glyceryl cocoate
Preservative	Improve product stability
Fragrance	Enhance consumer appeal

extensive use. In normal circumstances, product viscosity can be raised through the controlled addition of a compatible electrolyte. This group of surfactants does not easily lend itself to this method and alternative means of thickening, for instance, the use of materials such as PEG-55 propylene glycol oleate need to be considered.

A further way to enhance the characteristics of the primary surfactant is through the use of secondary surfactants such as amphoteric betaines and amine oxides. The most common of this class used is cocamidopropyl betaine, which enhances foam quality and provides some form of skin conditioning.

Although many nonionic surfactants are equally effective at removing excess oils, they are not widely used as primary materials in this medium. The reason is their poor foam production that most consumers associate with an effective product. More commonly found playing a secondary role, many nonionic products can enhance foam stability, leave a good skin feel, and may also have a thickening effect for the products. Among commonly used nonionics are sugar-based glucosides such as Decyl Glucoside, alkoxylated amides such as PEG 5 Cocamide, and alkanolamides such as Cocamide DEA.

If using diethanolamines such as Cocamide DEA, the formulator must use high-purity material and avoid using nitrating agents to prevent formation of nitrosamines.

A wide range of additional materials are found in surfactant systems, as shown in Table 5.

Solutions

While solutions are the simplest and easiest to produce formulation, consideration must be given to the way in which the end user will use the product and, therefore, whether this is the most effective format for delivering actives and benefits.

The major advantage of using solutions is the range of individual and mixtures of polar and nonpolar solvents that are available to the formulator from water through to oils. Due to the simplicity of many solutions, formulation interactions can be more carefully managed than in more complex systems such as emulsions.

There has been an increasing trend toward the use of wipe products that consists of a fibrous cloth soaked in a suitable solution. The formulator preparing solutions for this type of application must bear in mind the possible interactions with the cloth and the way in which the wipes will be used. This is important for packs offering multiple wipes that allow the user to reseal the pack after each removal. When choosing the solvent, the formulator should consider whether the volatility of their chosen solvent might cause unacceptable changes in the level and availability of the active. This may manifest itself in two ways. First, the loss of solvent may increase the concentration of active above the legally allowed level, or above the level at which it remains safe. Second, for crystalline solutes (which may or may not include the active), loss of solvent increases the risk of precipitation. This may result in injury to the end user, particularly if the product is intended for use around the eye area.

Gels

Gel formulations are particularly useful in acne treatments as they offer the possibility of delivering active ingredients in a totally oil-free manner. The majority of formulations will be water, alcohol, or mixtures of these materials, but formulators need to be aware that it is possible to gel oils, although this is unlikely to be used in this application. The exception to this is ointments, which it could be argued, are thickened oils, but the formulation of ointments is more complex and is dealt with in a later section.

In its simplest terms, a gel is a thickened solution, although the differing rheological qualities of gels from solutions offer formulators the possibility of improving application and ensuring better control of coverage than for solutions.

Carbomers are acrylic acid polymers available in a variety of grades, offering formulators a range of viscosities and textures with defined yield points that allow excellent spreading and rapid absorption during use. Standard grade carbomers lose viscosity in the presence of electrolyte, although hydrophobically modified grades with improved electrolyte tolerance are available. Due to the need to neutralize carbomers to achieve the gel structure, the range of actives that can be used is reduced compared with other gellants.

Xanthan gums are polysaccharides with high molecular weight that show much greater stability toward electrolytes. They have excellent suspending properties due to their pseudoplastic rheology. They will not produce clear gels easily and they are not as rapidly adsorbed onto the skin as carbomers.

Modified cellulose gums are similar in their chemistry to xanthan gums, but clear gels can be produced with certain grades. With a more lubricious feel than carbomers, they can be used on their own or in combination with carbomers to extend rub-in time.

Silicate systems are available from both natural and synthetic sources. The synthetic material produces clear water white gels that can be stabilized to produce products over a very wide pH range. Due to their anionic nature, they are incompatible with cationic materials.

Ointments

Although consumers may classify these products and creams as the same for the purpose of this section, an ointment is considered to be an oil base only with no water present. While this may seem unusual for a condition where excess oil is a major cause of the problem, as will be seen later, water-free conditions may be required to provide the best environment for the active.

Ointments, due to their oily nature, can be difficult to remove and leave the skin feeling greasy. For this application, formulators may consider the ointment to be the oil phase of an as yet unfinished emulsion, where the water used to wash the product off forms the final piece. Careful choice of ingredients will improve the rate of removal and with it the after use-skin feel. As always, there is a balance, in this case, between the desire for effective removal and the risk of irritation from the emulsifiers. There are a number of emulsifiers that offer a low irritation potential and their ability to form emulsions at low temperatures, including the polysorbate group.

Soap

Soap remains one of the most widely used personal washing products, and formulators should not discount this fact when considering topical treatments. Soap, while it has excellent cleansing properties, does not lend itself to efficient active delivery. The two major drawbacks with soap are that it is washed off and so the active concentration deposited may be small and its high pH can degrade certain actives, and cause a lower tolerability on more sensitive skin.

Alternatives to soap are Combi bars (combinations of soap and synthetic detergents) or Syndet bars, based wholly on synthetic detergents. Syndet bars offer the formulator more flexibility in that their pH is lower and can be modified by allowing a wider range of actives to be used. Soap, Combi, and Syndet formulations require specialist knowledge and equipment, and a number of companies offer contracted services in this area.

ACTIVE RAW MATERIALS
Retinoids

In this section, the range of materials being considered may be seen described as retinoids, retinoid types, or retinoid prodrugs. The appropriate description to use will depend on the individual compound being considered, but all the materials are used in topical treatments for acne, and are described in more detail elsewhere.

Retinoids are highly active, and from a formulator's viewpoint, often unstable compounds being affected variously by light, heat, and oxygen. There are a number of compounds that fall within this classification, including:

- Tretinoin, [Retin A® (Johnson & Johnson Corporation, New Jersey, U.S.A.)]
- Isotretinoin, [Accutane® (Hoffman-La Roche Inc., New Jersey, U.S.A.)]
- Adapalene, [Differin® (Galderma S.A., Lausanne, Switzerland)]
- Tazarotene, [Tazorac® (Allergan Inc., California, U.S.A.)]

For many, use in actinic lighting conditions should be avoided, and the raw material and finished product storage vessels should be flushed with nitrogen after use. In emulsion products, care should be taken during manufacture, both to avoid excess heat and to minimize incorporation of air that may lead to longer-term stability problems.

Retinoids are generally insoluble in water, but have varying solubility in alcohol, other solvents, and oils.

Products should be packed for storage and consumers in protective materials such as amber glass, metal, or plastic laminated tubes.

Benzoyl Peroxide

The clinical effectiveness of benzoyl peroxide is well-established and is discussed elsewhere. Benzoyl peroxide is a highly effective oxidizing agent, and contact should be avoided with reducing agents, metals (particularly transition metals), and organic materials to prevent the risk of fire and explosion. Peroxides break down when heated and are capable of rapidly continuing their decomposition even if the heat source is removed.

Insoluble in water and barely soluble in other solvents, it can most commonly be found in emulsion and gel formats. Ensuring adequate and equal dispersion throughout the formulation is critical. Milling with a colloid mill or high-shear mixers should be undertaken carefully to avoid high levels of heat generation. Mixing equipment should be of stainless steel manufacture and no transition metals, for example, copper collars, should be in contact with the product. Alternatively, benzoyl peroxide is dispersed well in a small amount of cooled bulk, under more controllable conditions before adding to the remainder of the product.

Products should be packed in airtight containers to maximize product life. Examples of products in use with this material include:

- Clearasil® Maximum Strength
- Benzac AC® Wash (Galderma Laboratories L.P., Texas, U.S.A.)
- Panoxyl® (Stiefel Laboratories Inc., Florida, U.S.A.)

Table 6 shows an example of a cream containing benzoyl peroxide.

TABLE 6 Sample Formulation Showing the Use of Benzoyl Peroxide

INCI designation	%w/w	Trade name	Supplier
Phase A			
Aqua (water)	60.50		
Methyl propanediol	5.0	MPDiol® Glycol	Lyondell
Allantoin	0.10		
Phase B			
Glyceryl stearate and PEG 100 stearate	3.0	Lipomulse 165	Lipo
Cetearyl alcohol and ceteareth-20	3.0	Lipowax D	Lipo
Cetearyl alcohol and cetearyl glucoside	2.0	Montanov 68	Seppic
Hexyldecanol	6.0	Eutanol G-16	Henkel KgaA
Cyclomethicone and dimethiconol	1.0	Dow Corning Fluid 1401	Dow Corning
Phase C			
Triethanolamine	0.3	Triethanolamine 99%	
Phase D			
Benzoyl peroxide	5.1	Lucidol 98%	Elf Atochem
Transcutol	5.0	Carbitol	
Propylene glycol and diazolidinyl urea and methylparaben and propylparaben	1.0	Germaben® II	ISP/Sutton
Alcohol denat	5.0	SD alcohol 40	
Polyquaternium-37 and propylene glycol dicaprylate/dicaprate and PPG-1 trideceth-6	3.0	Salcare SC96	Allied Colloids
Mixing instructions			
Premix phase D and leave to stand for 1 hr			
Heat phases A and B to 75°C			
Add phase B to phase A			
Add phase C			
Cool to 40°C			
Add remaining phases			
Adjust to pH 7.7 with citric acid if required			

Source: Courtesy of Lyondell Inc.

Salicylic Acid

The clinical effectiveness of salicylic acid is well-established and is discussed elsewhere. Salicylic acid is a white crystalline powder showing slight solubility in water but being freely soluble in alcohol. Salicylic acid is most active in its acid form, and formulators should use suitable buffer solutions in formulations to maintain the pH between 2 and 4.

Salicylic acid can be found in most of the formats described earlier under a number of brands, for example, Clearasil®, Clean & Clear®, and Neutrogena®.

Antibiotics

There are a variety of antibiotics used for topical applications and these include Tetracyclines and Macrolides such as Erythromycin. Although they each have unique physical properties and solubility, a common feature is their stability in aqueous solutions. It has been suggested that antibiotics such as erythromycin show increased loss of anti-microbial activity, over time, although this varies with product base (4). Varying pH can change this loss of activity, but, for products requiring extended shelf life of greater than a few weeks, alternative solvents or systems should be considered. Antibiotics are also adversely affected by heat and light.

For topical application gels, alcoholic solutions or ointments are the most commonly produced formats. Examples include:

- Akne-Mycin® [Erythromycin (Hermal Kurt Hermann GmbH, Reinbek, Germany)]
- Cleocin T® [Clindamycin (Pharmacia & Upjohn Company LLC, New Jersey, U.S.A.)]
- Topicycline® [Tetracycline (Shire LLC, Pennsylvania, U.S.A.)].

Resorcinol

Resorcinol is colorless to slightly pink–grey and is very reactive to light and air, turning red when oxidized.

The effectiveness of resorcinol has been recognized and claims that can be made through the use of this material are available (5).

Due to its good solubility in water and alcohol, resorcinol can be incorporated into a wide range of products, including emulsions, being stable to heat at normal emulsification temperatures and times. Manufacturing under vacuum reduces the risk of loss of activity, and products containing this material should be packed in materials with good oxygen barriers.

Examples of products containing resorcinol include Clearasil® Adult Care® Acne Treatment Cream.

Sulfacetamide

Sulfacetamide has been widely utilized for its antibacterial properties for a considerable period of time. In the sodium form, it is a white to off-white crystalline substance showing good solubility in water but reduced solubility in alcohol.

This material can be found in a 10% form in Klaron® (Aventis Pharmaceutical Inc., New Jersey, U.S.A.). Sulfacetamide has also been shown to be effective in combination with sulfur (6).

Azelaic Acid

Azelaic acid was first licensed for use in the United States in the late 1990s for mild-to-moderate inflammatory acne. While its exact mode of action remains unclear, it has antimicrobial properties and is active in reducing hyper keratinization. It has been reported to be active in a number of areas, including against hyper pigmentation, so there may exist a risk of skin lightening (7). Studies have suggested that it has similar activity to other active agents (8).

Azelaic acid is soluble in boiling water and alcohol and is, therefore, able to be formulated into a range of different product types.

Products containing this material include Azelex® (Allergan Inc., California, U.S.A.) and Finevin® (Schering Aktiengesellschaft, Berlin, Germany).

Sulfur

Sulfur is a yellow powder with a characteristic odor and should be stored away from light. It is practically insoluble in water, but shows some solubility in vegetable oils.

Due to its lack of solubility, sulfur must be well-dispersed. High-shear mixing appropriate for dispersing powders or making pastes prior to incorporation in the remainder of the formulation should be considered.

As it is a powder, the overall stability of the product will depend on the effective maintenance of the dispersion. This may be achieved through the appropriate choice of formulation and a good understanding of the rheology of the system to prevent migration and agglomeration of the powder. Although it may be acceptable to allow the consumer to remix the formulation through the process of shaking, the formulator should ensure that adequate dispersion is maintained throughout the shelf life of the product. Although not commonly used, products utilizing sulfur include Stiefel® Sulfur Soap (Stiefel Laboratories Inc., Florida, U.S.A.).

Sulfur is often used in combination with other ingredients, for example:

- With resorcinol in products such as Clearasil® Adult Care® Acne Treatment Cream
- With sulfacetamide in Sulfacet–R® (Aventis Pharmaceuticals Inc., New Jersey, U.S.A.).

Table 7 shows an example formulation utilizing sulfur and resorcinol.

STABILITY

Stability trials are used to identify problems that may affect the long-term quality and safety of the product. Due to the nature of the products under test, a number of testing regimes are possible. In this context, a distinction will be drawn between licensed (whether via prescribing requirements, monograph status, or OTC) and nonlicensed, where the product claims and/or ingredients are such that the product is more cosmetic in nature.

Informal Testing

During the normal course of product development, informal testing will be undertaken. This will normally be carried out at a limited number of locations not necessarily used for formal stability testing, for example, freeze-thaw testing. Testing may be undertaken in glass to allow easy visual assessment of formulation instability, for example, separation, discoloration. Active analysis may be performed, but is not the main focus of this testing.

TABLE 7 Sample Formulation Showing the Use of Sulfur and Resorcinol

INCI designation	%w/w	Trade name	Supplier
Phase A			
Glyceryl stearate	6.00	Lexemul 515	Inolex/S Black Group
Isopropyl myristate	3.00	Lexol IPM	Inolex/S Black Group
Stearic acid	2.00	Dervacid 3155	Undesa/S Black Group
Phase B			
Alcohol denat.	10.00	Ethanol DEB 96	
Bentonite	5.00	Bentonite	
Sulfur	2.00	Sulfur	
Phase C			
Aqua (water)	64.85	Deionized water	
Resorcinol	3.00	Resorcinol	Merck/S Black
Propylene glycol	3.00	Propylene glycol	
Triethanolamine		Triethanolamine 99%	Merck/S Black
Methylparaben	0.15	Methylparaben	Sharon Labs/S Black Ltd.
Mixing instructions			
Heat phase C to 65°C			
Premix phase B and add to phase C			
Heat phase A to 70°C			
Add phase A to phase C			

Source: Courtesy of S Black Ltd.

Formal Stability Testing

Prescribed, Monographed, and Over-the-Counter Drugs

For the purposes of this section, drug products are considered to be those that contain either drugs that must be prescribed by a physician or, in certain countries, by virtue of a monograph or OTC.

Where products are drugs, there are clear reasons for stability testing in a way that conforms to the ICH guidelines in place for drug products (9). These define:

- Number of batches to be tested
- Site of batch manufacture
- Testing protocols
- Degree of testing
- Shelf life allocation

ICH guidelines are updated on a regular basis, and formulators should use a stability-testing regime that conforms to the latest requirements.

Active ingredients are quantified by analysis using validated analytical methods and organoleptic assessment of the product for each temperature location at each time interval. Samples are removed from test and not replaced.

Due to the nature of the product, sign-off for sale and allocation of shelf life should be by an appropriately qualified person, as defined by the relevant legislation applicable in the country of intended sale.

Nonlicensed Products

There are no clear rules for stability testing of nonlicensed (Cosmetic) products at present. These products will be considered in the same way as mentioned earlier, that is:

- Number of batches to be tested
- Site of batch manufacture

- Testing protocols
- Degree of testing

The products to be formally tested will be determined by the degree of novelty. Where products have been developed from existing products, it is conceivable that only one laboratory-produced batch would be tested, but it is always good practice to carry out production trials and test samples generated.

An assessment should be carried out to determine the areas that would present most risk to the product stability. A typical testing regime is illustrated in Table 8.

Microbiological testing should also be carried out at regular intervals. Organoleptic testing would be the main test that is carried out, although it is prudent to carry out analysis for the presence of raw materials, where significant claims have been made. Sign-off for sale and allocation of shelf life should be done by someone who has sufficient experience and knowledge to make an objective assessment of the risk of this product failing to conform to its specification, or causing harm for its likely shelf life, and to conform to local regulation.

SAFETY EVALUATION

Safety of the finished product is a primary objective of the formulator. Consideration of the safety of the product should be an iterative process with consideration and review at all stages of the product's development.

Safety assessment takes place at three levels:

- Assessment of formulation raw materials and existing formulation adverse event/sales ratio
- Initial evaluation of the formulation to assess need for safety testing
- Assessment of formulation for suitability for in vivo trial or sale

New raw materials or materials being used in a novel way should be screened for potential safety issues. This will include detailed scrutiny of the Material Safety Data Sheet (MSDS), and the formulator should always discuss the implications with an expert in the field such as a toxicologist or medical practitioner. For licensed products, new raw materials (drugs and excipients) will require a full toxicological package to be provided to the appropriate regulatory body.

A record of adverse events that may have an impact on the safety should be maintained on all products sold. In some countries, this is a mandatory requirement and forms good practice if it is not. This serves two purposes:

- It allows ongoing assessment of the safety of the product to be made

TABLE 8 Nonlicensed Stability Testing Protocol

Testing location	Assessment periods
4°C	1, 3, 6, 9, 12, 24, and 30 months
25°C	1, 3, 6, 9, 12, 24, and 30 months
30°C	1, 3, 6, 9, 12, 24, and 30 months
40°C	1, 3, 6, and 9 months
Light cabinet	Two weeks

Note: Additional testing may be required, for example, high humidity and freeze-thaw dependent on the countries of sale and the product type.

■ It provides a means by which existing formulations can be assessed for safety before further development

The figures stored within the database should be used with the number of products sold to determine the degree of the potential problem and whether the base could be used. Monitoring of existing formulations allows reformulation to be rapidly undertaken, should adverse events rise to an unacceptable level. All reports related to safety issues should be investigated further, as it is important that only true adverse reactions are considered.

If a formulation is judged to be different from known base formulations, safety testing should be carried out. These may take the following forms:

■ In vitro tests for example:
  ● 3-D human skin model to measure the effects on cell viability.
  ● 3T3 NRU photo toxicity test to measure the number of cells that survive after exposure to the test chemical and UV light, compared with the number that survive after exposure to the chemical in the absence of UV light.
■ Transcutaneous electrical resistance (TER) procedure to measure skin corrosivity through electrical properties.
■ Repeat Insult Patch testing on human volunteers to assess the irritancy potential of the formulation. Such studies should always be undertaken under the supervision of medical practitioner and with appropriate ethical approval.
■ A user trial (controlled or uncontrolled) on a group of people.

Once the testing is complete, the product should be assessed to decide whether it is safe for sale. This may involve submission to a regulatory authority.

For products where this is not the case, assessment should be made by a suitably qualified and experienced assessor. There are published guidelines and requirements in certain countries as to the qualifications needed by these individuals (10,11). Formulators should always ensure that local regulations regarding this important aspect of developing a new product are met.

REPRODUCIBLE MANUFACTURE

Considerable effort is expended in ensuring that any formulation developed is safe, efficacious, and stable. As the product enters the marketplace, the formulation moves from the laboratory to larger production areas. The degree of control that the formulator can employ in the laboratory is significantly reduced, and considerations such as degree of mixing and heating and cooling rates become more significant.

Formulators should consider how the formulation will be manufactured at the time they produce their first laboratory sample, and recognize the difference between laboratory and scaled production in terms of raw materials and finished product.

Raw Material Considerations
A scale-up of formulation has two significant consequences for raw materials

■ Health and safety risk of the material
■ Handling of the material in bulk

In a laboratory setting, the risks posed by the majority of ingredients used in topical acne products are small and manageable. As scale-up occurs, the quantity of material increases and, as a result, the risk posed by materials that may be considered essentially nonhazardous in a laboratory setting increases. Powders or surfactants handled in larger quantities can pose a significantly higher risk. A risk assessment should always be undertaken and should take into account the quantity of material being handled, the environment in which it will be handled, and the extent to which negative effects could be ameliorated through training and the use of personal protective equipment.

Normal laboratory production usually entails handling of small quantities of raw materials in receptacles that allow easy removal. This may not be the case when the product is scaled up to full production size. Formulators should consider the way in which the material will be handled, the type of packaging in which it arrives, and whether any special handling equipment is required to enable it to be used safely and efficiently. Early discussion with appropriate personnel is essential if difficulties are to be avoided.

Product Considerations

Manufacture of bulk in a laboratory allows much greater intervention from the formulator than is possible in a production environment. The formulator should consider the method of manufacturing on a larger scale from first laboratory sample, through understanding the type of equipment that will ultimately be used. Production processes that are achievable in the laboratory are often not reproducible on a larger scale. These may include heating and cooling rates, and the type and amount of mixing experienced. Individual products will vary in the extent to which they are affected by these considerations, but as a general rule emulsions are likely to be the most susceptible.

The use of intermediate-sized mixing vessels in pilot facilities allows the formulator to assess the feasibility of manufacture and optimize the production method. Texture, efficacy, and stability are all attributes that may be affected during scale-up, and formulators should consider what testing needs to be carried out on pilot and full production batches before releasing the product for use by a wider population. As was seen earlier, there are clear requirements to test a range of pilot studies when considering stability and it is good practice, even when not legally required, to test batches produced in a production environment. Robust pilot studies leading to a consistent, reproducible method of manufacture are essential for the long-term success of the formulation.

INTELLECTUAL PROPERTY

A patent is designed to protect the intellectual property of an individual or organization, and can cover raw materials, product formulations, claims, and techniques. Patents may be filed in individual countries or as world patents, where a range of countries may be specified. Patents last up to 20 years, but the existence of published patent does not always mean that the patent is in force, as a fee must be paid each year to maintain continued validity.

Formulations should be screened by an appropriate expert in the field to identify potential patent infringements. This can save both considerable amount of time and money.

CONSUMER ACCEPTABILITY

As has been stated earlier, consumer acceptability is critical to the long-term success of the product. Trials to gauge consumer opinion should be an integral part of a products development. Products that use a prescribed drug can still be evaluated, but this will often be done on the base only during development and attributes confirmed during the follow-up clinical studies. Formulators should always confirm the regulatory requirements surrounding this type of trial before commencing any such trials.

Consumer trials may involve panels of volunteers trying products under controlled or uncontrolled conditions. This may take place in many locations such as shopping malls, public halls, and in consumers' homes. All trials use typical consumers to try products either once or over an extended period of time and give their opinion either through interview or via a written questionnaire.

An alternative approach is the use of sensory panels. These are small groups of volunteers who have shown a level of ability to be able to detect differences between products in a particular grouping, for example, fragrance, color, or touch. They may have undergone additional training to enhance this skill or to be able to describe their experience using a consistent language approach. Sensory testing offers a way of making a reproducible assessment of different products, often comparing test products to a known standard or control. The information provided allows the formulator to modify the in-use characteristics in critical areas. There are a number of ways in which such data can be presented; one such way is shown in Figure 6.

These types of tests can also be used to compare new formulations with current formulae, where changes need to be made, or with other products already marketed to assess their comparable attributes.

Sensory panels can be considered to offer a more consistent subjective assessment of product characteristics. The test will only be effective if the parameters chosen are those desired by the end consumer. When carrying out uncontrolled user trials, the wording of the questions should be neutral to avoid introducing bias, and so inducing the trial subjects to give the answer the formulator desires. Similar precautions should also be taken with controlled trials, where trial subjects are questioned as to their views. Inexperienced or biased trial supervisors risk

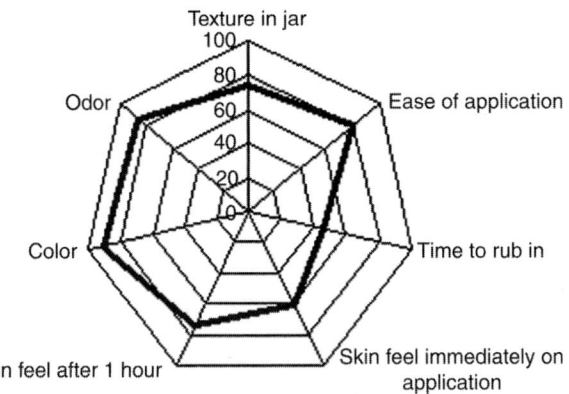

FIGURE 6 Spider graphs allow rapid assessment of key data. Multiple plotting of different products allows for the possibility of direct comparisons.

skewing the results in such a way that false positives are received that are not repeated when the general consumer uses the product.

Consultation with market research experts on conducting trials is important, as understanding the dynamics of such trials is key to meaningful results.

CLAIMS SUPPORT

It is a requirement that any claims made in relation to products are truthful. Formulators need to be aware when commencing formulation of the claims to be made and should consider the ways in which these could be delivered.

Care must be exercised in this area regarding the nature of the claim being made for the product. Formulators need to be clear of the local regulatory requirements surrounding the difference between claims that are purely cosmetic and those that may be considered to be medicinal.

Claims made for formulations fall into these broad categories:

- Claims made for specific or groups of raw materials.
- Claims made based on monograph requirements.
- Claims made based on the product function.
- Claims based on product performance.

Raw Materials
Raw material claims are made based either on the inclusion of an ingredient ("contains Chamomile"), its reported action ("contains Chamomile renowned for its soothing properties"), or testing ("contains alpha bisabalol, the active agent of Chamomile, which has been shown to reduce irritation").

Monograph
There are certain claims that are justified by recognition of the inclusion in legislation. Primary among these are the acne claims made in the U.S. monograph following the inclusion of a prescribed level of salicylic acid, sulfur, or resorcinol, or combinations of the latter two (5).

Product Function Claims
Such claims justify the function of a particular product, for example, shampoo and moisturiser.

Product Performance
Certain claims may only be attributable to the whole product rather than individual ingredients. Such claims usually quantify the action of the product function, for example, product X decreases sebum by 30%.

CLAIMS SUPPORT TESTING

With the exception of claims made for product function or based on ingredients included in monograph, some form of claim substantiation should be carried out. These may be labeled as clinical or claims substantiation trials but it is best practice to conduct any in vivo trial in accordance with Good Clinical Practice (GCP) principles and any additional local regulatory requirement.

Careful thought should be given to the type and nature of the trial, and this should only be carried out if the benefits justify the potential risks. Any information on the trial product should support the proposed trial and be able to be used to produce a trial protocol. This protocol should be reviewed and approved by an appropriate body.

The safety of the trial subjects is of paramount importance at all times and any trial should always be the responsibility of a qualified physician. Screening of any potential trial subject should take into account their health and the impact the trial may have on them. Informed consent should be obtained from every subject prior to participation in any trial.

Each individual involved in conducting a trial should be qualified and trained appropriately. All trial information should be gathered and used in a way that allows accurate analysis and conclusions to be drawn. Records should always be stored in a secure and confidential way and comply with any local regulatory requirement.

Trial products should be made in accordance with appropriate good manufacturing practice and used as stated in the approved protocol. There should be in place a method of auditing the trial to confirm that it was carried out according to the protocol.

ICH has produced guidelines on conducting clinical trials, and formulators will find important information that will allow them to perform high-quality studies (12). Although these guidelines are widely recognized, formulators should confirm before commencing clinical trials that local regulatory requirements have been satisfied.

For claims that are more cosmetic in nature, the European Cosmetic, Toiletries, and Perfumery Association publish guidance on the evaluation of the efficacy of cosmetic products (13).

SUMMARY

Topical anti-acne products covers a wide range of technology, regulatory, and product types. Good understanding of the fundamental formulation building blocks is essential in order to maximize the effectiveness of the range of ingredients available. A working knowledge of the activities that go to support the formulation enables the formulator to develop a clear strategy to deliver the desired stable, efficacious product with the minimum of problems.

This chapter has described many of the elements required to develop high-quality formulations that meet consumer's needs and expectations. The formulator is encouraged to use this only as a starting point and not to be afraid to carry out any experiment with the myriad of possible combinations of ingredients to delight new and existing users of topical acne products.

ACKNOWLEDGMENTS

The author would like to thank all those who helped in the preparation of this manuscript, with special thanks to Patrick Love, Steve Barton, Nick Moody, and Diane Pavis.

REFERENCES

1. Barton S. Formulation of Skin Moisturizers. In: Leyton, Rawlings, ed. Skin Moisturization. New York: Marcel Dekker, 2002: 547–584.
2. Knowlton J, Pearce S. Emulsions. In: Knowlton J, Pearce S, eds. Handbook of Cosmetic Science and Technology. 1st ed. Oxford: Elsevier Advanced Technology, 1993:108.
3. Searle J, Cognis (UK) Ltd. Do we need milder surfactants or is it a case of careful blending? SCS Formulate, Birmingham, Nov 2001.
4. Vandenbossche GMR, Vanhaecke E, De Muynck C, Remon JP. Stability of topical erythromycin formulations. Int J Pharm 1991; 67(2):195–199.
5. Code of federal regulations Title 21 Food and Drugs Part 333—Topical Anti-microbial Drug products for over-the-counter human use.
6. Breneman DL, Ariano MC. Successful treatment of acne vulgaris in women with a new topical sodium sulfacetamide/sulfur lotion. Int J Dermatol 1993; 32(5):365–367.
7. Thiboutot D. New treatments and therapeutic strategies for acne. Arch Fam Med 2000; 9(2):179–187.
8. Mackrides PS, Shaugnessy AF. Azelaic acid therapy for acne. Am Fam Physician 1996; 54(8):2457–2459.
9. Quality Guidelines on Stability Testing. International Conference on Harmonisation of Technical Requirements for Registration of Pharmaceuticals for Human Use. http://www.ich.org. Accessed April 2005.
10. European Community, The rules governing cosmetic products in the European Union. European Community 1999, Cosmetic Legislation Vol. 1.
11. Department of Trade and Industry, Cosmetic Products Regulations 1996, HMSO 1996.
12. Efficacy Guidelines. International Conference on Harmonisation of Technical Requirements for Registration of Pharmaceuticals for Human Use http://www.ich.org. Accessed April 2005.
13. The European Cosmetic, Toiletries and Perfumery Association: Guidelines for the Evaluation of the Efficacy of Cosmetic Products. http://www.colipa.com/. Accessed April 2005.

18 In Vitro Models for the Evaluation of Anti-acne Technologies

John Bajor
Department of Research and Development, Home and Personal Care Division, Unilever PLC, Trumbull, Connecticut, U.S.A.

INTRODUCTION

Acne is the disease manifesting from a multifactorial process involving the pilose-baceous appendages, and although the exact mechanism is unknown, four biological mechanisms are believed to play critical roles in the formation of a lesion:

1. increased sebum production,
2. aberrant keratinocyte proliferation and differentiation,
3. enhanced bacterial growth and metabolism, and
4. irritation and inflammation.

Acne is unique to humans, and although animals can be induced to form come-dones, there is no representative in vivo model aside from humans, which incorpor-ates the above-mentioned factors. Furthermore, of the four types of pilosebaceous appendages described by Kligman (1), only the sebaceous pilosebaceous unit, which contains a large sebaceous gland and a small vellus hair, has the propensity to develop acne. Even so, acne is still a remarkably rare event, with only a small per-centage of follicles being diseased at any single time.

A detailed structural analysis of the follicular plug, or comedone, that can develop into an acne lesion reveals a compacted agglomeration of desquamated follicular keratinocytes, bacteria, sebaceous gland products/remnants, and hair fibers. Finally, the static condition of the comedone allows for a favorable growth environ-ment for bacteria, such as *Proprionibacterium acnes* and *Staphylococcus epidermidis* that can lead to inflammation.

Although no in vivo or in vitro model exists to examine the entire complexity of lesion formation, several in vitro models are available to evaluate technologies targeting specific biological mechanisms occurring in acne. This review is aimed at disclosing the types of in vitro models available to evaluate technologies that may alleviate or prevent acne lesion formation.

EVALUATION OF TECHNOLOGIES TARGETING THE SEBACEOUS GLAND

The sebaceous gland of the skin is the part of the pilosebaceous unit, which secretes a unique lipid mixture of triglycerides, wax esters, and squalene during pro-grammed differentiation (2).

The sebaceous gland consists solely of one epithelial cell type, the sebocyte. Sebocyte migration out of the gland's basal layer and full differentiation requires approximately two weeks, during which time the cells increase in volume 100- to 150-fold and become lipid-filled (3–6). Lipid secretion into the follicular duct then occurs via a holocrine mechanism, and hence destroying the sebocyte. Therefore, the absolute rate and amount of sebum secretion is dependent upon sebaceous gland density and size, metabolic activity of the sebocytes, and lipogenic capacity of the ductal reservoir.

The movement of sebum through the follicular canal and onto the epidermal surface allows for interaction with bacterial and epidermal lipases that can degrade the triglyceride fraction partially or completely to free fatty acids (7–9).

Most of the literature documenting sebaceous gland physiology has resulted from the use of human volunteer subjects or animal models. Several in vitro models have been developed for further understanding sebocyte physiology, which are based on two technologies: the in situ culture of the human sebaceous gland and the in vitro culture of sebocytes in a monolayer with and without fibroblast feeder support.

Sebaceous Gland Organ Culture Maintenance

Culture of the entire sebaceous gland offers several advantages in comparison to sebocyte monolayer culture. For example, as the three-dimensional architecture is maintained, proliferation and lipid synthesis can be simultaneously examined in the basal and differentiated cell layers, respectively. An additional advantage over animal models lies in the fact that delivery of potential sebum suppressive compounds to the gland is not hindered, so absolute biological efficacy can be evaluated.

Sebaceous glands can be isolated by dissection of human skin (surgical waste, donor, cadaver, etc.) by a variety of methods including microdissection (10) and shearing (11). Once obtained, the glands are placed directly in growth medium (or can be floated by placement upon nitrocellulose filters) and incubated at 37°C in the presence of carbon dioxide (12). Studies using intact sebaceous glands with and without the attached dermal/epidermal components have been utilized to measure lipogenesis rates in subjects with acne (13) and the effect of substrates on lipid rates and patterns (14–16). Acetate was determined to be the most preferred substrate resulting in maximal incorporation into newly formed lipids. Pappas et al. (17) reported that the sebaceous gland selectively utilizes the 16:0 fatty acid for incorporation into wax esters and elongated fatty acids such as 18:0. As a control, acetate was incorporated into all of the cellular and secreted lipids.

During prolonged incubation at the air/liquid interface, newly formed sebocytes tend to differentiate similarly as interfollicular keratinocytes taking on a flattened phenotype with minimal lipid synthesis occurring. Through a thorough investigation of factors impeding differentiation, Guy et al. (18,19) reported that many of the common growth medium components, such as phenol red, HEPES buffer, epidermal growth factor (EGF), and serum, reduced overall lipogenesis. In the absence of phenol red (which is known to have estrogen-like properties) and EGF, the intact sebaceous gland can be maintained for up to two weeks without significant necrosis (Fig. 1). DNA, protein synthesis, and lipogenesis rates remained consistent over the maintenance period.

In the presence of estradiol (600 pM) and 13-*cis*-retinoic acid (1 μM), lipogenesis rates were decreased on average by 36% and 48%, respectively (Fig. 1). Histologically, a thickening of the undifferentiated cell layer accompanied by luminal keratinization was evident.

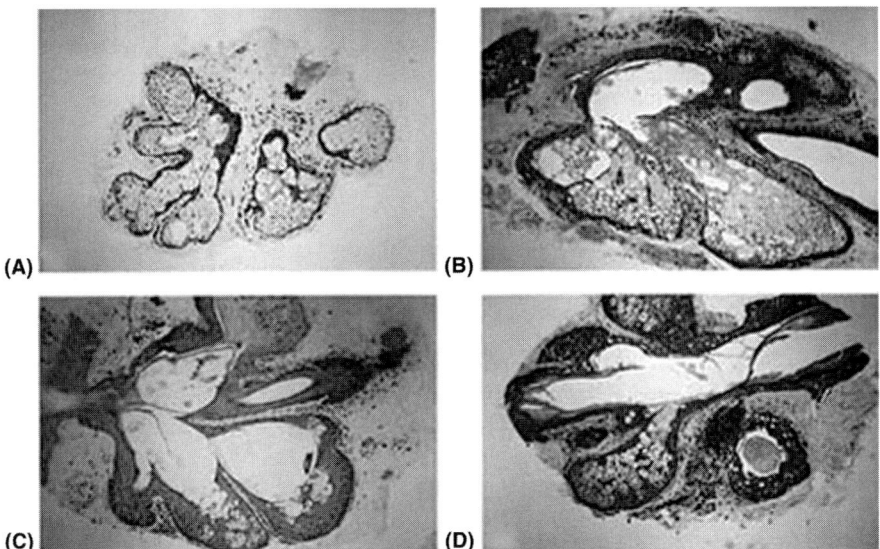

FIGURE 1 Organ culture of the human sebaceous gland. Sebaceous glands can be maintained in culture over seven days with no discernable loss in proliferation or lipid synthesis. (**A**) Freshly isolated human sebaceous gland. (**B**) Sebaceous gland maintained in culture for seven days. (**C**) As in (**B**), but supplemented with 600 pM 17-β-estradiol. Rates of cell division are comparable to control but lipid synthesis is decreased on average by 41%. (**D**) As in (**B**), but supplemented with 1 μM 13-*cis*-retinoic acid. Rates of cell division and lipid synthesis are decreased by 36% and 48%, respectively. *Source*: From Ref. 19.

Surprisingly, testosterone and dihydrotestosterone (DHT) had no effect on enhancing lipogenesis in the cultured glands, possibly because the glands were already at maximal lipogenesis rates. This finding implied that androgens are not necessary for the short-term stimulation of glandular function or, alternatively, that the growth conditions for sebaceous gland maintenance have been fully optimized.

Additionally, peroxisome proliferator activated receptors (PPARs) have been shown to be important in the regulation of lipid metabolism in adipose and liver cells. PPARs are nuclear hormone receptors and sebocytes express the subtypes α, β, and γ that appear to play important roles in proliferation and differentiation. Downie et al. (20,21) investigated the role of PPAR and additional nuclear hormone receptor ligands on sebaceous gland proliferation and differentiation.

PPARα, PPARβ, PPARγ, retinoid-X-activated receptor α, liver-X-activated receptor α, and pregnane-X-receptor, but not farnesoid-X-activated receptors, were all detected in fresh and seven-day maintained glands. The PPAR ligands arachidonic acid, BRL-49653, clofibrate, prostaglandin J2, eicosatetraynoic acid (EYTA), leukotriene B4, linoleic acid, linolenic acid, oleic acid, and WY-14643 all inhibited lipid synthesis, whereas bezafibrate, juvenile hormone III, and farnesol were ineffective. With the exception of EYTA at 10 μM, no effects on gland proliferation were evident (20,21).

The sebaceous gland in situ model is also applicable for the culture of sebaceous glands isolated from animals. Toyoda and Morohashi (22) performed organ culture on sebaceous glands obtained from mice to evaluate the effects of neuropeptides (calcitonin gene-related peptide, substance P, vasoactive intestinal polypeptide, and neuropeptide Y) in addition to nerve growth factor. Sebaceous glands treated with substance P resulted in accelerated lipid synthesis over the control glands by increasing the rate of proliferation and differentiation postulating that stress could participate in the pathogenesis of acne.

Sebocyte Monolayer Culture

Although the advantages of sebaceous gland organ culture are evident, the procedure is time-consuming and dependent on continued sources of viable tissue for additional glands. Cell culture offers an alternative over organ culture maintenance, as large numbers of cells can be processed and frozen back allowing multiple experiments to be performed on a similar cell lineage. However, continued holocrine destruction of sebocytes also necessitates a stem cell population required for maintenance. Stem cells are self-renewing and are capable of generating large numbers of differentiated progeny throughout an individual's life span (23). Stem cells can also generate a transit amplifying population, which has a high probability of postmitotic differentiation. Within the human sebaceous gland, transit amplifying cells have been detected (24,25). For a recent review on hair follicle stem cells, refer to Lavker et al. (26).

The in vivo data appeared consistent with early in vitro experiments that failed to yield viable sebocytes during extended culture conditions (27–29). This resulted in a similar but less stringent need as organ culture for ample biopsies to supply sufficient sebocytes for experimentation.

Several laboratories have successfully cultured human sebocytes in the presence of fibroblast support and in serum-free conditions to examine the effects of serum, growth factors, and biopsy location (30–33). Sebocyte culture provides an excellent model to change local environmental growth conditions (i.e., hormones, vitamins, carbohydrates, etc.) and to evaluate lipogenesis inhibitors in a higher throughput mode than that which could normally be obtained through the use of organ culture maintenance. This can be accomplished either through extended culture to evaluate gross morphological changes (i.e., sebocyte size, keratin expression patterns, and lipid vacuole content) or through rapid evaluation using radiolabeled substrates. Tritiated thymidine will be incorporated into the cells as a marker for proliferation, whereas radiolabeled glucose and/or acetate can be used as tracers for lipid synthesis.

Two procedures are suitable for generating sebocyte monolayer cultures. In the explant outgrowth method, isolated sebaceous glands are attached to culture plates by limited drying followed by addition of growth medium. Fibroblast-feeder support can later be added, but this appears not to be necessary. After several days of incubation, proliferative basal sebocytes are seen as visible outgrowths from the gland (Fig. 2).

Alternatively, a much more common approach is to digest sebaceous glands by limited trypsin proteolysis and plate the released cells in mass culture upon a fibroblast feeder layer. After several days, colonies of attached cells will begin to proliferate into small colonies that can be further cloned and/or passed.

During the proliferative stage, sebocytes are indistinguishable from keratinocytes expressing keratins 5 and 14. Upon reaching confluence, the cells take on a sebocytic phenotype as they enlarge, express keratins 4, 7, and 13, and become

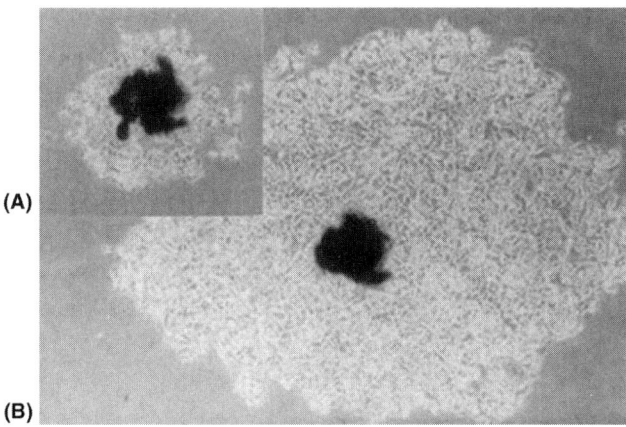

(A)

(B)

FIGURE 2 Primary culture of human sebocytes derived from explant growth. Human sebocytes can be propagated in monolayer culture by outgrowth of sebaceous glands through in vitro explant culture. (**A**, inset) Colony size at day 5. (**B**, main photograph) Colony size at day 10. *Source*: From Ref. 31.

lipid filled. Detection of an intracellular lipid droplet is evident by retention of lipophilic dyes such as Nile red, oil red O, or Sudan black (Fig. 3). Sebocytes, in comparison to cultured keratinocytes, synthesize and accumulate considerably more intracellular lipids at comparable stages of differentiation (Fig. 4), and analysis by thin layer chromatography (TLC) reveals similar classes of sebum-specific lipids as those made de novo (Fig. 5).

Although sebocytes can be cultured for an extensive passage number (34), there may be a tendency for sebaceous cells to de-differentiate to varying degrees, especially in regard to sebum specific lipids. The rate-limiting step in squalene synthesis shifts, as the cells tend to accumulate higher levels of cholesterol, which is then esterified into cholesterol esters. This de-differentiation appears to have been corrected by Zouboulis et al. (35), when freshly isolated cells were immortalized by transfection with a PBR-322 based plasmid containing the coding region of the simian virus-40 large T antigen. These sebocytes have been passaged over 50 times with no discernable loss of phenotype (Fig. 6).

Regardless of the culture conditions being utilized, sebocyte monolayer culture has been used successfully to answer many questions regarding cell metabolism and lipid synthesis, specifically the androgen metabolism and retinoid pathways.

Fujie et al. (31) reported that the androgens testosterone and DHT stimulated the proliferation as well as the lipid synthesis of sebocytes in a dose-dependent manner with maximal effects occurring at 10^{-9} and 10^{-10} M, respectively. Zouboulis et al. (32) found that testosterone stimulated facial sebocyte proliferation by 50% at 10^{-6} M and DHT at 10^{-8} M. In the presence of the antiandrogen spironolactone, sebocyte proliferation was reduced by 50% at 10^{-7} M and additionally, the stimulatory effect seen with DHT was neutralized. Spironolactone has been successfully used as a treatment for acne (36,37), suggesting that the inhibitory effects of antiandrogens may be occurring at the cellular level.

The stimulatory effect seen with androgens in sebocyte monolayer culture is in contrast to the results seen in organ culture in which no effects were evident. This

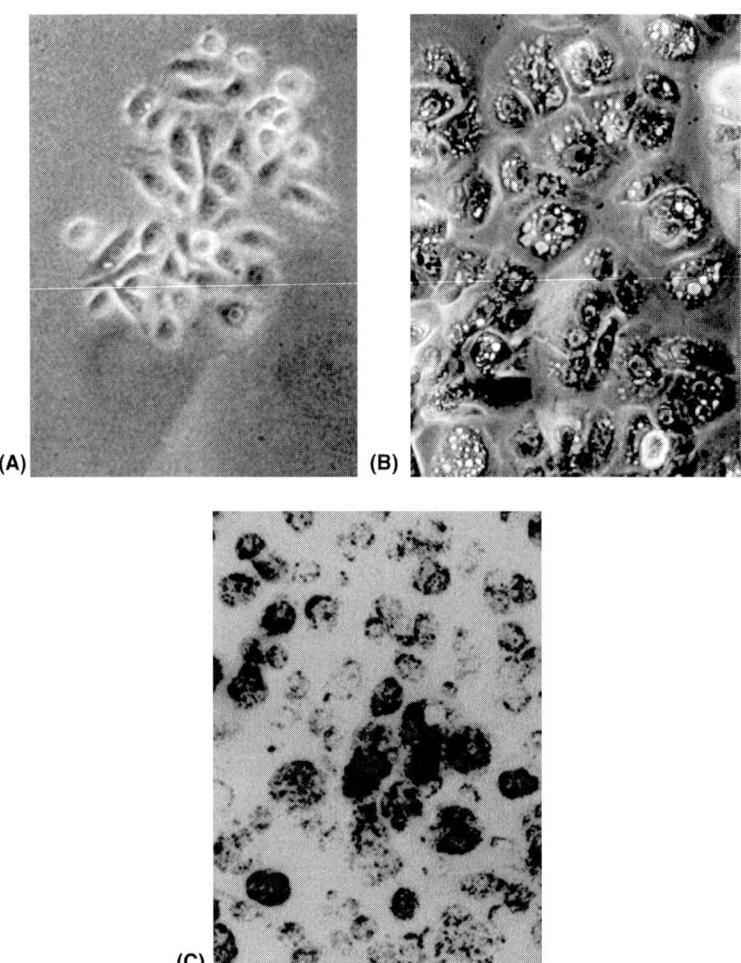

FIGURE 3   The in vitro culture of human sebocytes. Human sebocytes can be cultured in vitro under a variety of conditions including the presence/absence of serum, phenol red, and fibroblast support to attain sebocyte-specific differentiation characteristics. (**A**) Preconfluent human sebocytes cultured in vitro in serum-free medium in the absence of fibroblast support. (**B**) Sebocytes cultured in phenol red-free and serum-free medium at seven days postconfluence. Note the accumulation of intracellular lipid droplets. (**C**) Sebocytes at seven days postconfluence stained with oil red O confirming the presence of intracellular lipids.

may be due to a dilution of inherent androgens, as sebocytes multiply to a greater extent in monolayer culture. However, it has been documented that sebocytes are able to synthesize testosterone from adrenal precursors in parallel to an inactivation process to maintain androgen homeostasis (38). Alternatively, the presence of ingredients in the growth medium such as phenol red, which has inhibitory activity via estrogen-like properties, may account for the stimulatory effects seen with androgens. It is suggested that all experiments with cultured sebocytes be performed using phenol red-free medium under reduced lighting conditions for optimal benefits.

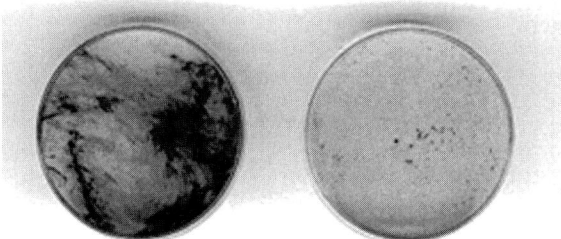

FIGURE 4 Oil red O staining of sebocyte and keratinocyte cultures. Upon reaching confluence, sebocyte differentiation involves synthesis and accumulation of intracellular lipid droplets. (*Left*): Human sebocytes cultured in vitro for seven days postconfluence in serum-free/phenol red-free medium (60 mm^2 area). Note the extensive oil red O staining within the dish confirming the presence of lipids. (*Right*): Similar aged culture of human keratinocytes stained with oil red O. Note the absence of significant intracellular lipids.

It is well-known that oral administration of 13-*cis*-retinoic acid reduces sebaceous gland size and lipid synthesis, whereas the all-*trans* and 9-*cis* isomers of retinoic acid are significantly less effective. Therefore, cultured sebocytes have also been utilized as a model to further understand retinoid responsiveness and potential mechanism of action.

Tsukada et al. (39) reported that isomerization of 13-*cis*-retinoic acid to all-*trans* retinoic acid occurs in SZ-95 sebocytes, subsequently providing the biological benefit. No isomerization was evident in HaCaT keratinocytes and the reverse

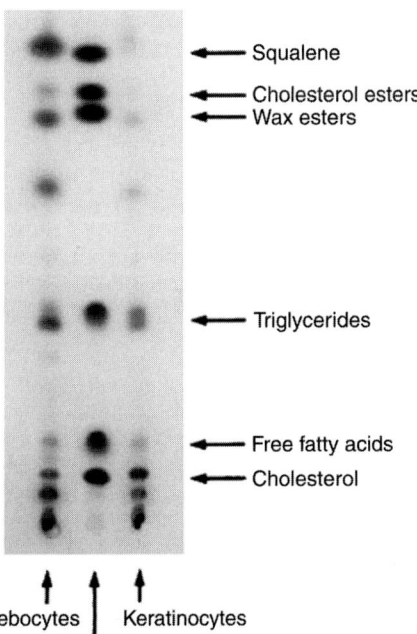

— Squalene

— Cholesterol esters
— Wax esters

— Triglycerides

— Free fatty acids

— Cholesterol

Sebocytes | Keratinocytes
Lipids standards

FIGURE 5 Thin layer chromatography (TLC) of neutral lipids. TLC of neutral lipids extracted from sebocytes and epidermal keratinocytes. Note the enhanced detection of sebocyte-specific lipids including wax esters and squalene. *Source*: From Ref. 31.

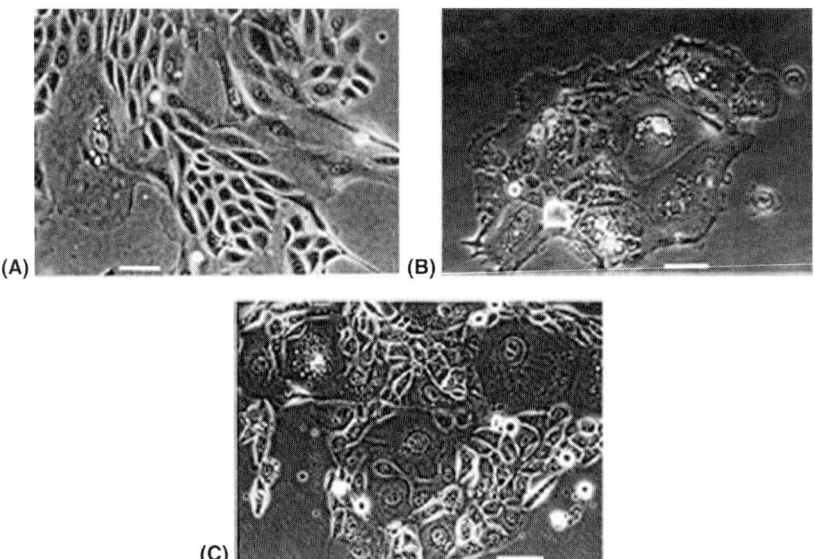

FIGURE 6   Culture of immortalized sebocytes. Human facial sebocytes can be immortalized to retain sebocyte-specific differentiation characteristics by transfection with simian virus-40 large T antigen. The resulting cell line (SZ-95) was further cloned and extensively passaged with no discernible loss of features. (**A**) Preconfluent cultures of human sebocytes prior to transfection. (**B**) First passage of SZ-95 immortalized sebocytes. (**C**) SZ-95 immortalized sebocytes at 50th passage. Note the appearance similar to sebocytes from first passage. *Source*: From Ref. 35.

conversion of all-*trans* to 13-*cis*-retinoic acid was not evident in sebocytes. Both 13-*cis* and all-*trans* retinoic acid suppressed mRNA expression of cytochrome P450-1A2, and in addition, 13-*cis*, all-*trans*, and 9-*cis*-retinoic acid reduced sebocyte proliferation on average by 40% at 10^{-7} M. Retinoids also do not appear to effect the programmed cell death of human sebocytes (40).

In additional studies, Zouboulis et al. (41,42), using nontransfected sebocytes, reported that 13-*cis*-retinoic acid reduced radiolabeled acetate incorporation by 48%, whereas all-*trans* and acitretin only reduced incorporation by 38% and 27%, respectively.

Additional reports using immortalized sebocytes have also been documented to measure expression of steroidal enzymes (43), PPARs, and transcriptional factors (44), in addition to melanocortin receptors and the effects of select interleukins (ILs) (45). Finally, the patent databases are an excellent source of reviewing intellectual property on sebum suppressive technologies.

Rat Preputial Sebocyte Monolayer Culture

The rodent preputial gland has also been used as a model for the human sebaceous gland. These specialized glands open to the surface on either side of the urethral meatus, and secretions are involved in territorial marking and mating behavior (46).

Using techniques similar to that used with human sebaceous glands, rat preputial glands can be isolated, digested, and cultured upon a fibroblast feeder layer to produce monolayer cultures (47,48) that can be manipulated and studied. Rosenfield (49) reported on the relationship of sebaceous cell stage with growth in culture in that fully differentiated sebocytes are not capable of attachment and proliferation, whereas early differentiated cells are. Subsequent studies by Laurent et al. (48) documented the requirement of serum and growth factors to enhance growth and that preputial sebocytes also expressed cytokeratin-4 and formed fewer cornified envelopes than keratinocytes. The effects of estrogen on preputial cell behavior (50) and characterization of the cultured cells (51,52) along with the mechanism of androgen action (53) and effects of PPARs (54) have also been reported.

Preputial cells differentiate in a similar process, but to an overall lesser extent than human sebocytes even in the presence of androgens (Fig. 7). Rosenfield et al. (55) discovered that preputial cells cultured in vitro lack the presence of PPAR ligands that will induce lipid droplet formation. The effect of PPAR ligands was found to be distinct and additive to the effect seen with androgens in increasing lipid droplet formation.

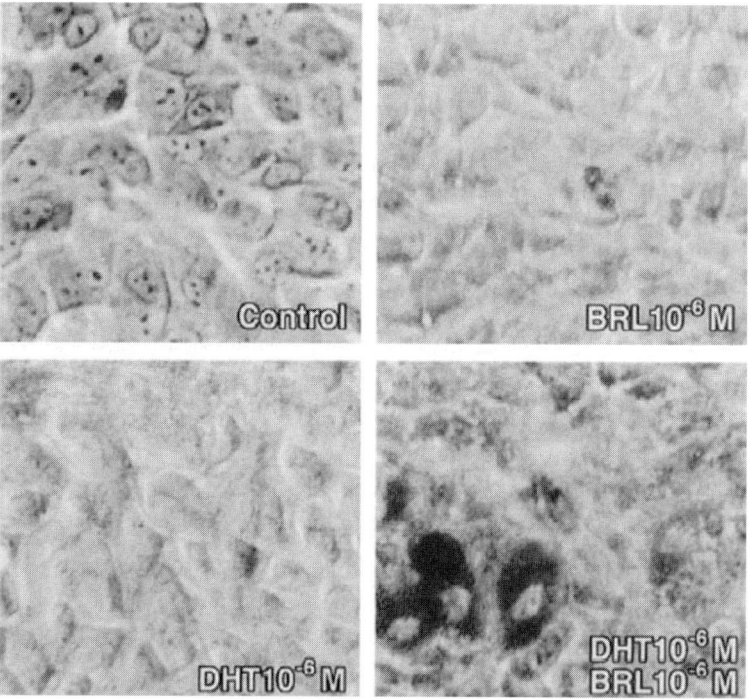

FIGURE 7 Differentiation of preputial sebocytes. Preputial sebocytes can be cultured in vitro with 3T3-fibroblast support. Differentiated sebocytes containing lipids are positively identified via staining with oil red O. (*Top left*): Oil red O staining of preputial sebocytes cultured in vitro for nine days in which 11% of the culture has differentiated into lipid-forming colonies. (*Lower left*): Oil red O staining of preputial sebocytes cultured in the presence of 10^{-6} M dihydrotestosterone (DHT) in which 25% of the culture has differentiated into lipid-forming colonies. (*Top right*): Oil red O staining of preputial sebocytes cultured in the presence of 10^{-6} M peroxisome proliferator activated receptor γ ligand BRL-49653 in which 66% of the culture has differentiated into lipid-forming colonies. (*Lower right*): Oil red O staining of preputial sebocytes cultured in the presence of 10^{-6} M DHT and BRL-49653 in which 80% of the culture has differentiated into lipid-forming colonies. *Abbreviation*: DHT, dihydrotestosterone. *Source*: From Ref. 53.

Kim et al. (56), furthermore, investigated the effect of retinoids on preputial cell growth and differentiation. All-*trans* retinoic acid and retinoic acid receptor agonists resulted in a decrease in cell number, colony size, and number of lipid-forming colonies. Kim concluded that retinoic acid receptors and retinoid-X-receptors play select roles in sebocyte proliferation and differentiation.

Other In Vitro Sebaceous-Cell-Based Models

Animal models such as the hamster flank organ and hamster ear have been developed to study the effects of anti-acne and sebum-suppressive capabilities of compounds and formulations in vivo. Following application, the target areas are excised, weighed, and processed for histological examination. In other animal models, monitoring of sebum secretions follows intravenous or oral administration of sebum-suppressive agents.

The hamster auricle sebaceous gland has been successfully cultured and utilized as a model for human sebaceous glands. Glands are isolated and cells are grown on a 3T3 fibroblast-feeder layer using standard protocols. Ito et al. (57), Sato et al. (58), and Akimoto et al. (59) have reported that the amount of lipid produced increases following the peak of sebocyte proliferation and that androgens stimulate, whereas retinoic acid, EGF, and vitamin D_3 suppress overall activity.

EVALUATION OF TECHNOLOGIES TARGETING THE PILOSEBACEOUS DUCT

The pilosebaceous duct is lined by a stratified, squamous epithelium, and consists of keratinocytes that undergo a similar, but distinct, terminal differentiation process compared to the keratinocytes that comprise the interfollicular epidermis. The upper fifth of the duct is identical to the interfollicular portion; however, the remaining portion, the infrainfundibulum, is histologically different. In the infrainfundibulum, the granular layer is frequently absent and the keratinocytes contain a tremendous amount of glycogen. In addition, the stratum corneum is only two to three layers thick and will desquamate into the central part of the pilosebaceous duct where mixing with sebum and bacteria occurs (1).

Ductal hypercornification results initially in the formation of microcomedones, eventually leading to the production of a comedonal lesion resulting from the accumulation of corneocytes in the pilosebaceous duct. This is believed to be the result of enhanced keratinocyte proliferation, enhanced desquamation, inadequate squame separation, or a combination of factors thereof. Individuals with acne have more cornified material in their ducts when compared with control subjects (60).

Organ Culture of the Infrainfundibulum

Keratinocyte cell culture of the interfollicular epidermis is well-established, and procedures are available to expand cell populations in serum containing and serum-free medium in the presence and absence of fibroblast-feeder support (61–63). In addition, three-dimensional models are also well-characterized to simulate a living skin equivalent. Using these models, it is possible to monitor the cultures to examine the effects on keratinocyte proliferation and differentiation using a variety of end-point markers.

In contrast, the culture of the infrainfundibulum is less established and only one laboratory has reported on the use of the infundibula as a model for acne (64–66). Using a procedure similar to that used for isolating sebaceous glands, pilosebaceous ducts can be isolated by micro-dissection of keratomed layers of skin. Interestingly, it was found that only subjects with high rates of sebum secretion contained pilosebaceous ducts large enough for positive identification and isolation.

Isolated infundibula have been successfully cultured in serum-free medium containing essential growth factors for up to seven days (66). During this culture period, morphology of the duct is retained, although desquamated corneocytes are not eliminated via the follicular canal (Fig. 8). Rather, the keratinocytes/corneocytes accumulate in the lumen, whereas the keratinocytes express markers consistent with those found in the basal and suprabasal layers.

In the presence of 1 *ng*/mL of IL-1α, the infundibula were found to hypercornify resulting in a darkly stained appearance (Fig. 8). The resulting scaling was histologically similar to the changes seen in a comedonal lesion in vivo and addition of an excessive amount of IL-1α receptor blocker prevented this hypercornification process from occurring. This is of note, as IL-1α is found in high concentrations in open comedones (67–69). The addition of 5 *ng*/mL EGF or transforming

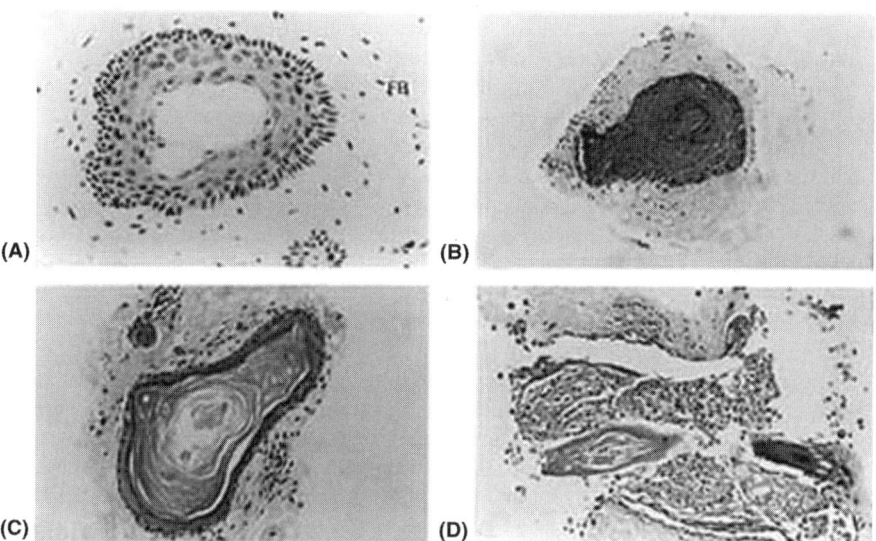

FIGURE 8 Cross-sections of infundibula isolated and maintained in vitro. Infundibula from human pilosebaceous follicles can be isolated and cultured in vitro with retention of viability and architecture as a model for acne. (**A**) Freshly isolated infundibulum depicting stratified squamous epithelium with dispersed fibroblasts in dermal portion. (**B**) Infundibulum maintained in vitro for seven days depicting visible stratum granulosum and stratum corneum in the central regions. (**C**) Infundibulum maintained in vitro for seven days in the presence of 1 *ng*/mL Il-1α depicting scaling phenotype in central lumen. (**D**) Infundibulum maintained in vitro for seven days in the presence of 5 *ng*/mL epidermal growth factor depicting loss of architecture. *Source*: From Ref. 66.

growth factor-α resulted in a disorganized appearance of infundibular morphology, although individual cellular integrity was retained. Looking at the retinoids, 13-*cis*-retinoic acid (1 µM) supplemented into the medium resulted in a significant fall in the rate of DNA synthesis after seven days maintenance which can be interpreted as an inhibition of new ductal cell growth.

In a subsequent report, the effects of inflammatory cytokines on the infundibulum were evaluated. The addition of 100 U of interferon-γ, 10 ng/mL of tumor necrosis factor-α or 10 ng/mL IL-6 resulted in the expression of intercellular adhesion molecule-1 which was not seen with IL-1α treatment.

Although the organ culture of the infundibulum suffers from the same constraints as sebaceous gland organ culture, the advantages over keratinocyte monolayer culture lend support as an additional model for the understanding and treatment of acne.

As previously mentioned, keratinocyte cell culture procedures are well-established and it is beyond the scope of this chapter to disclose the numerous references related to epidermal biology. However, the use of keratinocyte monolayer models in further understanding acne is reported in subsequent areas of this review.

EVALUATION OF TECHNOLOGIES TARGETING ENZYMES INVOLVED IN ANDROGEN METABOLISM AND LIPID SYNTHESIS
Enzyme Assays for In Vitro Androgen Metabolism

Human skin is a collection of androgen-responsive tissues, which have been recognized to contain a wide variety of enzymes capable of metabolizing topically applied drugs and endogenous substrates supplied by the body.

One of the most important classes of hormones affecting the pilosebaceous appendage, and more specifically the sebaceous glands, is the sex steroids secreted by the testes and ovaries in response to pituitary gonadotrophic hormones (70). In general, androgens stimulate sebaceous gland activity, whereas estrogens have a suppressive function (70,71). Androgens are the best-known stimulators of the sebaceous glands, and are responsible for the development and enlargement of the glands that occur at puberty (72). Castration results in sebaceous gland atrophy accompanied by an overall decrease in sebum production (73). The most effective androgens possess a 17β-hydroxyl group that includes testosterone, 5α-DHT, 5α-androstene-3β, and 17β-diol.

The enzymes involved in androgen metabolism in follicles that have been identified using biochemical and histological techniques include 3β-hydroxysteroid dehydrogenase (3β-HSD), 17β-HSD, and 5α-reductase. A schematic diagram of the pathways of cutaneous androgen metabolism and the converting enzymes involved has been effectively conveyed by Chen et al. (74) in Figure 9.

The reduction of testosterone to DHT by the enzyme 5α-reductase is one of the most important reactions involved in androgen metabolism. DHT is a more potent androgen than testosterone due to its greater affinity for the androgen receptor and enhanced stability. DHT is generally considered responsible for increased sebum production, as increased local formation of DHT has been documented in acne (75) and by increasing the size of the sebaceous gland (73). Two subtypes of 5α-reductase have been identified.

The Type I isozyme has an optimal pH of 6 to 9 and has been found localized in skin from the scalp, chest, dermal papilla, and sebaceous gland regions (76).

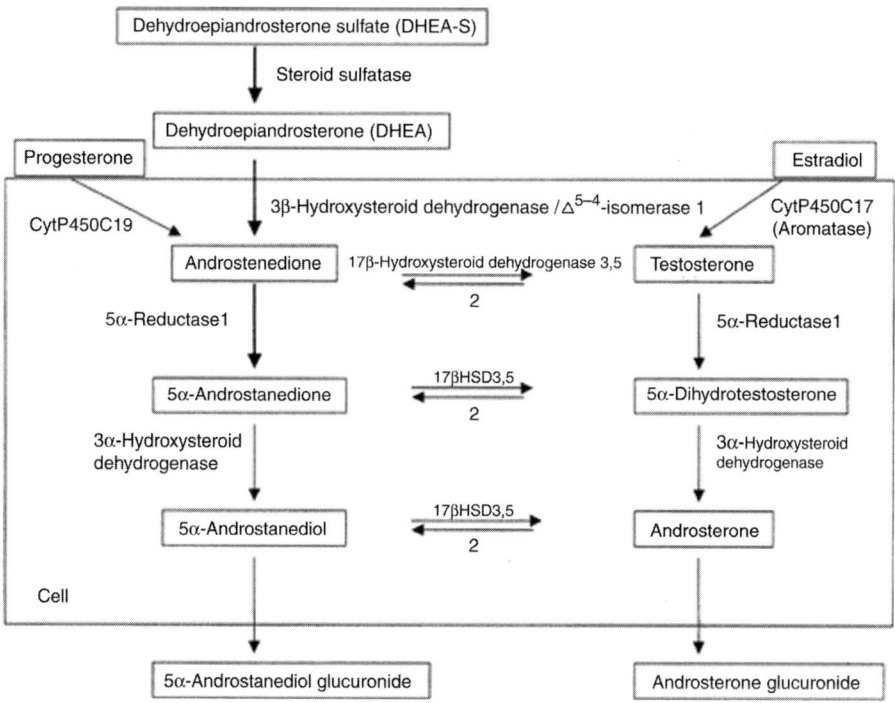

FIGURE 9 Pathways of cutaneous androgen metabolism and the converting enzymes. *Abbreviations*: DHEAS, dehydroepiandrosterone sulfate; 17β-HSD, 17β-hydroxysteroid dehydrogenase. *Source*: From Ref. 74.

Activity was found to be greater in acne-bearing facial skin and in sebaceous glands than in other cells of similar location. Activity was also higher in glands in the facial region than glands in other bodily regions. In a subsequent study (77), keratinocytes cultured from the infrainfundibulum demonstrated greater 5α-reductase activity than those obtained from the interfollicular epidermis. Overall activity was highest in the sebaceous gland followed by the duct, infrainfundibulum, and lastly the epidermis. Acne-bearing skin was found to produce 2 to 20 times more DHT than normal skin, and facial skin produced more DHT than normal back skin.

The Type II isozyme has an acidic pH optimum and is present in the epididymis, seminal vesicles, prostate, and the inner root sheath of the terminal hair follicle (78).

Specific target assays for 5α-reductase are problematic in nature as the enzyme is difficult to extract and the substrate testosterone is water insoluble. Nonetheless, several assays are available to monitor androgen metabolism in cell/tissue homogenates or in living cell/tissue culture systems. The enzymatic assay for conversion of testosterone to DHT involves adding testosterone (usually radiolabeled) together with a cell or tissue homogenate in the presence of NADPH. Inhibitors can be added and after a set period of time, the steroids formed are isolated and separated either by TLC, HPLC, or GC (79).

Complementary to using skin homogenates, activity of enzymes involved in androgen modulation can be assessed using cell monolayer cultures and living skin equivalents. Although keratinocyte methods for cultivation of each are well-established, cell culture may be of limited use for evaluating water-insoluble compounds or formulations. For the latter, the use of a reconstituted three-dimensional living skin model has been reported by Bernard et al. (80) and Slivka (81).

Harris et al. (82) reported on the expression of 5α-reductase in COS cells, whereas Sugimoto et al. (83) constructed 5α-reductase expression vectors that were transfected into a human adrenal carcinoma cell line. Type I 5α-reductase was strongly inhibited by the chloride salts of cadmium, copper, and zinc (inhibition constant or K_i less than 5 μM), moderately by nickel and iron (K_i less than 250 μM), and no inhibition by manganese, magnesium, calcium, or lithium. Only the Type II isozyme was inhibited by copper at 11 μM. Additionally, minimal effects were seen when the chloride counter ion of zinc was replaced with sulfate, chloride, or acetate, with acetate being the least effective.

In general, 5α-reductase inhibitors are classified into two categories: steroidal and nonsteroidal, and there is very little overlap in efficacy between the two different isozymes. In fact, many of the Type II inhibitors have little to no effect on sebum production in vivo. This is possibly the result because the two enzymes have only 50% homology in amino acid sequences. The gene for Type I isozyme is located on chromosome 5, whereas the gene for Type II isozyme is located on chromosome 2 (84).

Using foreskin keratinocytes (85), testosterone was utilized as a substrate in the production of 5α-reduced metabolites including DHT (5α-reductase), androstenedione (17β-HSD Type II), androsterone, and androstanediol (3α-HSD activity). A similar pattern was reported with fibroblasts, although scalp skin fibroblasts metabolized testosterone only to a limited extent. Using cultured keratinocytes obtained from the infrainfundibulum and epidermis (86), Thiboutot et al. found that mean enzyme activities were slightly higher in the acne group, but not statistically different from the control group. Overall activity was greatest in the infrainfundibulum.

Altenburger and Kissel (87) cultured the human keratinocyte cell line HaCaT as a model to express the enzyme systems involved in testosterone metabolism, which were subsequently identified by LC/MS. HaCaT cells were found to predominantly express the Subtype I isoform of 5α-reductase. Similar studies have been reported utilizing keratinocyte cultures derived from breast skin (88), in cultured fibroblasts (89), and living skin equivalents (90).

Assays for the Rate-Limiting Enzymes Involved in Cholesterol and Fatty Acid Synthesis

In the formation of squalene and cholesterol, 3-hydroxy-3-methylglutaryl-coenzyme A (HMG-CoA) is the rate-limiting enzyme involved in the cholesterol synthesis pathway. As reported by Shapiro et al. (91) and Smythe et al. (92), radiolabeled HMG-CoA is added to skin homogenates containing NADP (as a necessary cofactor) along with glucose-6-phosphate and glucose-6-phosphate dehydrogenase to form radiolabeled mevalonate. The reaction then involves a spontaneous conversion of mevalonate to mevalonolactone, which can then be separated by TLC and quantified.

Using this assay with isolated sebaceous gland homogenates, Smythe et al. (92) reported that HMG-CoA activity decreased with subject age, and enzyme activity was inactivated via phosphorylation.

In the study of fatty acid synthesis, acetyl-coenzyme A carboxylase (acetyl-CoA) has been identified as a rate-limiting step. This assay involves adding radio-labeled bicarbonate to skin homogenates in the presence of ATP and acetyl-CoA. Total radioactivity incorporated is then quantified via direct scintillation counting.

All of the enzyme assays described are amenable for high throughput screening to assess compounds that may modulate lipid synthesis.

EVALUATION OF TECHNOLOGIES TARGETING THE RESIDENTIAL MICROBIAL FLORA

It is not clear why *P. acnes, S. epidermidis,* and other microbes colonize sebaceous follicles and why no correlation is evident between the *P. acnes* population and the acne grade of the subjects in question (93), but antimicrobial therapy provides excellent clinical relief, especially for inflamed lesions.

Proprionibacterium acnes is an anaerobic, pleomorphic diphtheroid bacillus that produces propionic and acetic acids during normal metabolism. These and other bacteria also produce biologically active extracellular products including phosphatases, hyaluronidase, proteases, and neuraminidase, all of which may increase the permeability of the follicular epithelium. Bacteria can also produce low molecular weight chemotactic factors that can recruit polymorphonuclear leukocytes. In the process of phagocytosis of bacteria, hydrolases are liberated, which further disrupts the integrity of the wall (94). *Proprionibacterium acnes* can also stimulate both the classic and alternative pathways of complement activation, leading to the production of neutrophil chemotactic factors, which attract additional leukocytes resulting in further inflammation (95).

An antimicrobial agent is a chemical that kills or inhibits the growth of bacteria and other microbes. Agents that kill bacteria are bactericidal, whereas those that do not kill but only inhibit further growth are known as bacteriostatic. Many compounds are both bacteriostatic and bactericidal depending on the concentration being tested. Additionally, compounds may be bacteriolytic in which agents induce death by cellular lysis. An example of a bacteriolytic agent is the antibiotic penicillin. In general, antimicrobial agents should be selected on the basis of targeting specific cell types such as bacteria instead of mammalian cells that can be tested in vitro by confirmation in keratinocyte or fibroblast monolayer cultures.

Antimicrobial activity is measured by determining the smallest amount of an agent that will inhibit the growth of a specific organism otherwise known as the minimum inhibitory concentration (MIC). Two methods are commonly utilized to determine the MIC for a particular agent: the tube dilution technique and the agar diffusion method.

Test Tube Method (Tube Dilution Technique)
A series of culture tubes containing microbial growth medium with varying levels of the test compound are inoculated and incubated. A culture tube in which growth does not occur is evident by an absence of turbidity. This is an estimate as variables such as pH, oxygen level, temperature, and inoculum size can modulate the effect.

Agar Diffusion Method
Petri plates containing an agar medium are evenly inoculated with the antimicrobial agent. Known amounts of the antimicrobial agents are added to filter

paper discs, which are then placed in contact with the surface of the agar. During incubation, the test compound will diffuse from the filter paper into the agar and a zone of inhibition will be created indicating the overall potency of the test compound.

EVALUATION OF TECHNOLOGIES TARGETING IRRITATION AND INFLAMMATION

Skin irritation is the culmination of a complex inflammatory process involving epidermal keratinocytes, dermal fibroblasts, endothelial cells, and invading leukocytes in which early symptoms may consist of swelling, redness, and itching continuing to scaling and erythema (96). Histologically, irritation involves both the epidermis and dermis with inflammatory infiltrates entering from the microvasculature and chemical mediators being released by a variety of cell types inhabiting the area.

The major function of the keratinocytes is not only to provide a barrier and structural integrity of the pilosebaceous follicle, but also to play a pivotal role in the inflammatory process through the release/response to surrounding cytokines. On the other hand, the central role of bacteria in acne is to incite inflammation (97). Cytotoxins are compounds that stimulate chemotactic activity and are produced by *P. acnes* and other microbes within the follicle, which diffuse through the follicular wall and attract neutrophils (98). These chemical mediators can then go on to activate macrophages, neutrophils, natural killer cells, and other cells inducing the production of additional cytokines. Important mediators of inflammation include histamine, leukotrienes, interleukins, prostaglandins, and neuropeptides. Neutrophils then produce enzymes and generate free oxygen radicals that will result in disruption of the follicle. Inflamed papules, pustules, and nodules develop when comedones rupture and extrude their contents into the dermis rather than onto the surface of the skin.

The standard approach for assessing skin irritation is based on the Draize method (99), which involves applying a single dose of test material to shaved albino rabbits. The formation of an erythema response is determined by visual inspection of the skin over a set time course after removal of the patch. Over the last 60 years, many laboratories have developed in vitro models for a substitute of the Draize method with variable success. These models are based on in vitro monolayer culture of fibroblasts or keratinocytes or construction of a three-dimensional living skin equivalent.

Cell Cytotoxicity Assays

Monolayer cultures of epithelial cells are usually used as the first in vitro screen for the evaluation of toxicity and inflammatory potential of agents. There are several types of assays available that can be used with keratinocyte and fibroblast monolayer cultures, which differ in their end-point measurement. In general, cells are treated with test compounds during the active proliferation stage in which cytotoxicity can be readily detected.

Neutral Red Uptake Assay
Neutral red is a nontoxic dye selectively retained by lysosomes of living cells. A good correlation has been found between the amount of neutral red retained and

the overall viability of the culture. The assay is limited to a neutral pH but can measure inhibitors over a wide range of concentrations (100,101).

Trypan Blue Assay
Cells with intact membranes exclude the dye trypan blue and remain uncolored, whereas cells with damaged membranes allow the dye to penetrate and be retained. Trypan blue is normally an "all or none" response in that partially damaged cells may not retain the blue color (101,102).

MTT Assay
The dye MTT [3-(4,5-dimethylthiazol-2-yl)-2,5-diphenyl tetrazolium bromide] is converted from the oxidized to the reduced form by an NADP-dependent reaction catalyzed by succinate dehydrogenase. In the oxidized form, MTT is yellow and turns blue/black upon reduction (103,104). This reaction is dependent upon overall mitochondrial activity and agents that increase activity will also increase MTT reduction.

Alamar Blue^{TM}
The Alamar Blue^{TM} assay involves the addition of a fluorogenic redox indicator to growing cells in culture. The oxidized form of Alamar Blue^{TM} has minimal fluorescence; however, upon entering living cells, the dye becomes reduced and turns bright red (105). Fluorescence is measured at 530/590 nm (excitation/emission) and is a direct reflection of cell viability.

Release of Cytosolic Enzymes
Lactate dehydrogenase is released into the culture medium in the later stages of cell death. The reaction is based on the conversion of pyruvate to lactate and is measured at 340 nm (101).

Three-Dimensional Living Skin Equivalents
Current living skin equivalents are the most complex in vitro models available; however, they are also limited in their composition. Although most contain the major skin structural cell types (keratinocytes and fibroblasts) along with dermal matrix components (collagen), they do not contain the other cell types and vascular components which are also important contributors to the skin inflammatory mechanism.

However limited, these models do reproduce many of the characteristics of normal human epidermis. Ponec et al. (106) performed a detailed study on the variability among commercial living skin equivalents. Tissue architecture was examined using light and electron microscopy along with immunohistochemistry for specific markers. High-performance TLC was additionally used to assess lipid composition. Of the three commercially available models examined along with an in-house prepared model, all generated a stratified epidermis, keratohyalin granules, and the formation of a stratum corneum (Fig. 10).

Faller and Bracher (107) determined the reproducibility of irritation responses using three commercially available three-dimensional models along with an in-house model using MTT and measurement of IL-1α as markers. IL-1α is a major inflammatory mediator released by both corneocytes and keratinocytes upon irritant challenge and potentiates further effects in macrophages, neutrophils, and

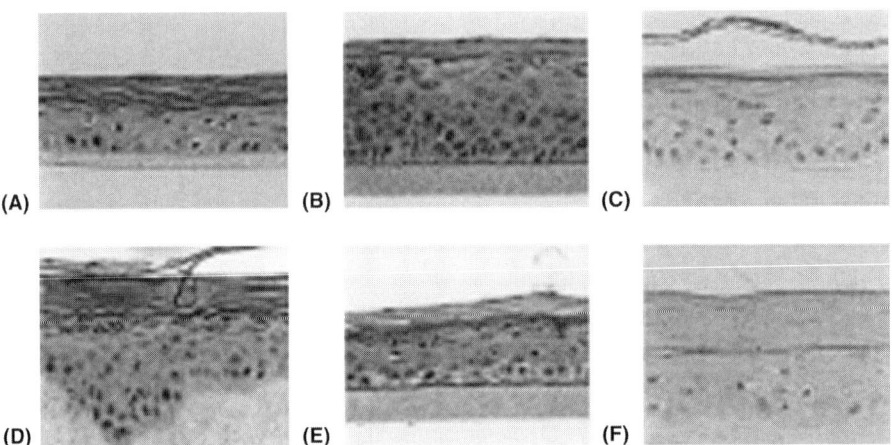

FIGURE 10 Histological appearance of reconstructed skin models. Histological sections of reconstructed skin models in which each demonstrate a stratified epidermis, the presence of keratohyalin granules, and the formation of a stratum corneum. (**A**) Skinethic, (**B**) Epiderm Epid-200-HCF, (**C**) Episkin irritation model, (**D**) reconstructed epidermis on a de-epidermized dermis, (**E**) EpiDerm penetration model, and (**F**) Episkin penetration model. *Source*: From Ref. 106.

fibroblasts. IL-1α is believed to be the active species in the skin and is known to trigger the arachidonic acid cascade that converts arachidonic acid into a variety of inflammatory metabolites (108). For a review of cytokines produced by keratinocytes, see Grone (109). Faller and Bracher (107) found that the models tested had high degrees of variability between different suppliers, especially with regard to the release of IL-1α, although variability among cultures from the same supplier was less.

Sugibayashi et al. (110) examined the kinetics of cytotoxicity by several irritants using in vitro skin equivalents and found that the rate of skin irritation closely mirrored the application concentration, intrinsic toxicity of the agent, and the barrier function of the skin. Other laboratories detailing three-dimensional living skin equivalents have been recently reported by Faller et al. (111), Portes et al. (112), Fentem et al. (113), and Gay et al. (114).

In addition to looking at inflammatory markers, it is important to also assess cellular toxicity, most commonly by measuring leakage of lactate dehydrogenase from keratinocytes and fibroblasts into the surrounding medium. Time course assays are normally performed following application. Examples of use of these models are documented by Lee et al. (115) using cultured human fibroblasts for screening of skin toxicity against surfactants using Neutral red and Alamar blue. Coquette et al. (116) looked at IL-1α and IL-8 expression and release in living skin equivalents for irritation predictability. Bernhofer et al. (117) emphasized the involvement of fibroblasts in modulating inflammatory responses as a result of signals from the keratinocytes.

An immediate response of the skin to irritants is the release of arachidonic acid from keratinocytes followed by subsequent metabolism into pro-inflammatory prostaglandins such as PGE2 (118). This eicosanoid response is induced by a number of irritants including IL-1α (119). Water-soluble extracts of comedones have the ability to induce inflammation in most subjects, whereas insoluble keratinous material will promote inflammation in all subjects (120). Also reported by Puhvel and Sakamoto (121) was that lipids extracted from pooled comedones had chemotactic activity for neutrophils in vitro using an assay monitoring cellular migration on agarose plates. Allaker et al. (122) examined culture supernatants from three *Propionibacterium* species and *S. epidermidis* for smooth muscle contracting compounds as an indicator of inflammatory activity. Webster et al. (123) reported that *P. acnes* stimulated lysosomal release in the presence, but not in the absence, of serum. This stimulatory activity has been shown to be the result of *P. acnes'* ability to activate and induce cytokine production by cells of the mononuclear phagocyte system (124).

SUMMARY AND FURTHER THOUGHTS

The factors involved in the pathogenesis of acne are depicted in Figure 11 (125), and although the remission of acne remains a mystery (125,126), several technologies have been developed for the topical control of acne identified through single in vitro assays or a combination of different models.

Benzoyl peroxide has been reported to have multiple effects including bacteriostatic activity, mild comedolytic activity, enhancement of local blood flow, and the release of free radical oxygen. Benzoyl peroxide is an organic peroxide that is bactericidal against *P. acnes* along with additional anti-inflammatory activity (127). There is a wide range of antimicrobial activity against multiple species and resistance does not occur. Hegemann et al. (127) investigated the release of reactive oxygen species regulated by protein kinase C (PKC) and calmodulin from human neutrophils; although benzoyl peroxide inhibited PKC activity (IC_{50} of 1.35 mM), there was no activity against calmodulin, suggesting that the

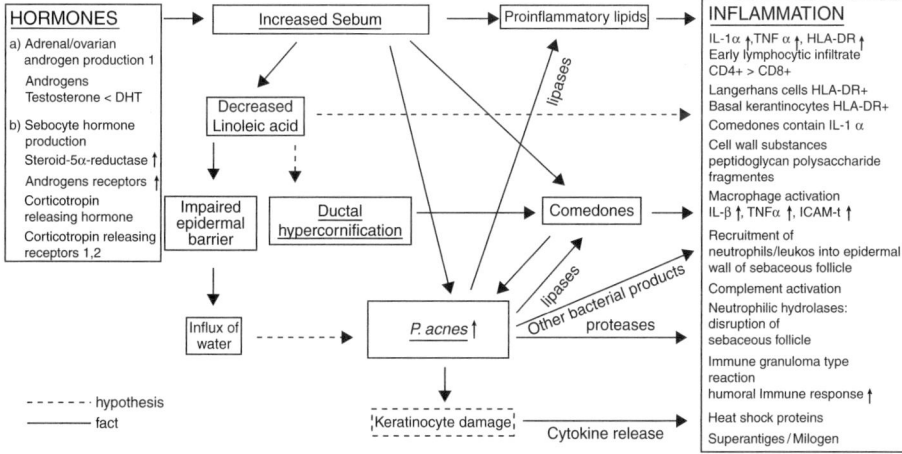

FIGURE 11 Synopsis of factors involved in the pathogenesis of acne. Factors involved in the pathogenesis of acne are increased sebum production, ductal cornification, bacterial colonization, and inflammation. *Abbreviations*: HLA-DR, human leukocyte antigen-D related; ICAM, intercellular adhesion molecule; IL, interleukin; TNF, tumor necrosis factor. *Source*: From Ref. 125.

anti-inflammatory activity of benzoyl peroxide was not mediated by PKC or calmodulin.

Babich et al. (128) used a human keratinocyte cell line to evaluate the cytotoxicity of benzoyl peroxide. As determined by uptake of Neutral red, irreversible cell death was evident after a one-hour exposure to 0.15 mM and greater concentrations of benzoyl peroxide, whereas reductions in proliferation were seen at concentrations from 0.02 to 0.08 mM. Stress and damage as evident by vacuolization and LDH release were seen after four hours at 0.05 mM levels. As a control, the IC_{50} of benzoic acid was 29.5 mM.

Similar degrees of cytotoxicity were found with other organic peroxides suggesting that the cytotoxicity of benzoyl peroxide may be related to the generation of reactive oxidative free radicals. King et al. (129) found that benzoyl peroxide, as a free radical generating compound, acts as a tumor promoter in mouse skin by causing DNA strand breaks and base modifications in cultured murine keratinocytes. Matsui et al. (130) also found that benzoyl peroxide inhibited both human and murine PKC in a cell-free system, although there was no translocation evident from the cytosol to the membrane when tested in cultured human keratinocytes. Other reports investigating the mechanism of action of benzoyl peroxide include Valacchi et al. (131) who examined the depletion of vitamin E and IL-1α gene expression in HaCaT keratinocytes, Burkhart et al. (132) who reported increases in free radical activity in combination with antibiotics, and Lawrence et al. (133) in that benzoyl peroxide interferes with metabolic cooperation with cultured keratinocytes.

Another compound that has been utilized for the topical control of acne is salicylic acid. Salicylic acid reduces inflammation by inhibiting the synthesis of prostaglandins that are generated in inflamed tissues. Salicylic acid also inhibits the conversion of arachidonic acid to PGE2, which is catalyzed by the enzyme cyclooxygenase. Salicylic acid also inhibits comedogenesis by promoting desquamation of the follicular epithelium. Additional agents that have been used to treat acne include sulfur for the treatment of inflammatory acne lesions through keratolysis activity and azelaic acid, a dicarboxylic acid that has both antibacterial and antikeratinizing activity (134,135).

In addition to the models and assays described in this review, other in vitro models have been developed around the hair follicle. Although these models were not developed to look at acne per se, they may be of interest for specific cell types. Blume et al. (136) reported on the monolayer culture of keratinocytes isolated from terminal hair follicles that express glycoproteins during proliferation (gp38) and differentiation (gp80). These glycoproteins are absent in normal interfollicular keratinocytes. Limat and Noser (137) also reported on the serial cultivation of keratinocytes from the outer root sheath of hair follicles.

Lenoir-Viale et al. (138) documented the effects of retinoic acid on an in vitro model reconstructed from the outer root sheath of human hair follicles, whereas Hoeller et al. (139) divulged an improved method on the construction of in vitro skin equivalents from human hair follicles and fibroblasts. Additionally, Michel et al. (140) has developed a tissue-engineered human skin equivalent containing hair follicles.

The in situ organ culture of the entire pilosebaceous appendage has further been developed by Kealey's laboratory to monitor hair growth. This model appears to be the most complex, as it contains the entire follicle including the sebaceous gland (141–143).

Katz and Taichman (144) reported on the development of a two-chamber culture model in which proteins secreted by keratinocytes could be isolated and characterized. In this model, a fully differentiated keratinocyte epithelium is grown on plastic inserts apart from fibroblasts in the lower chamber.

In conclusion, multiple in vitro models are available for the identification of technologies to alleviate or prevent the formation of acne lesions. By using these models, it is possible to determine the mechanism of action of lead candidates.

REFERENCES

1. Kligman AM. An overview of acne. J Invest Dermatol 1974; 62:268–287.
2. Stewart ME, Downing DT. Chemistry and function of mammalian sebaceous lipids. Adv Lipid Res 1991; 24:263–301.
3. Epstein EH, Epstein WL. New cell formation in human sebaceous glands. J Invest Dermatol 1966; 46:453–458.
4. Plewig G, Christophers E, Braun-Falco O. Proliferative cells in the human sebaceous gland: labeling index and regional variations. Acta Derm 1971; 51:413–422.
5. Tosti A. A comparison of the histodynamics of sebaceous glands and epidermis in man: a microanatomic and morphometric study. J Invest Dermatol 1974; 62:147–152.
6. Downing DT, Strauss JS. On the mechanism of sebaceous secretion. Arch Dermatol Res 1982; 272: 343–349.
7. Nicolaides N, Wells GC. On the biogenesis of the free fatty acids in human skin surface fat. J Invest Dermatol 1957; 29: 423–433.
8. Freinkel RK. Origins of free fatty acids in sebum I: the role of coagulase negative staphylococci. J Invest Dermatol 1968; 50:186–188.
9. Marples RR, Kligman AM, Lantis LR, et al. The role of the aerobic microflora in the genesis of fatty acids in human surface lipids. J Invest Dermatol 1970; 55:173–178.
10. Hay JB, Hodgkins MN. Distribution of androgen metabolizing enzymes in isolated tissues of human forehead and axillary skin. J Endocrinol 1978; 79:29–39.
11. Kealey T, Lee CM, Thody AJ, et al. The isolation of human sebaceous glands and apocrine sweat glands by shearing. Br J Dermatol 1986; 114:181–188.
12. Ridden J, Ferguson D, Kealey T. Organ maintenance of human sebaceous glands: in vitro effects of 13-cis retinoic acid and testosterone. J Cell Sci 1990; 95:125–136.
13. Cooper MF, McGrath H, Shuster, S. Sebaceous lipogenesis in human skin. Br J Dermatol 1976; 94:165–172.
14. Downie MMT, Kealey T. Lipogenesis in the human sebaceous gland: glycogen and glycerophosphate are substrates for the synthesis of sebum lipids. J Invest Dermatol 1998; 111:199–205.
15. Middleton B, Birdi I, Heffron M, et al. The substrate determines the rate and patterns of neutral lipid synthesized by isolated human sebaceous glands. FEBS Lett 1988; 231:59–61.
16. Cassidy DM, Lee CM, Laker MF, et al. Lipogenesis in isolated human sebaceous glands. FEBS Lett 1986; 200:173–176.
17. Pappas A, Anthonavage M, Gordon JS. Metabolic fate and selective utilization of major fatty acids in human sebaceous gland. J Invest Dermatol 2002; 118:164–171.
18. Guy R, Ridden C, Kealey T. The improved organ maintenance of the human sebaceous gland: modeling in vitro the effects of epidermal growth factor, androgens, estrogens, 13-cis retinoic acid, and phenol red. J Invest Dermatol 1996; 106:454–460.
19. Guy R, Kealey T. The organ-maintained human sebaceous gland. Dermatology 1998; 196:16–20.
20. Downie MMT, Sanders DA, Maier LM, et al. Do PPARs have a Regulatory Function in the Human Sebaceous Gland? Keystone Symposia: The PPARs—A Transcription Odyssey, 2001.

21. Downie MMT, Sanders DA, Stock DM, et al. The PPAR ligands ETYA, WY 14643, LY 171883, clofibrate, BRL 49653 and prostaglandin J2 inhibit sebaceous lipogenesis whereas the PPAR ligand bezafibrate is ineffective (abstr). J Invest Dermatol 2000; 115:552.

22. Toyoda M, Morohashi M. Pathogenesis of acne. Med Electron Microsc 2001; 34:29–40.

23. Lajtha LG. Stem cell concepts. Differentiation 1979; 14:23–24.

24. Cotsarelis G, Sun TT, Lavker RL. Label retaining cells reside in the bulge area of pilosebaceous unit: implications for follicular stem cells, hair cycle and skin carcinogenesis. Cell 1990; 61:1329–1337.

25. Lavker RM, Miller S, Wilson C, et al. Hair follicle stem cells: their location, role in hair cycle, and involvement in skin tumor formation. J Invest Dermatol 1993; 101:16s–26s.

26. Lavker RM, Sun TT, Oshima H, et al. Hair follicle stem cells. J Invest Dermatol Symp Proc 2003; 8:28–38.

27. Xia L, Zouboulis C, Detmar M, et al. Isolation of human sebaceous glands and cultivation of sebaceous gland-derived cells as an in vitro model. J Invest Dermatol 1989; 93:315–321.

28. Zouboulis CC, Xia L, Detmar M, et al. Culture of human sebocytes and markers of sebocytic differentiation in vitro. Skin Pharmacol 1991; 4:74–83.

29. Yang JS, Lavker RM, Sun TT. Upper human hair follicle contains a subpopulation of keratinocytes with superior in vitro proliferative potential. J Invest Dermatol 1993; 101:652–659.

30. Doran TI, Baff R, Jacobs P, et al. Characterization of human sebaceous cells in vitro. J Invest Dermatol 1991; 96:341–348.

31. Fujie T, Shikji T, Uchida N, et al. Culture of cells derived from the human sebaceous gland under serum-free conditions without a biological feeder layer or specific matrices. Arch Dermatol Res 1995; 288:703–708.

32. Zouboulis CC, Akamatsu H, Stephanek K, et al. Androgens affect the activity of human sebocytes in culture in a manner dependent on the localization of the sebaceous glands and their effect is antagonized by spironolactone. Skin Pharmacol 1994; 7:33–40.

33. Akamatsu H, Zouboulis CC, Orfanos CE. Control of human sebocyte proliferation in vitro by testosterone and 5-alpha-dihydrotestosterone is dependent on the localization of the sebaceous glands. J Invest Dermatol 1992; 99:509–511.

34. Bajor JS, Siegel DM, Kleinberg I, et al. The in vitro proliferative potential of the human sebocyte (abstr). J Invest Dermatol 1994; 102:564.

35. Zouboulis CC, Seltmann H, Neitzel H, et al. Establishment and characteristics of an immortalized human sebaceous cell line (SZ95). J Invest Dermatol 1999; 113:1011–1020.

36. Messina M, Manieri C, Rizzi G, et al. A new therapeutic approach to acne: an antiandrogen percutaneous treatment with spironolactone. Curr Ther Res 1983; 34:319–324.

37. Muhlemann MF, Carter GD, Cream JJ, et al. Oral spironolactone: an effective treatment for acne vulgaris in women. Br J Dermatol 1986; 115:227–232.

38. Fritsch M, Orfanos CE, Zouboulis CC. Sebocytes are the key regulators of androgen homeostasis in human skin. J Invest Dermatol 2001; 116:793–800.

39. Tsukada M, Schroder M, Roos TC, et al. 13-*cis* retinoic acid exerts its specific activity on human sebocytes through selective intracellular isomerization to all-*trans* retinoic acid and binding to retinoid acid receptors. J Invest Dermatol 2000; 115:321–327.

40. Wrobel A, Seltmann H, Fimmel S, et al. Differentiation and apoptosis in human immortalized sebocytes. J Invest Dermatol 2003; 120:175–181.

41. Zouboulis CC, Korge B, Akamatsu H, et al. Effects of 13-*cis*-retinoic acid, all-*trans*-retinoic acid, and acitretin on the proliferation, lipid synthesis and keratin expression of cultured human sebocytes in vitro. J Invest Dermatol 1991; 96:792–797.

42. Zouboulis CC, Xia L, Korge B, et al. Cultivation of Human Sebocytes *In Vitro*: Cell Characterization and Influence of Synthetic Retinoids. Retinoids: 10 Years on. Basel: Karger. 1991:254–273.

43. Thiboutot D, Jabara S, McAllister JM, et al. Human skin is a steroidogenic tissue: steroidogenic enzymes and cofactors are expressed in epidermis, normal

sebocytes, and an immortalized sebocyte cell line (SEB-1). J Invest Dermatol 2003; 120:905–914.

44. Chen W, Yang CC, Sheu HM, et al. Expression of peroxisome proliferator-activated receptor and CCAAT/enhancer binding protein transcription factors in cultured human sebocytes. J Invest Dermatol 2003; 121:441–447.
45. Bohm M, Schiller M, Stander S, et al. Evidence for expression of melanocortin-1 receptor in human sebocytes *in vitro* and *in situ*. J Invest Dermatol 2002; 118:533–539.
46. Deplewski D, Rosenfield R. Role of hormones in pilosebaceous unit development. Endocr Rev 2000; 21:363–392.
47. Potter JER, Prutkin L, Wheatley VR. Sebaceous gland differentiation. I: separation, morphology and lipogenesis of isolated cells from the mouse preputial gland tumor. J Invest Dermatol 1979; 72:120–127.
48. Laurent SJ, Mednieks MI, Rosenfield RL. Growth of sebaceous cells in monolayer culture. In Vitro Cell Dev Biol 1992; 28A:83–89.
49. Rosenfield RL. Relationship of sebaceous cell stage to growth in culture. J Invest Dermatol 1989; 92:751–754.
50. Alves AM, Thody AJ, Fisher C, et al. Measurement of lipogenesis in isolated preputial gland cells of the rat and the effect of oestrogen. J Endocrinol 1986; 109:1–7.
51. Wheatley VR, Potter JER, Lew G. Sebaceous gland differentiation. II: the isolation, separation and characterization of cells from the mouse preputial gland tumor. J Invest Dermatol 1979; 73:291–296.
52. Wheatley VR, Brind JL. Sebaceous gland differentiation. III: the uses and limitations of freshly isolated mouse preputial gland cells for the in vitro study of hormone and drug action. J Invest Dermatol 1981; 76:293–296.
53. Rosenfield RL, Deplewski D, Kentsis A, et al. Mechanism of androgen induction of sebocyte differentiation. Dermatology 1998; 196:43–46.
54. Rosenfield RL, Deplewski D, Greene ME. Peroxisome proliferator-activated receptors and skin development. Horm Res 2000; 54:269–274.
55. Rosenfield R, Kentsis A, Deplewski D, et al. Rat preputial sebocyte differentiation involves peroxisome proliferator-activated receptors. J Invest Dermatol 1999; 112:226–232.
56. Kim MJ, Ciletti N, Michel S, et al. The role of specific retinoid receptors in sebocyte growth and differentiation in culture. J Invest Dermatol 2000; 114:349–353.
57. Ito A, Sakiguchi T, Kitamura K, et al. Establishment of a tissue culture system for hamster sebaceous gland cells. Dermatology 1998; 197:238–244.
58. Sato T, Imai N, Akimoto N, et al. Epidermal growth factor and 1α,25-dihydroxyvitamin D3 suppress lipogenesis in hamster sebaceous gland cells in vitro. J Invest Dermatol 2001; 117:965–970.
59. Akimoto N, Sato T, Sakiguchi T, et al. Cell proliferation and lipid formation in hamster sebaceous gland cells. Dermatology 2002; 204:118–123.
60. Holmes RL, Williams M, Cunliffe WJ. Pilosebaceous duct obstruction and acne. Br J Dermatol 1972; 87:327–332.
61. Rheinwald JG, Green H. Serial cultivation of strains of human epidermal keratinocytes: the formation of keratinizing colonies from single cells. Cell 1975; 6:331–334.
62. Randolph RK, Simon M. Characterization of retinol metabolism in cultured human epidermal keratinocytes. J Biol Chem 1993; 268:9198–9205.
63. Leigh IM, Lane EB, Watt FM. The culture of human epidermal keratinocytes. In: Leigh IM, Lane EB, Watt FM, eds. The Keratinocyte Handbook. Cambridge: Cambridge University Press, 1994:43–51.
64. Guy R, Ridden C, Barth J, et al. Isolation and maintenance of the human pilosebaceous duct: 13-cis retinoic acid acts directly on the duct in vitro. Br J Dermatol 1993; 128:242–248.
65. Guy R, Kealey T. The effects of inflammatory cytokines on the isolated human sebaceous infundibulum. J Invest Dermatol 1998; 110:410–415.
66. Guy R, Kealey T. Modeling the infundibulum in acne. Dermatology 1998; 196:32–37.
67. Ingham E, Eady A, Goodwin CE, et al. Pro-inflammatory levels of interleukin-1a like bioactivity are present in the majority of open comedones in acne vulgaris. J Invest Dermatol 1992; 98:895–901.

68. Antilla HIS, Reitamo S, Saurant JH. Interleukin-1 immunoreactivty in sebaceous glands. Br J Dermatol 1992; 127:585–588.

69. Hauser C, Surat JH, Schmitt A, et al. Interleukin-1 is present in normal human epidermis. J Immunol 1986; 136:3317–3221.

70. Strauss JS, Pochi PE. The hormonal control of human sebaceous gland. In: Montagna W, Ellis R, Silver A, eds. Advances in the Biology of the Skin: The Sebaceous Glands. Oxford: Pergamon Press, 1963:220–254.

71. Rony HR, Zakon SJ. Effects of androgens in the sebaceous glands of human skin. Arch Dermatol Syphilol 1943; 48:601–604.

72. Thody AJ, Shuster S. Control and function of sebaceous glands. Phys Rev 1989; 69:383–416.

73. Ebling FJ, Ebling E, McCaffery V, et al. The response of the sebaceous glands of the hypophysectomized-castrated male rat to 5α-dihydrotestosterone, androstenedione, dehydroepiandrosterone and androsterone. J Endocrinol 1971; 51:181–190.

74. Chen WC, Thiboutot D, Zouboulis CC. Cutaneous androgen metabolism: basic research and clinical perspectives. J Invest Dermatol 2002; 119:992–1007.

75. Sansone G, Reisner RM. Differential rates of conversion of testostcrone to dihydrotestosterone in acne and in normal human skin: a possible pathogenic factor in acne. J Invest Dermatol 1971; 56:366–372.

76. Thiboutot DM, Harris G, Iles V, et al. Activity of the type I 5α-reductase exhibits regional differences in isolated sebaceous glands and whole skin. J Invest Dermatol 1995; 105:209–214.

77. Thiboutot DM, Knaggs H, Gilliland K, et al. Activity of type I 5α-reductase is greater in the follicular infrainfundibulum compared with the epidermis. Br J Derm 1997; 136:166–171.

78. Itami S, Kurata S, Sonoda T, et al. Characteristics of 5α-reductase in cultured human dermal papilla cells from beard and occipital scalp hair. J Invest Dermatol 1991; 96:57–60.

79. Takayasu S, Wakimoto H, Itami S, et al. Activity of testosterone 5α-reductase in various tissues of human skin. J Invest Dermatol 1980; 74:187–191.

80. Bernard F, Barrault C, DeGuercy A, et al. Expression of type I 5α-reductase and metabolism of testosterone in reconstructed human epidermis (skinethic®): a new model for screening skin-targeted androgen modulators. Int J Cosmet Sci 2000; 22:397–407.

81. Slivka SR. Testosterone metabolism in an *in vitro* skin model. Cell Biol Toxicol 1992; 8:267–276.

82. Harris G, Azzolina B, Baginsky W, et al. Identification and selective inhibition of an isozyme of steroid 5α-reductase in human scalp. Proc Natl Acad Sci USA 1992; 89:10787–10791.

83. Sugimoto Y, Lopez-Solache I, Labrie F, et al. Cations inhibit specifically type I 5α-reductase found in human skin. J Invest Dermatol 1995; 104:775–778.

84. Amichai B, Grunwald MH, Sobel R. 5α-Reductase inhibitors—a new hope in dermatology? Int J Dermatol 1997; 36:182–184.

85. Munster U, Hammer S, Blume-Peytavi U, et al. Testosterone metabolism in human skin cells in vitro and its interaction with estradiol and dutasteride. Skin Pharmacol Appl Skin Physiol 2003; 16:356–366.

86. Thiboutot D, Knaggs H, Gilliland K, et al. Activity of 5-alpha-reductase and 17-beta-hydroxysteroid dehydrogenase in the infrainfundibulum of subjects with and without acne vulgaris. Dermatology 1998; 196:38–42.

87. Altenburger R, Kissel T. The human keratinocyte cell line HaCaT: an in vitro cell culture model for keratinocyte testosterone metabolism. Pharm Res 1999; 16:766–771.

88. Milewich L, Kaimal V, Shaw CB, et al. Epidermal keratinocytes: a source of 5α-dihydrotestosterone production in human skin. J Clin Endocrinol Metab 1986; 62:739–746.

89. Pinsky L, Kaufman M, Straisfeld C, et al. Lack of difference in testosterone metabolism between cultured skin fibroblasts of human adult males and females. J Clin Endocrinol Metab 1974; 39:395–398.

90. Ernesti AM, Swiderek M, Gay R. Absorption and metabolism of topically applied testosterone in an organotypic skin culture. Skin Pharmacol 1992; 5:146–153.
91. Shapiro DJ, Imblum RL, Rodwell VW. Thin layer chromatographic assay for HMG-CoA reductase and mevalonic acid. Anal Biochem 1969; 31:383–390.
92. Smythe CDW, Greenall M, Kealey T. The activity of HMG-CoA reductase and acetyl-CoA carboxylase in human apocrine sweat glands, sebaceous glands, and hair follicles is regulated by phosphorylation and by exogenous cholesterol. J Invest Dermatol 1998; 111:139–148.
93. Leyden JJ, McGinley KJ, Mills OH, et al. Proprionibacterium levels in patients with and without acne vulgaris. J Invest Dermatol 1975; 65:382–384.
94. Winston MH. Acne vulgaris: pathogenesis and treatment. Pediatr Dermatol 1991; 38;889–903.
95. Shalita AR, Wei LL. Inflammatory acne. Dermatol Clin 1983; 1;361–364.
96. DeLeo VA. Cutaneous irritancy. Frazier JM, ed. In Vitro Testing: Applications to Safety Evaluation. New York: Marcel Dekker 1992:191–203.
97. Holland KT, Ingam E, Cunliffe WJ. A review: the microbiology of acne. J App Bacteriol 1981; 51:195–215.
98. Ingham E. The immunology of *Propionibacterium acnes* and acne. Curr Opin Infect Dis 1999; 12:191–197.
99. Draize JH, Woodard G, Calvery HO. Methods for the study of irritation and toxicity of substances applied topically to the skin and mucous membranes. J Pharmacol Exp Ther 1944; 82:377–390.
100. Filman DJ, Brawn RJ, Dandliker WB. Intracellular supravital stain delocalization as an assay for antibody-dependent complement-mediated cell damage. J Immunol Methods 1975; 6:189–207.
101. Eun HC, Suh DH. Comprehensive outlook of in vitro tests for assessing skin irritancy as alternates to draize tests. J Dermatol Sci 2000; 24:77—91.
102. De Haan P, Heemskerk AE, Gerritsen A, et al. Comparison of toxicity tests on human skin and epidermoid (A431) cells using free fatty acids as test substances. Clin Exp Dermatol 1993; 18:428–433.
103. Mosmann T. Rapid colorimetric assay for cellular growth and survival: application to proliferation and cytotoxicity assays. J Immunol Methods 1983; 65:55–63.
104. Denizot F, Lang R. Rapid colorimetric assay for cell growth and survival. J Immunol Methods 1986; 89:271–277.
105. Nakayama GR, Caton MC, Nova MP, et al. Assessment of the alamar blue assay for cellular growth and viability *in vitro*. J Immunol Methods 1997; 204:205–208.
106. Ponec M, Boelsma E, Gibbs S, et al. Characterization of reconstructed skin models. Skin Pharmacol Appl Skin Physiol 2002; 15(suppl):4–17.
107. Faller C, Bracher M. Reconstructed skin kits: reproducibility of cutaneous irritancy testing. Skin Pharmacol Appl Skin Physiol 2002; 15(suppl):74–91.
108. Peplow PV. Actions of cytokines in relation to arachidonic acid metabolism and eicosanoid production. Prostaglandins Leukot Essent Fatty Acids 1996; 54:303–317.
109. Grone A. Keratinocytes and cytokines. Vet Immunol Immunopathol 2002; 88:1–12.
110. Sugibayashi K, Watanabe T, Hasegawa T, et al. Kinetic analysis on the *in vitro* cytotoxicity using living skin equivalent for ranking the toxic potential of dermal irritants. Toxicol In Vitro 2002; 16:759–763.
111. Faller C, Bracher M, Dami N, et al. Predictive ability of reconstructed human epidermis equivalents for the assessment of skin irritation of cosmetics. Toxicol In Vitro. 2002; 16:557–572.
112. Portes P, Grandidier MH, Cohen C, et al. Refinement of the Episkin® protocol for the assessment of acute skin irritation of chemicals: follow-up to the ECVAM prevalidation study. Toxicol In Vitro 2002; 16:765–770.
113. Fentem JH, Briggs D, Chesne C, et al. A prevalidation study on in vitro tests for acute skin irritation: results and evaluation by the management team. Toxicol In Vitro 2001; 13:57–93.
114. Gay R, Swierek M, Nelson D. The living sin equivalent as a model *in vitro* for ranking the toxic potential of dermal irritants. Toxicol In Vitro 1992; 6:303–315.

115. Lee JK, Kim DB, Kim JI, et al. *In vitro* cytotoxicity tests on cultured human skin fibroblasts to predict skin irritation potential of surfactants. Toxicol In Vitro 2000; 14:345–349.

116. Coquette A, Berna N, Vandenbosch A, et al. Analysis of interleukin-1α and interleukin-8 expression and release in *in vitro* reconstructed human epidermis for the prediction of *in vitro* skin irritation and/or sensitization. Toxicol In Vitro 2003; 17:311–321.

117. Bernhofer L, Seiberg M, Martin K. The influence of the response of skin equivalent systems to topically applied consumer products by epithelial-mesenchymal interactions. Toxicol In Vitro 1999; 13:219–229.

118. Needleman P, Turk J, Jakschik B, et al. Arachidonic acid metabolism. Ann Rev Biochem 1986; 55:69–102.

119. Pentland A, Mahoney M. Keratinocyte prostaglandin synthesis is enhanced by IL-1. J Invest Dermatol 1990; 94:43–46.

120. Puhvel SM, Sakamoto M. An in vivo evaluation of the inflammatory effect of purified comedonal components in human skin. J Invest Dermatol 1977; 69:401–406.

121. Puhvel SM, Sakamoto M. The chemoattractant properties of comedonal components. J Invest Dermatol 1978; 71:324–329.

122. Allaker RP, Greenman J, Osbourne RH. The production of inflammatory compounds by *Propionibacterium acnes* and other skin organisms. Br J Dermatol 1987; 117:175–183.

123. Webster GF, Leyden JJ, Tsai CC, et al. Polymorphonuclear leukocyte lysosomal release in response to *Propionibacterium acnes* in vitro and its enhancement by sera from inflammatory acne patients. J Invest Dermatol 1980; 74:398–401.

124. Ingham E, Walters CE, Eady EA, et al. Inflammation in acne vulgaris: failure of skin micro-organisms to modulate keratinocyte interleukin-1α production *in vitro*. Dermatology 1998; 196:86–88.

125. Jappe U. Pathological mechanisms of acne with special emphasis on *Propionibacterium acnes* and related therapy. Acta Derm Venereol 2003; 83:241–248.

126. Downie MMT, Sanders DA, Kealey T. Modeling the remission of individual acne lesions in vitro. Br J Derm 2002; 147:869–878.

127. Hegemann L, Toso SM, Kitay K, et al. Anti-inflammatory actions of benzoyl peroxide: effects on the generation of reactive oxygen species by leukocytes and the activity of protein kinase C and calmodulin. Br J Dermatol 1994; 130:569–575.

128. Babich H, Zuckerbraun HL, Wurzburger BJ, et al. Benzoyl peroxide cytotoxicity evaluated in vitro with the human keratinocyte cell line, RHEK-1. Toxicology 1996; 106:187–196.

129. King FK, Egner PA, Kensler TW. Generation of DNA base modification following treatment of cultured murine keratinocytes with benzoyl peroxide. Carcinogenesis 1995; 17:317–330.

130. Matsui MS, Mintz E, DeLeo VA. Effect of benzoyl peroxide on protein kinase C in cultured human epidermal keratinocytes. Skin Pharmacol 1995; 8:130–138.

131. Valacchi G, Rimbach G, Saliou C, et al. Effect of benzoyl peroxide on antioxidant status, NF-kB activity and interleukin-1α gene expression in human keratinocytes. Toxicology 2001; 165:225–234.

132. Burkhart CN, Specht K, Neckers D. Synergistic activity of benzoyl peroxide and erythromycin. Skin Pharmacol Appl Skin Physiol 2000; 13:292–296.

133. Lawrence NJ, Parkinson EK, Emerson E. Benzoyl peroxide interferes with metabolic co-operation between cultured human epidermal keratinocytes. Carcinogenesis 1989; 5:419–421.

134. Russell JJ. Topical therapy for acne. Am Fam Physician 2000; 61:357–366.

135. Matsuoka LY. Acne and related disorders. Clin Plast Surg 1993; 20:35–41.

136. Blume U, Schon M, Zouboulis CC, et al. Vellus hair follicle-derived keratinocyte culture: a new experimental model in human hair research. Skin Pharmacol 1994; 2:27–32.

137. Limat A, Noser FK. Serial cultivation of single keratinocytes from the outer root sheath of human scalp hair follicles. J Invest Dermatol 1986; 87:45–48.

138. Lenoir-Viale MC, Galup C, Darmon M, et al. Epidermis reconstructed from the outer root sheath of human hair follicle: effect of retinoic acid. Arch Dermatol Res 1993; 285:197–204.

139. Hoeller D, Huppertz B, Roos TC, et al. An improved and rapid method to construct skin equivalents from human hair follicles and fibroblasts. Exp Dermatol 2001; 10:264–271.
140. Michel M, Dheureux N, Pouliot R, et al. Characterization of a new tissue-engineered human skin equivalent with hair. In Vitro Cell Dev Biol 1999; 35:318–326.
141. Philpott MP, Green MR, Kealey T. Human hair growth in vitro. J Cell Sci 1990; 97:436–471.
142. Sanders DA, Philpott MP, Nicolle FV, et al. The isolation and maintenance of the human pilosebaceous unit. Br J Derm 1994; 131:166–176.
143. Kealey T, Philpott M, Guy R. Human pilosebaceous culture. Methods Mol Biol 1997; 75:101–115.
144. Katz AB, Taichman LB. Epidermis as a secretory tissue: an in vitro tissue model to study keratinocyte secretion. J Invest Dermatol 1994; 102:55–60.

Index